D1503996

ELECTRONIC HEALTH RECORDS AND COMMUNICATION FOR BETTER HEALTH CARE

Studies in Health Technology and Informatics

Editors

Volume 87

Earlier published in this series

Vol. 59. I.A.F. Stokes (Ed.), Research into Spinal Deformities 2
Vol. 60. M. Di Rienzo, G. Mancia, G. Parati, A. Pedotti and A. Zanchetti (Eds.), Methodology and Clinical Applications of Blood Pressure and Heart Rate Analysis
Vol. 61. R.A. Mortensen (Ed.), ICNP® and Telematic Applications for Nurses in Europe
Vol. 62. J.D. Westwood, H.M. Hoffman, R.A. Robb and D. Stredney (Eds.), Medicine Meets Virtual Reality
Vol. 63. R. Rogers and J. Reardon, Recommendations for International Action
Vol. 64. M. Nerlich and R. Kretschmer (Eds.), The Impact of Telemedicine on Health Care Management
Vol. 65. J. Mantas and A. Hasman (Eds.), Textbook in Health Informatics
Vol. 66. The ISHTAR Consortium (Eds.), Implementing Secure Healthcare Telematics Applications in Europe
Vol. 67. J. Oates and H. Bjerregaard Jensen (Eds.), Building Regional Health Care Networks in Europe
Vol. 68. P. Kokol, B. Zupan, J. Stare, M. Premik and R. Engelbrecht (Eds.), Medical Informatics Europe '99
Vol. 69. E.B. Barber, F.-A. Allaert, B. Blobel and C.P. Louwerse (Eds.), Security Standards for Healthcare Information Systems
Vol. 70. J.D. Westwood, H.M. Hoffman, G.T. Mogel, R.A. Robb and D. Stredney (Eds.), Medicine Meets Virtual Reality 2000
Vol. 71. J.T. Ottesen and M. Danielsen (Eds.), Mathematical Modelling in Medicine
Vol. 72. I. Iakovidis, S. Maglavera and A. Trakatellis (Eds.), User Acceptance of Health Telematics Applications
Vol. 73. W. Sermeus, N. Kearney, J. Kinnunen, L. Goossens and M. Miller (Eds.), WISECARE
Vol. 74. O. Rienhoff, C. Laske, P. van Eecke, P. Wenzlaff and U. Piccolo (Eds.), A Legal Framework for Security in European Health Care Telematics
Vol. 75. G.O. Klein (Ed.), Case Studies of Security Problems and their Solutions
Vol. 76. E.A. Balas, S.A. Boren and G.D. Brown (Eds.), Information Technology Strategies from the United States and the European Union
Vol. 77. A. Hasman, B. Blobel, J. Dudeck, R. Engelbrecht, G. Gell and H.-U. Prokosch (Eds.), Medical Infobahn for Europe
Vol. 78. T. Paiva and T. Penzel (Eds.), European Neurological Network
Vol. 79. A. Marsh, L. Grandinetti and T. Kauranne (Eds.), Advanced Infrastructures for Future Healthcare
Vol. 80. R.G. Bushko (Ed.), Future of Health Technology
Vol. 81. J.D. Westwood, H.M. Hoffman, G.T. Mogel, D. Stredney and R.A. Robb (Eds.), Medicine Meets Virtual Reality 2001
Vol. 82. Z. Kolitsi (Ed.), Towards a European Framework for Education and Training in Medical Physics and Biomedical Engineering
Vol. 83. B. Heller, M. Löffler, M. Musen and M. Stefanelli (Eds.), Computer-Based Support for Clinical Guidelines and Protocols
Vol. 84. V.L. Patel, R. Rogers and R. Haux (Eds.), MEDINFO 2001
Vol. 85. J.D. Westwood, H.M. Hoffman, R.A. Robb and D. Stredney (Eds.), Medicine Meets Virtual Reality 02/10
Vol. 86. F.H. Roger France, I. Mertens, M.-C. Closon and J. Hofdijk (Eds.), Case Mix: Global Views, Local Actions

ISSN: 0926-9630

Electronic Health Records and Communication for Better Health Care

Proceedings of EuroRec '01

Edited by

François Mennerat

Président, PROREC-France, Paris, France

Amsterdam • Berlin • Oxford • Tokyo • Washington, DC

ISBN 1 58603 253 4 (IOS Press)
ISBN 4 274 90511 X C3047 (Ohmsha)
Library of Congress Control Number: 2002105611

Publisher
IOS Press
Nieuwe Hemweg 6B
1013 BG Amsterdam
The Netherlands
fax: +31 20 620 3419
e-mail: order@iospress.nl

Distributor in the UK and Ireland
IOS Press/Lavis Marketing
73 Lime Walk
Headington
Oxford OX3 7AD
England
fax: +44 1865 75 0079

Distributor in the USA and Canada
IOS Press, Inc.
5795-G Burke Centre Parkway
Burke, VA 22015
USA
fax: +1 703 323 3668
e-mail: iosbooks@iospress.com

Distributor in Germany, Austria and Switzerland
IOS Press/LSL.de
Gerichtsweg 28
D-04103 Leipzig
Germany
fax: +49 341 995 4255

Distributor in Japan
Ohmsha, Ltd.
3-1 Kanda Nishiki-cho
Chiyoda-ku, Tokyo 101-8460
Japan
fax: +81 3 3233 2426

PRINTED IN THE NETHERLANDS

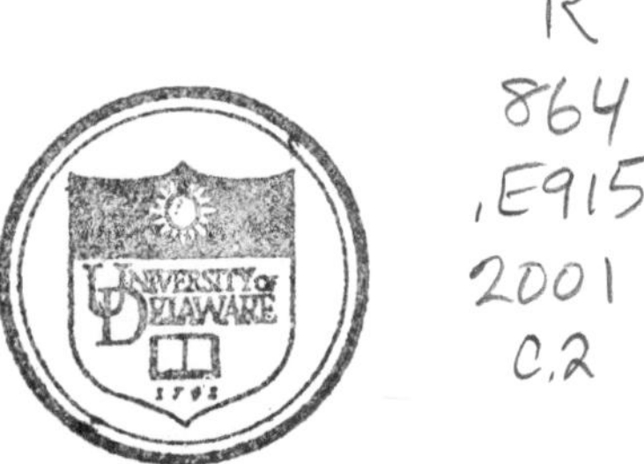

Preface

The annual **EuroRec Working Conference** has become the traditional gathering of all the partners involved on the scene of Electronic Health Records (EHRs). Twenty countries, ranging from South to North, from East to West, and from Europe and beyond, have been represented in its 2001 edition.

Naturally, a EuroRec conference follows the overall objectives of the European **PROREC initiative**: to promote the use of EHRs, in order to support the delivery of good quality health care.
What are the blockages impending the practical and effective implementation of communicating EHRs, both in hospital and in ambulatory care (general practice, ambulatory secondary health care, community care)? The issue has multiple facets that have to be dealt with at the same time.

While the existence of relevant technical specifications is acknowledged as of utmost importance, ahead or beyond the technical concern lie key issues that are of cultural, economic, ethical, and political nature: each one of these specific lines must be paid great attention to.
"Which incentives, which business model, which solutions for communicating EHRs in hospital and ambulatory care?" These key questions have been the thread for a series of specific workshops that have taken place over the two conference days, each one addressing a specific topic:

Does the use of EHRs reveal a cultural gap?
EHRs have to find their right place in the face to face dialogue between patients and health care professionals. To what extent does their introduction bring significant changes in the everyday process of health care delivery? How much does it interfere with the face to face dialogue between patients and health care professionals? Would educational programmes facilitate the transition?

An ethical concern: security, privacy and data protection
The outburst of the telematics era and of the internet raises new fears that privacy might prove increasingly difficult to protect. Confidentiality and security issues are now put on the front line.
How can privacy be protected? How can confidentiality and security issues be dealt with? Which control is granted to patients over the transfer, interchange, and use of their personal health data stored in EHRs? Are there limitations to the concept of a virtual patient record?

An economic concern: are there business models?
For the industry, what can be the return on investment for the development of new communicating EHR products? For the managers, and for the end users, what can be the return on investment for the purchase, learning, and use of communicating EHRs?
Today, in most countries, there is no business model for communicating EHRs, because there is no business model for integrated care (nor for co-ordinated care and continuity of care either).

A political concern: managing the change
Communicating EHRs are at the core of integrated health care networks. How and by whom are they to be organised, implemented, managed and controlled? Beyond the conventional and fashionable speech, is there a true interest in continuity of care?
Which incentives for an enhanced communication process between health care agents, based on EHRs? Eventually, who will pay for it? How, and how much? In most countries, end users still prove unwilling to do so. To support their marketing efforts, the pharmaceutical drugs industry is partly interested in retrieving data that reflect the clinical activities. Are public authorities ready to take the challenge?

The technical concern
What are the current specifications and standards, encompassing terminology and security issues that support EHR communication?
What is the importance of the European pre-standard ENV 13606 "EHRcom" for the future of communication between dissimilar systems?
What is the actual perspective for solutions based on open source developments?
A special "Industry Forum" has also been provided, where selected software developers and vendors have been invited to express their views, and present innovative and performing solutions.

May the speakers, chairpersons, and all those who have brought any contribution of a kind or another to the success of this EuroRec '01 conference, be thanked again here.

Each EuroRec conference gets something special.
Even with the endeavour of the authors of the papers that form this book, the proceedings can in no way be sufficient to capture and recall the exceptional atmosphere of these two days of active work and warm friendship.

Let me grasp this opportunity to invite all the readers of this book to join in the PROREC initiative, and attend the future EuroRec Working Conferences, that will undoubtedly be even greater successes.
They prove the right place to initiate or strengthen partnerships between the various parties whose endeavour concur to the implementation and actual use of top quality EHCR systems throughout Europe. EuroRec conferences represent a special opportunity to meet, to exchange ideas and experiences, to acquire a better knowledge of market trends, new policies at national and European levels, new initiatives, and on-going projects.

We all look forward to meeting you over the coming years.

Dr. François Mennerat MD PhD
Chairman of PROREC-France

Contents

Electronic Health Records and Communication
for Better Health Care
F. Mennerat (Ed.)
IOS Press, 2002

Welcome at EuroRec 2001

François MENNERAT, MD PhD
Chairman of ProRec-France
mailto:presidence@prorec-france.org

Ladies and Gentlemen, Dear Colleagues,

It is a great pleasure for me to welcome you at EuroRec '01, the 4th European Working Conference on Electronic Health Records, .especially in this beautiful city of Aix.

On behalf of the Board of ProRec-France, the members of which are striving for your satisfaction and comfort over these two days, I wish to greet heartily the representatives of authorities, the speakers, Chairpersons, and particularly the participants from overseas who have made their way to Aix. To my knowledge, 20 nations are represented here today, thus making this conference a true international one.

We are deeply grateful to our sponsors for their appreciated help in making a success of this conference.

Thus EuroRec '01 is the 4th European Working Conference on Electronic Health Records. The previous ones have taken place

- in November 1997 in Paris, at a time when ProRec-France did not exist yet
- in October 1998 in Rotterdam, where it was hosted by EPRiMP, the "Electronic Patient Records in Medical Practice" conference organised by IMIA, the International Medical Informatics Association
- in May 1999 in Seville, the same week as TEPR "Towards Electronic Patient Record", the annual conference organised in Orlando by Peter Waegemann
- unfortunately, 2000 had to be skipped
- and this year, in 2001, ProRec-France is in charge of organising the EuroRec conference, and now we are here in this beautiful city of Aix-en-Provence.

What is ProRec?

"ProRec" stands for "Promotion Strategy for the European Healthcare Record", and ProRec-France is the French ProRec Centre, a non-profit society founded in 1998 according to the French law on non-profit association enacted in 1901, the centenary of which is being celebrated throughout France this very year.

Where does ProRec come from?

ProRec results from two successive European projects:

- **MEDIREC** in 1994-1995
  A 18 months Concerted action of the AIM programme from the 3rd European Framework Programme of Research and Development (1991-1994), that had led to the "Lisbon Declaration"[1] and paved the way to the following
- **PROREC** in 1996-1998
  A 36 months project of the Health Telematics programme from the 4th European Framework Programme of Research and Development (1994-1998), that has led to the foundation of several ProRec Centres, among others ProRec-France

It is worth noting that in turn, over the 5th European Framework Programme of Research and Development (1998-2002), ProRec-France is now involved along with its natural partners from Belgium, Germany, Hungary, Italy, the Netherlands, Portugal, Slovenia, and Spain in **WIDENET**, an accompanying measure of the IST-Health programme, to long 36 months (December 2000 – November 2003).
Following this project, there might well be something between 9 and 15 ProRec Centres: Belgium, Spain, France, Hungary, the Netherlands, Germany, Slovenia, Portugal, Italy are already in existence, or on the agenda.
Denmark, Greece, Romania, Bulgaria, Sweden, and —why not?— the UK might follow soon.
And to establish a durable link between them all, the European Institute of Health Records and Management —the *EuroRec Institute*— will be created, to federate the ProRec Centres, and perform those activities that are relevant at the European level.

What are the objectives and actions of ProRec?

The broad objective assigned to ProRec is to identify, and subsequently try and help solve the issues opposing or slowing down the process of widely implementing high quality EHRs[2] throughout Europe.
This implies addressing any issues directly related to EHRs, as well as some others that could be seen as collateral ones, such as e.g. terminology, patient or providers identification, or linkage to knowledge bases and practice guidelines.

An EHR system is not merely a sub-system within a broader Health Information System. An EHR system is firstly a professional tool at the disposal of clinicians and patients, for the sake of the latter. Their aim is to help patients and health care providers find the most possible satisfying answer to their needs and concerns , not payers and managers.
EHR systems are very specific in that they are meant to support the core activity of any Health Systems: provide timely and duly personalised quality health care —curative or preventive— to those persons who actually need it. In this perspective, management and payment issues, practice evaluation, and even possibly epidemiology, do appear as relatively secondary, if not ancillary activities.
It has thus been found that a key to success for ProRec is to act predominantly at the ground

[1] To be recalled in annex.
[2] EMR, EPR EHCR, EHR: the terminology is variable and somehow confusing; there is a need for clarification and consensus on a yet seemingly unstable typology.

level —"think European (the market), act local (the needs)"— by:

- taking account of local specificity and implementing national or regional ProRec Centres;
- bringing together and involve field actors: those who actually use an electronic record as a professional tool, together with those who will actually provide the necessary solutions.

Practically, the ProRec Centres together are committed, among other activities, to:

- set up and maintain an index of Electronic Health Records systems providers
- establish a set of quality criteria against which any software can be assessed by future users and purchasers.

The thread of EuroRec '01

Quality criteria for EHR systems are multiple. The most prominent one (that possibly covers most others) is interoperability.
The issue of widespread use of interoperable electronic health records is manifold.
The keys are to be sought in various directions.
We have chosen this year to highlight five of them: particularly cultural, ethical, economic, political, and technical.

Cultural:

The use of an EHR induces a change in behaviour of both doctors and patients. To what extent does it interfere with the patient-doctor normal relationship, and the face to face dialogue between patients and health care professionals? Is it necessarily for worse? Would educational programmes facilitate the transition?

Ethical:

Fears exists, probably not totally unjustified, that the use of communicating EHR systems increases the risk of confidentiality breach. The issue of personal data protection needs to be tackled in a convincing way. Which rights are granted to patients over the storage, transfer, interchange, and re-use of their personal health data? How does the concept of a virtual patient record impact this concern? What about the traceability of clinical data. What about identifiers of health care professionals, health care organisations, and patients?

Economic:

Solution providers struggle to find workable business models. Users —free-standing or hospital departments—, and managers encounter also tremendous difficulties in finding theirs for purchasing and using quality communicating EHR systems.
Which business models can be found for communicating EHR systems? What can the return on investment be for:-

the industry,
the managers (e.g. of hospitals),
and the healthcare professionals —free-standing or practising in hospital departments

on the development, purchase, and use of quality communicating EHR systems?

Is there an economic future for integrated care, and is this part of the solution?

Political:

Granted that the widespread use of EHR systems should bring improvement in the quality of health care, explicit policies should be set up, based on change management techniques. Who will drive the business redesign throughout the health system? Which incentives should be introduced for an enhanced communication process between health care agents? Who will pay, and how much? Communicating EHR systems are at the core of integrated health care networks. How, and by whom, are they to be organised, implemented, managed and controlled? How to foster continuity of care?

Technical:

EHR communication cannot but rely on standards in the fields of data representation and architecture, terminology, security, etc. CEN/TC251, GEHR, HL7: where are we? What is the way for a global standard, that would undoubtedly help the market forces to take off?

Over the two conference days, this set of five issues will be addressed in five dedicated workshops. All attendees are kindly (though firmly...) invited to take an active part in incurring debates. If they are willing to back their address by some kind of a visual presentation, they can present one or two slides, provided that they advise one of the chair-persons of their intent before the workshop commences.

Also, on Tuesday, a special "Industry Forum" will take place where several software developers will make live presentations of innovative and performing solutions.

And over this conference, demonstrations of communication between dissimilar systems based on ENV 13606 "EHRcom" standard, or GEHR specifications are to be organised on the stand of ProRec.

On behalf of all ProRec Centres we wish you a fruitful conference, and a very nice time in this beautiful city of Aix.

Annex: The MEDIREC Lisbon Declaration

It is recommended that the Member States through the Commission promote a framework for action within Europe to further develop common aspects of the Electronic Health Care Records based on the following:

1. The EHCR is the nucleus of the relationship between the patient, the HC delivery system and all its professionals. As such, a EHCR should be the core of the new generation of Health Information Systems.

2. The main objective of the use of any EHCR must be to improve quality in care by having the record and its associated information always available for the HC professionals when needed at the point of care.

3. The use of EHCR's should lead to direct benefits for the professionals by making their work more efficient. This will arise from supporting the diagnostic process, enhancing HCR accuracy and completeness, improving medical knowledge and disease management, and allowing better preventive care and patient handling.

4. Within HC systems, either at European, national, regional or local level, the use of appropriate EHCR's will also contribute to adequate planning and resource management, facilitation of the continuity of care, registration of healthcare interventions, improvement of epidemiological and morbidity information, and hence, a more cost-effective care process.

5. The European citizen shall by means of any EHCR have (1) guaranteed right of access to the HC he is entitled for, (2) right of access to his individual data and related services, (3) the effective protection of his right of free circulation with respect to the confidentiality of his individual data.

6. Further actions and developments on EHCR's should be based upon standards and consensus that ensure interoperability, and allow EHCR's coming from different origins to be reliable, communicable, recognisable and comparable.

7. A role of the Health Telematics European Industry is to tackle the need for the development of new products in a huge growing market, offering the enabling technology to fulfil user requirements. Multimedia, 3D images, interchange formats, message contents, linguistic barriers and suitable user interfaces are among the challenges to be developed in a framework of confidentiality and security for patient data.

8. The use of EHCR's will require the adequate management of "cultural changes" in all parties involved towards, amongst others, technological innovations, patterns of practice, education and training. Active participation of all parties, including European, national, regional and local Health Authorities in the definition and promotion of the use of EHCR's is mandatory.

9. The effective co-operation between all interested parties including users, professionals, authorities, industry, standardisation bodies and others at a European level and through a process of managed convergence towards European EHCR's, would benefit from the set-up of an appropriate Structure based on existing organisations that could promote that mission.

10. In order to achieve these goals and to encompass the future, Member States individually and through the Commission should encourage common efforts and policies through adequate resource allocation, focusing on the European EHCR, and leading us to patient-centred HC systems.

*Electronic Health Records and Communication
for Better Health Care
F. Mennerat (Ed.)
IOS Press, 2002*

Interference with the patient-doctor relationship – The cultural gap? Lessons from observation

Dr Nick Booth
Dr Paul Robinson
Sowerby Centre for Health Informatics at Newcastle, UK.

Despite widespread advances in design and production of electronic health care record systems, there is still a lack of progress to paperless and networked health information in most European countries.

In this article I want to discuss a taxonomy of modes of interference with the clinical process associated with electronic health record introduction. Much of the work at SCHIN is concerned with research into electronic health records at the point of care. This is partly because of the origins of SCHIN as a primary care focussed health informatics research centre. Since the mid 1990s however, SCHIN has widened its scope to both primary and hospital care situated clinical systems, including an interest in DSS, Networking and communication, messaging, architecture and standards, and terminology and classification. It is in this context that the discussion is grounded. SCHIN now includes a large research team including medical informaticians and practising clinicians, knowledge authors and pharmacists, technical and software specialists and sociologists.

In particular the paper will discuss experiences in two current projects, the Durham and Darlington electronic health record project (DuDEHR) and the Information in the consulting room project (iiCR). The iiCR project is described later in the paper.

The DuDEHR project

The DuDEHR project concerns system architecture for a national shared health information service, and is based on a fundamental ethical and legal framework. It sets out to engage clinicians, managers, IT staff and patients in an iterative design process, using animated enterprise models as a stimulus for discussion. The whole project is underpinned by a thread of ethnological research, examining the methods which clinicians and associated staff use in handling health information in clinical situations, and comparing theory with observed practice.

We have created a taxonomy of interference modes with clinical care associated with a move from paper systems. It should be noted however that such failure modes are not always associated with electronic systems exclusively. Nevertheless we feel that this taxonomy is a helpful illustration of the problems arising from the widespread adoption of ICT promoted by pressure in national health services to improve efficiency and quality of health care delivery. It spans the technical, social and organisational domains and introduces problems associated with the cognition in the consultation.

User interface	Security –Login –Whose keys? –Trust Location and interface –Palm or desktop Intuitive/ergonomics Network speed
Data quality issues	Local agreement –Consistency of use of terminology/classification/free text/paper –Multidisciplinary team –Local audit Organisational issues –Mandatory clinical governance –Cross boundary integrated care pathways –Information model inconsistencies
Architecture/information model	UK primary care – three major systems, three different record architectures –Need a semantically stable interchange standard –Clarity and consistency about context in terminology –In a shared information service we need also: **Provenance:** Examples of data attributes required over WAN based EHR Name of actor and place of work –Role and qualification –Responsibilities –Purpose of data collected –Which system collected on –Certification of results of investigations Patient information consent status
Organisational issues	Prime purpose of the system –Who bought it? Policy imposes process –Data entry requirement – any feedback? Implied alteration of clinical method –Decision support –Care pathways –Sharing evidence with patient

Configurability / reconfigurability	Embedded DSS or ICPs –Can it be edited for local use or new circumstances/evidence Organisational change / team configuration Interference with mandated change Clinicians can reconfigure –With paper if necessary –And without the computer
Individual human factors	Patient –Suspicious of computer –Concerned about confidentiality –Distracted in the consultation? Clinician –Uncomfortable with technology –Reluctant to change and accommodate –Underused –Or a dangerous distraction?.....

The iiCR project

This project uses a model of interpersonal communication (Kurtz and Silverman) as a frame through which we have looked at the impact of computer use during the consultation in primary care. Whereas there are many pressures on Medical Practitioners to use the computer during consultations, it is recognised that computer use has the potential to damage the interpersonal communication, reduce rapport and so adversely affect the health outcomes that derive from the episode. The aim of the research was to identify communication skills that enable the practitioner to maintain rapport with the patient and also use the computer in the consultation. Having identified these skills, we are now developing a training package to disseminate them.

We asked selected General Practitioners to video tape a surgery. The doctors that we approached were all involved in Post Graduate Medical Education and they all judged themselves to be proficient at using the computer during the consultation. The research team looked at all the consultations from each doctor. One or two consultations from each tape were transcribed verbatim using a Conversation Analysis method.

Briefly, the findings were that:

1. this group used paper a lot
2. Practitioners prefer to type when the patient is not watching them
3. there is a wide variation between practitioners of how willing they are to share information with the patient (and visual access to the screen).

Two themes emerge from this work. The first is Multitasking. While people are able to accomplish several tasks at once, e.g. drive a car, talk to passenger, listen to radio etc, we do not think that they are able to concentrate on two things at once. Particularly, they are not able to concentrate on a complex interaction with the computer and attend to the patient at the same time.

There are several instances of this on the tapes that we observed. Consequently, a key skill that we identified for the training package is the ability to structure the consultation to avoid trying to do two things at once.

The other issue is the way that the computer brings all sorts of medical knowledge into the consulting room. Traditionally doctors have gained expert knowledge away from the place of work (at medical school, conferences, in libraries etc). Electronic media now make expert knowledge available in the consultation. This means that the traditional transaction in the consultation "what can I tell you about this?" will be replaced by "what can we find out about this?"

We think that this has profound implications for the future of practice.

References

Durham EHR Project: http://www.schin.ncl.ac.uk/DurhamEHR
IiCR project http://www.schin.ncl.ac.uk/iicr

Electronic Health Records and Communication for Better Health Care
F. Mennerat (Ed.)
IOS Press, 2002

Trust me, I'm a patient! The effect of an EHR on *my* consultation

Dr. Nikki Shaw
Senior Research Associate.
Centre for Health Services Research.
University of Newcastle upon Tyne. 21 Claremont Place.
Newcastle upon Tyne. NE3 1SX. United Kingdom.
Chair:
European Federation of Medical Informatics Working Group 7
(Primary Care Informatics)
& WONCA Informatics (Europe)
Email: nikki.shaw@dial.pipex.com

Abstract. A general assumption has been made within the health care community that the introduction of an Electronic Health Record (EHR) is beneficial and improves clinical care [1]. However, it is my contention as both a Health Informatician, and more importantly a patient, that this assumption is not supported by evidence, either scientific or anecdotal. However, to my mind of more importance than this is the complete lack of understanding about how using an EHR effects my consultation. This paper discusses this issue and identifies four lessons to be learned by the EHR community.

1 Background

The use of an EHR is most widely experienced in English General Practice where computerisation can be traced back to the 1970's with the Department of Health sponsored Ottery St. Mary project. This project produced the first "paperless" general practice system [2]. This development was built upon over the years until, in 1989, Direct Reimbursement for the purchase of computers in General Practice commenced. This change in policy, alongside the introduction of the new GP contract in 1990, culminated in a growth in the use of computers in general practice from 20% in 1989 to 79% in 1993 [3] and commonly believed to be 98% in the present day.

Various nationally led initiatives (Table 1) have provided support for the further development of EHRs in general practice. However, a brief survey of published literature provides little evidence that this development, and its associated expense (c. £47 million pounds per year [4]), is supported by evidence that establishes the value to patients of such systems.

Table 1:
Initiatives that have supported the development of UK GP Computerisation

- The introduction of GP fundholding
- Publication of the 1992 Information Management & Technology (IM&T) strategy [NHSE, 1992]
- The establishment of the Requirements for Accreditation (RFA) programme
- GP/FHSA links
- The development of READ codes
- The publication of the UK National Standard EDIFACT Messages
- The publication of the British Medical Association's (BMA) nine principles for medical data security

2 The Evidence

2.1 The effect of an EHR on the consultation

The published evidence supporting the use of an EHR in consultation does appear to be promising as three primary benefits of EHR use during the patient consultation have been identified [5, 6]:

1. The EHR saves doctor's time.
2. The EHR helps doctors select medication.
3. The EHR provides quick access to up-to-date information.

At first appearance, this sounds like utopia. However, how do any of these 'benefits' affect my consultation? Does the fact that an EHR saves doctors time mean that I get to spend any more time with my doctor? No! In fact, consultation times are currently pared to an absolute minimum in most English surgeries with 7-minute appointments being the norm.

"The EHR helps doctors select medication". The effect of this on my consultation is nil. It may help the doctor select medication. However, going on my recent experiences this doesn't mean that they will pick the best medication for me as an individual. Admittedly I have a complex set of allergies and intolerances, however it was noticeable that when my doctor couldn't prescribe the EHR recommended medication for me recently it was to the paper BNF and myself (an informed patient) that he turned to for advice. For after all, who is better placed than the patient to decide what side effects they are willing to suffer?

"The EHR provides quick access to up-to-date information". One wonders where this information is being found. If across the internet or within an intranet [7] (E.g.: NHSnet) and without a great deal of experience in finding information it can take you longer to find what you want than it would to simply reach up to a bookshelf and look it up for yourself or to telephone a colleague.

The counter argument to these suggestions is that EHR provided information is more up-to-date? Is this actually the case? How often is the content of your EHR system updated? It was noticeable a few years ago that accurate information was being provided to patients about the OCP scare by popular magazines before GPs had even been officially informed (by the Government, let alone their EHR) that there was a potential problem.

As for internet/intranet based information how do you know that the information provided is valid or even when it was last updated? Many sites do not provide this information.

2.2 The effect of an EHR on patients

Lets turn our attention to the patients themselves for a moment. The prevailing concern expressed by patients is that of confidentiality [5, 6, 8, 9]. In particular, patients are worried about the possibility of the next patient viewing their records on screen [6]. Furthermore, patients find it disturbing not knowing what their doctor is doing when they work on the computer [5] and wished to be able to view their own clinical details, on screen, during the consultation. The perceived competence of the doctor with using the EHR has also found to be of concern with doctors themselves finding the experience stressful and patients reporting, higher levels of post consultation stress [10].

Of grave concern is the fact that back in the 1980's [11] and mid 1990's [12] patients reported being less willing to speak frankly about personal matters to their general practitioner if they used a computer and that they would change to another doctor if their general practitioner did use a computer in their consultation. Unfortunately, this work does not appear to have been followed up and it is unknown whether patients did actually migrate between GP's if their own started using a computer.

The most damning finding regarding the use of an EHR is that they have no effect. Surely, the entire purpose of an EHR is to improve patient care? This can be demonstrated by a number of studies that reported that patients ratings of:

- Doctor attentiveness and rapport,
- Information provision by the doctor,
- Their own post consultation stress and satisfaction
- Their intended compliance

were not significantly affected by the use of a computer in their consultation [4, 5, 9, 10].

In fact, what has been repeatedly emphasised by patients is that it is the interpersonal aspects of the doctor-patient relationship, such as the doctor looking up when they entered the room, speaking to them and maintaining eye contact, and not appearing to be preoccupied with the computer [6] that mattered. Of particular concern is the stated view that if the doctor was perceived to lack sufficient confidence and skill when using the computer then the patient's confidence in the doctor would be reduced [6].

Curiously though, whilst most patients seem to feel that using an EHR does not affect the duration of the consultation [9] this has not actually been found to be the case in reality with consultations using an EHR taking an average of 90-148 seconds longer [4, 13, 14].

2.3 The effect of an EHR on patient outcomes

There is virtually no evidence to support the theory that the use of an EHR in general practice improves patient care. In fact, the little evidence that there is, is contradictory and tends towards stating that it is difficult to demonstrate [15].

Even the commonly held belief that computerised prompt systems improves clinical compliance [13] with preventative measures is underpinned by contradictory evidence [1, 16]. Despite this, the prevailing assumption is still that the use of an EHR will lead to improved patient care [17], and that by providing a continuously improving EHR better care will automatically follow [13]. A contingency of health professionals (size as yet unknown) remains to be convinced [18, 19].

What is also of interest is that despite the fact that nearly three-quarters of practices surveyed in 1997 thought that their EHR system had helped them improve their delivery of care [20] thirty seven per cent of respondents felt that their system had either not affected their delivery of patient care or that it got in the way of that delivery of care.

A logical deduction from this is that clinical systems must be perceived as improving patient care through methods not associated with the consultation itself, which supports the belief that computerised clinical systems have greater benefit for administration purposes than for direct clinical care [21, 22]. It is of interest then that studies [4, 19] suggest that despite assertions to the contrary [20] doctors actually use the computer far less during the consultation than that commonly assumed. In fact, the commonest function for which the EHR is used is prescribing [4, 23].

3 Discussion

If, as the evidence suggests, EHR systems are under-utilised by health care practitioners [4, 23] the reasons for this must be understood.

The primary reason must be the lack of evidence of their use leading to an improvement in patient care. If EHR systems are ever to be fully utilised they must be made to be beneficial to the practitioner at the point of care for the individual patient.

Whilst, it is accepted that administration, management and research and audit [24, 25] are useful activities; it is not these activities that are important when a patient walks into the consultation. At the point of consultation the health professional needs to know the medical history of that patient, the best management for that patient's condition and be able to provide the facets of the doctor-patient relationship upon which we have come to rely. They do not need to know how many patients they have in their practice with the same condition, only how best to treat that condition and how they have treated this patient previously.

4 Conclusions

EHR systems have probably come too far to turn back and address what should have been answered prior to widespread implementation: *'How does an EHR improve patient care at the individual patient level?'*

Society has come to rely on computers throughout all aspects of life and healthcare is no different. However, we can learn from other disciplines and our own mistakes. It is well known that many promising and technologically feasible proposals have failed to fulfil their promise because of a failure to acknowledge the socio-political realities of an application area [26]. Now is the time to learn from these realities and address these non-technical issues before we repeat the same mistakes again.

Firstly, damage limitation exercises must be enacted immediately. Already, the long recognised benefit to patient care of the primary care cradle-to-grave record is being eroded. No longer does a patient's notes get passed from one GP to another in their entirety. Now it depends on multiple factors as to how much of the record a practice receives and in what format. Modern day notes often consist of no more than page after page of computer printouts that are either summarised or disregarded on arrival at the new practice and a new computerised record commenced. As the patient moves round the country, this cycle repeats. This can only be rectified by the different EHR system suppliers moving even faster than they already are, to develop the systems necessary to exchange records between disparate clinical systems, in a secure and confidential manner, whilst maintaining their integrity and meaning.

Secondly, the systems themselves must support the dual role that they must now perform. They must provide clinical benefit to the health professional for direct patient care whilst at the same time they must encourage use in such a way that data recorded can be used with confidence for clinical audit/governance at an aggregate level. For it is only when existing EHR systems are simple enough to make their use second nature, like the stethoscope, that we will we be able to ensure that their use leads to improved patient care [4].

Thirdly, we must learn from our history. The recently revised English Information Strategy [27] placed an increased emphasis on the development of the EHR. Once again, an assumption has been made that an increased use of technology will lead to an improvement in the quality of patient care. To date, there is little evidence of this in anything other than a contrived research setting [22]. We must provide the evidence that supports or disproves this assumption so that a judgement can be made in full possession of all the facts.

Finally, we must educate and train not only our health care professionals [28] but also our patients. For example, despite the reservations expressed by patients about the possibility of the next patient seeing their records on screen, it is not actually common for patients to be able to view their own records, let alone any one else's [5]. This raises the whole issue of disclosure and it is well known that patients do not necessarily want full disclosure and that there are certainly some entries, such as personal comments or life expectancy that they definitely do not wish to see [6].

This is no different for patients and health care providers using an EHR than it is for those using paper records. In fact, none of the education and training issues raised by the use of an EHR in consultation, with the exception of basic computing skills, are new. They are the same issues that have been faced by health care professionals since the time of Hypocrites [29]. What is new is that under the guise of introducing technology these issues are at last being identified and addressed.

Acknowledgements

The author wishes to make it clear that the views expressed are personal and not necessarily representative of her employing bodies.

Dr N T Shaw is funded as a National Health Service Executive (North West Region) Research & Development Post-Doctoral Training Fellow. The support of the National Health Service Executive (North West Region) Research & Development department and Oldham Primary Care Group is therefore gratefully acknowledged.

References

1. NHS Executive (1998) Information for Health: An information strategy for the modern NHS 1998-2005. IMG Reference Number A1103. ISBN 0 95327190 2
2. Fogarty L. (1997) Primary care informatics development – One view through the miasma. Journal of informatics in Primary Care January 1997. pp2-11
3. Chisholm S. Gillies A. (1994) A snapshot of the computerisation of general practice and the implications for training. Auditorium 3:1 pp21-26
4. Richards H.M. Sullivan F.M. Mitchell E.D. Ross S. (1998) Computer use by general practitioners in Scotland. British Journal of General Practice 48 pp1473-1476
5. Brown J. (1998) The computer in the general practice consultation: a literature review. Health Informatics Journal. 4 pp106-108
6. Ridsdale L. Hudd S. (1994) Computers in the consultation: the patients' view. British Journal of General Practice 44 pp367-369
7. Kidd M (2001) General Practice on the Internet Aust Fam Physician 30(4):359-61
8. Als A.B. (1997) The desk-top computer as a magic box: patterns of behaviour connected with the desk-top computer; GPs' and patients' perceptions. Family Practice V14:1 pp17-23
9. Rethans J.J. Höppener P. Wolfs G. Dierderiks J. (1988) Do personal computers make doctors less personal? BMJ 296 pp1446-1448

10. Brownridge G. Herzmark G.A. Wall T.D. (1985) Patient reactions to doctors' computer use in general practice consultations. Soc. Sci. Med. 20:1 pp47-52
11. Potter A.R. (1981) Computers in general practice: the patients' voice. Journal of the RGP 31 pp683-685
12. Greatbatch D. et al (1995) How do desk-top computers affect the doctor-patient interaction? Family Practice V12:1 pp32-36
13. Sullivan F. Mitchell E. (1995) Has general practitioner computing made a difference to patient care? A systematic review of the published reports. BMJ 311 pp848-852
14. Mitchell E, Sullivan F (2001) A descriptive feast but an evaluative famine: systematic review of published articles on primary care computing during 1980-1997
15. Gillies A. Rawlings G (1998) Can computers improve the health of the nation? Health Informatics Journal 4 pp109-112Yano E.M. et al (1995) Helping practices reach primary care goals. Arch Intern Med 155 pp1146-1156
16. Yano EM et al (1995) Helping practices reach primary care goals Arch Intern Med 155:1146-1156
17. Bolton P. (1995) Clinical Decision Making: Are computers really helpful? Australian Family Physician V24:5 pp882-885
18. Miller A. Jeffcote R. (1997) Practice nurses and computing: some evidence on utilisation, training and attitude to computer use. Health informatics Journal V3:1 pp10-16
19. Balas E.A. et al (1996) The clinical value of computerized information services: A review of 98 randomized clinical trials. Arch Fam Med V5 pp271-278
20. NHS Executive (1998) Evaluation of GP Computer Systems 1997: National Report. January 1998
21. Campbell S.M. Roland M.O. Gormanly B. (1996) Evaluation of a computerised appointment system in general practice. 46 pp477-478
22. Tyrer F. Hambleton I. Lawrenson R. Pierce M. (1996) Building a research database from computerised general practice records. Journal of informatics in primary care. September 1996. Pp8-13
23. Ahmed M.A. Berlin A. (1997) IT in general practice: current use and views on future development. Journal of Informatics in Primary Care. November 1997. pp5-8
24. Ellis N. T. (1997) 'An information based approach to clinical audit in the UK National Health Service', PhD Thesis, University of Central Lancashire, September 1997. 2 Vols
25. Ellis N. T. (1999) Telemedicine & Information for Health: The Impediments to Implementation. HC'99 Information At The Heart Of Clinical Practice March 22-24 1999, Conference Presentation
26. Regan B.G. (1991) Computerised information exchange in healthcare. The Medical Journal of Australia. V154 pp140-144
27. NHS Executive (2001) Building The Information Core
28. Liaw ST, Marty JJ (2001) Learning to consult with computers Med Educ 35(7):645-51
29. Shaw N T (2001) Going Paperless: A guide to computerisation in primary care Radcliffe Medical Press

Electronic Health Records and Communication for Better Health Care
F. Mennerat (Ed.)
IOS Press, 2002

IS4ALL: A Working Group promoting universal design in Health Telematics

Constantine Stephanidis[1,2] and Demosthenes Akoumianakis[1]
[1]*Institute of Computer Science*
Foundation for Research and Technology - Hellas
Science and Technology Park of Crete Heraklion, Crete, GR-71110 Greece
and
[2]*Department of Computer Science*
University of Crete

Georges de Moor[3,4]
[3]*University Hospital Ghent*
Department of Medical Informatics and Statistics
De Pintelaan 18, Gent 9000, Belgium
and
[4]*Microsoft Healthcare Users Group Europe (MS-HUGe)*
Zomerstraat 25; B-9270 Laarne-Kalken, Belgium

Abstract. In this article, we present an overview of the work being carried out by the EC-funded project IS4ALL (IST-1999-14101). Specifically, we describe the methodological frame of reference, which drives the project's objective to introduce universal access principles into the design of Health Telematics applications and services. Health Telematics is chosen due to some distinctive characteristics, such as the variety of end users involved, the changing healthcare contexts of use and the penetration of new computer-mediated activities, which re-shape the way in which healthcare practices are structured and organized.

1. Introduction

IS4ALL (Information Society for All) – is an EC-funded project aiming to advance the principles and practice of Universal Access in Information Society Technologies, by establishing a wide, interdisciplinary and closely collaborating network of experts (Working Group) to provide the European Information Technology and Telecommunications (IT&T) industry in general, and Health Telematics in particular, with a comprehensive code of practice on how to appropriate the benefits of universal design.

Universal design is the term used to reflect a particular perspective upon the design of interactive products and services that respects and values the dimensions of diversity intrinsic in human capabilities, technological environments and contexts of use. The universal design movement has its roots in the conscious effort to address the special requirements of the ageing population and users with disabilities. Initial areas of application have been mainly concerned with the design of landscapes and built environments. More recently, universal design became respected and practised in architecture, interior design, civil engineering, etc [1].

In the 1990's, universal design obtained a broader connotation and attracted considerable interest in the field of IT&T. Several projects were carried out (for a review see [2]) in an attempt to address technical issues, raise awareness and advance an understanding of the challenges pertaining to the appropriation of the benefits of universal design in IT&T. In the field of Human-Computer Interaction (HCI), universal design has addressed the shortcomings in traditional HCI design practices to cope with the different dimensions of diversity [2, 3, 4, 5]. To this end, universal design has been the focal issue of concern in the context of an International Scientific Forum[1] and several research and development projects over the past decade [2, 3, 4, 5].

These experiences have created the compelling need to establish on a more formal basis a wider, interdisciplinary and closely collaborating "network of experts" (Working Group) to provide the Information Society Technologies industry with a comprehensive code of practice detailing how to appropriate the benefits of universal design. This is currently being pursued in the context of the European Commission[2] funded project IS4ALL[3] (Information Society for All).

2. The Focus

IS4ALL concentrates on the European Health Telematics industry and seeks to develop appropriate instruments to facilitate this industry towards approaching, internalising and exploiting the benefits of universal access. The particular domain of Health Telematics of interest to IS4ALL is the users interaction with Electronic Patient Records (EPRs). Users in this context comprise a broad and diverse community of humans interacting with segments of an EPR, including the medical community as well as end users. Moreover, such interaction may be carried out using different technological platforms (e.g., desktop machines, Internet appliances, mobile equipment), in a variety of contexts of use. Specifically, emerging interaction platforms, such as advanced desktop-oriented environments (e.g., advanced GUIs, 3D graphical toolkits, visualisers), and mobile platforms (e.g., palmtop devices), enabling ubiquitous access to electronic data from anywhere, and at anytime, are expected to bring about radical improvements in the type and range of Health Telematics services. Accounting for the accessibility, usability and acceptability of these technologies so as to facilitate universally accessible applications and services requires an early and explicit focus on the broad range of issues that pertain to universal access.

Toward this objective, IS4ALL will develop a comprehensive *code of practice* (e.g., enumeration of methods, process guidelines) consolidating existing knowledge on Universal Access in the context of Information Society Technologies, as well as *concrete recommendations* for emerging technologies (e.g., emerging desktop and mobile platforms), with particular emphasis on their deployment in Health Telematics. IS4ALL will also undertake a mix of *outreach activities* to promote Universal Access principles and practice, including workshops and seminars targeted to mainstream IT&T industry.

---

[1] The International Scientific Forum "Towards an Information Society for All' was launched in 1997, as an international ad hoc group of experts sharing common visions and objectives, namely the advancement of the principles of Universal Access in the emerging Information Society. The Forum held three workshops to establish interdisciplinary discussion, exchange of knowledge, dissemination, and international co-operation. The 1st workshop took place in San Francisco, USA, August 29, 1997, and was sponsored by IBM. The 2nd took place in Crete, Greece, June 15-16, 1998. The 3rd took place in Munich, Germany, August 22-23, 1999. The latter two events were partially funded by the European Commission. The Forum has produced two White Papers [3, 4].

[2] For an overview of the European Commission perspective and of the 5th Framework Programme on Information Society Technologies (IST), the reader may visit the web site: http://www.cordis.lu/ist/overv-1.htm#objective

[3] http://is4all.ics.forth.gr

3. The Approach

The technical approach to be followed in IS4ALL builds on a scenario-based perspective to requirements engineering. IS4ALL scenarios are perceived as narrative descriptions of computer-mediated human activities in a Health Telematics environment. A Health Telematics environment may be bound to a clinic within the hospital, a ward within a clinic or even to the end user's business or residential environment. Working with scenarios in IS4ALL entails several steps.

3.1 Generating the scenario

Scenarios can be developed at different levels. They can range from vision-oriented statements of intended actions to concrete experiences with an implemented artifact. IS4ALL makes use of scenarios, which describe existing practices or *use cases* in a Health Telematics environment. Such scenarios are developed in collaboration with Health Telematics professionals or end users who declare how a task is being performed. The typical modality in which these scenarios are developed are narratives, accompanied with (paper or system) mock-ups of a system in use. The development of such a scenario involves a certain degree of iteration between IS4ALL and the people / experts responsible for drafting the scenario. These iterations mainly clarify elements of the scenario through structured "question & answer" sessions.

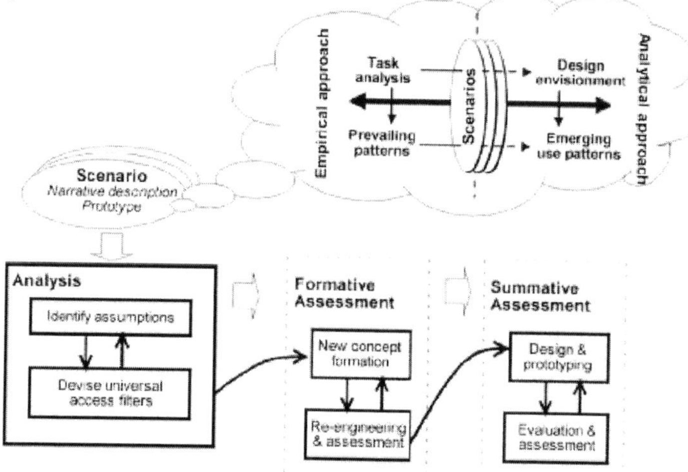

Figure 1: Working with scenarios – steps and phases

Since scenarios may or may not have an explicit focus on universal access, a key question is to devise suitable mechanisms or techniques for working with these scenarios to derive useful insights for the purposes of the project. This entails a reference model or a structured guide towards introducing universal access principles in the agenda of the Healthcare Telematics practitioners (see Figure 1).

3.2 Identifying breakdowns and envisioning new design alternatives

This is an analytical step (see shaded part of Figure 1), which involves a conscious effort to unfold, record and reflect upon implicit/explicit claims or assumptions embodied in the original scenario. For example, by inspecting (parts of) the current implementation of the user interface to the integrated electronic health record of HYGEIAnet, one can derive several implicit assumptions, such "the user interface is designed for desktop access", or "the user interface is designed for users with fine spatial control, fine eye-hand coordination, ability to pull and push targets, ability to initiate movement on demand, etc." Relaxing some of these assumptions facilitates insight into novel usage contexts. Articulating concrete proposals for these novel usage contexts is a critical step towards introducing universal access principles.

3.3 Scenario screening

Scenario screening refers to the task of articulating concrete specifications for envisioned contexts of use, thus fostering an iterative re-engineering process of the initial scenario towards universal access. A prime concern of IS4ALL is to define and document techniques, which can be used for scenario screening. These techniques may be informal – based on intuition – or formal means through which designers can reason about tentative scenarios. One approach, which seems to be popular, entails the definition of universal access filters, which lead designers to explore alternative pathways towards deriving accessible solutions to potential design breakdowns. Universal access filters may take several forms. The most popular is that of questions, which seek to provide insights into how a particular task is to be carried out (by a user, using a particular access terminal in a context of use). Figure 2 depicts a revised version of the illustration in Figure 1, which denote the role of universal access filters.

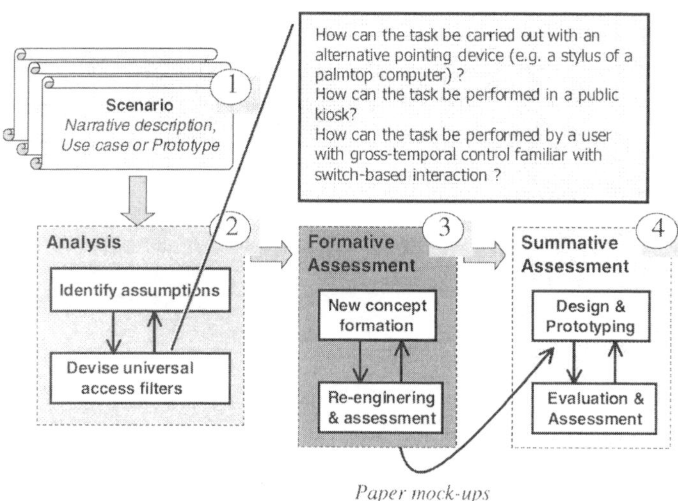

Figure 2: Using universal access filters

What is important to note is that universal access filters are useful when there is a tentative design to be assessed. In such cases, they help designers identify potential break down or shortcomings in the use of the product by certain user groups. Moreover, they can be used as a basis for argumentation during design, thus fostering an analytical insight to universal design. Nevertheless, accessibility filters do not provide answers or design concepts; rather they motivate the designers to think about a problem or certain aspects of the problem. Another shortcoming is the fact that they are usually experience-based, thus relying on intuition rather than a formal basis. This means that there may be needed several categories of filters to inform and facilitate an all-inclusive design process (or universal design).

4. Discussion

In the previous sections, we have described recent progress in IS4ALL with particular emphasis on scenario development. In the context of the project, scenarios constitute the primary means for eliciting requirements for universal access in Health Telematics, and in particular EHRs. In many ways, the approach is similar to the trend towards requirements engineering with scenarios, which has become popular in Software Engineering communities. Nevertheless, there are distinct differences between the IS4ALL work and other similar approaches in the treatment and articulation of scenarios. For IS4ALL, scenarios offer a preliminary design resource and a common reference ground for design deliberations. These deliberations should aim to unfold critical design issues, which bind the original scenario (i.e., the target users, the underlying technology and the context of use). Such binding conditions subsequently form the primary means of a re-engineering process, which extends the original scenario with insights from universal access. This re-engineering process is referred to as *scenario screening* and is depicted in the diagram of Figure 3.

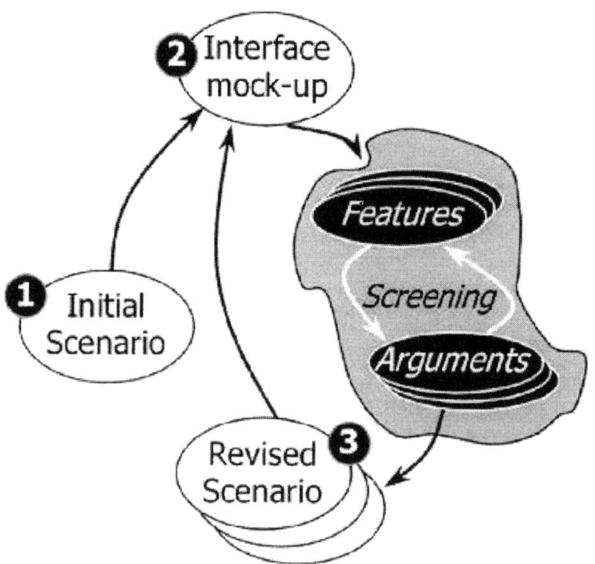

Figure 3: Elements of a re-engineering approach to facilitate scenario screening for universal access

Scenario screening serves the purpose of extrapolating the universal access design considerations relevant to a particular scenario. Work has already begun aiming to use a designated set of scenarios as design resources to guide the development of a code of practice, which would enable Health Telematics application developers to systematically identify the elements of an artifact, which can become subject to universal access re-engineering. In particular, the IS4ALL project is working on three distinct scenarios reflecting diverse usage contexts, universal access requirements and prospective solutions.

One scenario is drawn from HYGEIAnet [10], the regional Health Telematics network of Crete and in particular the services designed around the Virtual Electronic Patient Record. The current version of these services are desktop-oriented and IS4ALL is exploring alternatives for the WWW, and various network-attachable devices, including a WAP phone and iPAQ. The second scenario is based on the EC-funded project WARDINHAND [11]. This project develops a ward-bound information system accessible through a palm device. The final scenario is inspired from the EC-funded project C-CARE [12] and describes how concepts from this project are hosted by a national EDI for medical data in Belgium. In the future, these scenarios will be further developed to depict, through prototypes and mock-ups, new work patterns resulting from universal access insights. These developments will be periodically documented in future reports as well as in the project's web site.

Acknowledgements

IS4ALL is a multidisciplinary Working Group co-ordinated by the Institute of Computer Science of the Foundation for Research and Technology – Hellas (ICS-FORTH), Greece. The membership includes: Microsoft Healthcare Users Group Europe (MS-HUGe); the European Health Telematics Association (EHTEL); Consiglio Nazionale delle Ricerche – Istituto di Ricerca sulle Onde Elettromagnetiche (CNR-IROE) Italy; Fraunhofer-Gesellschaft zur Foerderung der angewandten Forschung e.V. - Forschungszentrum Informationstechnik GmbH (FhG-FIT), Germany; Institut National de Recherche en Informatique et Automatique – Laboratoire lorrain de recherche en informatique et ses applications (INRIA), France; and Fraunhofer-Gesellschaft zur Foerderung der angewandten Forschung e.V. - Institut fur Arbeitswirtschaft und Organisation (FhG-IAO), Germany.

The IS4ALL consortium would also like to explicitly acknowledge the co-operation with HYGEIAnet [10] and the IST-funded projects WARDINHAND [11] and C-CARE [12] for the purposes of constructing reference scenarios.

References

1. Mace, R. L., Hardie, G. J., and Plaice, J. P. (1991). Accessible environments: Toward universal design. In W. Preiser, J. Vischer and E. White (Eds.) Design interventions: Toward a more human architecture. New York: Van Nostrand Reinhold.
2. Stephanidis, C. and Emiliani, P-L. (1999). "Connecting" to the information society: a European perspective, *Technology and Disability Journal*, 10(1), pp. 21-44.
3. Stephanidis, C., Salvendy, G., et al., (1998). Toward an Information Society for All: An International R&D Agenda. *International Journal of Human-Computer Interaction*, Vol. 10(2), pp. 107-134.
4. Stephanidis, C., Salvendy, G., et al., (1999). Toward an Information Society for All: HCI challenges and R&D recommendations. *International Journal of Human-Computer Interaction*, Vol. 11(1), pp. 1-28.
5. Stephanidis, C. (Ed.), (2001). User Interfaces for All – Concepts, Methods and Tools. Mahwah, NJ: Lawrence Erlbaum Associates (ISBN 0-8058-2967-9).
6. Story, M. F., 1998. *Maximising Usability: The Principles of Universal Design*. Assistive Technology, vol. 10 (1), pp. 4-12.
7. HFES/ANSI 200, 1997. Draft HFES/ANSI 200 Standard, Section 5: Accessibility. Santa Monica, USA, Human Factors and Ergonomics Society.
8. Akoumianakis, D., Stephanidis, C., 1999. Propagating experience-based accessibility guidelines to user interface development. Ergonomics, 42 (10), pp. 1283-1310.
9. Savidis, A., Paramythis, A., Akoumianakis, D., Stephanidis, C., 1997. *Designing user-adapted interfaces: the unified design method for transformable interactions*. In the Proceedings of the ACM Conference on Designing Interactive Systems: Processes, Methods and Techniques (DIS'97), Amsterdam, The Netherlands, 18-20 August, New York, ACM Press, pp. 323-334.
10. http://www.hygeianet.gr/
11. http://www.wardinhand.org
12. http://dbs.cordis.lu/fep-cgi/srchidadb?ACTION=D&SESSION=16152001-10-25&DOC=19&TBL=EN_PROJ&RCN=EP_RCN_A:55034&CALLER=PROJ_IST)

Electronic Health Records and Communication
for Better Health Care
F. Mennerat (Ed.)
IOS Press, 2002

Health Information Change Management Lessons Learned from a Third of a Century of Change Introduction

Dr John S Bryden
Glasgow, G41 5AA
Scotland, UK
jsb@johnsbryden.com

Abstract. This paper concentrates on the disincentives that discourage particularly doctors from readily adopting new health informatics techniques and suggests that health project management is a different model of management from that used in other industries.

Je veux vous remercier de votre invitation si gentille à vous parler. Je suis John Bryden, médecin de santé publique, informaticien de santé.

I am John Bryden, a consultant in public health who has been managing change in health informatics for almost 35 years.

For an audience that is largely French it is worth explaining that Public Health Doctors in Scotland are quite different from your *médecins inspecteurs départementaux.* These Scots doctors are National Health Service (NHS) medical managers and in health informatics innovation may be routinely the managers of health informatics change.

Most of the participants here come from conservative professions which resist change.

Most subscribe to the views attributed to Gaius Petronius Arbiter in the court of Nero around 50 AD.

We trained hard ..
But it seemed that every time we were beginning to form up into teams
We would be reorganised.
I was to learn later in life that we tend to meet any new situation by reorganising; and a wonderful method it can be for creating the illusion of progress
while producing confusion, inefficiency, and demoralisation.

The particular techniques of change management described here apply to medical doctors but are equally applicable to most of the health professions.

The fundamental education of doctors turns them into effective independent decision makers. The more senior they are the stronger become their decision making abilities.

They are accustomed to being the team leaders in clinical care and are in most societies legally responsible for that care.

Clinical goals may be quite different from political or health service management goals.

Doctors do not fit in with classical industrial or business management techniques.

Managing change in other organisations where the management is hierarchical can frequently be by direction.

Such authoritarian approaches are doomed to failure with health professionals.

This congress is discussing the electronic health record and the management of the change this introduces. It is arguable that these are the kind of techniques that should be used to introduce any form of change in health services.

This paper will discuss some of the techniques that should be adopted to encourage successful change management and some case studies including one which failed.

1. Health Project Management

Sometimes health informatics projects may seem to be like trying to herd cats.

The essential is enthusiastic leadership.

That leader must identify the key opinion leaders ensuring that the "Why" of the project is well understood. It must be understood "why" the project is being introduced, what are its health goals and what health gain there will be for society and for patients.

The danger of medical informatics devotees must not be underestimated. They can be too uncritical of unsatisfactory systems and particularly mislead suppliers of the non-acceptability of hardware and software and by their fervour hide groundswells of discontent.

2. Project Specification

Clinical goals must be identified as well as management objectives

Realistic aims are essential. Limitations of current software must be identified and accepted.

Care is multiprofessional. Systems must serve all professions. Their individuality must be respected.

Adequate infrastructure must be planned and included in the costings. A full on-going training/education programme must be well planned. It must be an ever "revolving door" both to keep staff refreshed and new staff briefed. The costing of this must include not only the teaching costs but also to ensure that there is staff "cover" when people are absent on the courses.

Despite formal "lowest tender" procedures too cheap a price may mean inadequate attention to the clinical needs.

In all of this project management there should be persistant leadership and from a leader who is able to resist popular and political pressures and shows continuing willingness to listen to and learn from users.

The trouble is that this may lead to the problems of financial control when the system development becomes iterative.

3. Workshop Questions

Who will drive the development? This has two levels:

- The implementation management – which has to be as described previously.
- The on-going running of the system – this has to be at a lower level of skill but keeping all the previous points in mind.

How will continuity of care be fostered? This must be within the project specification described above.

Incentives for improving communications. These must have been part of the build-up of the project management and system specification.

Who will pay and how much and for what. Every country has its own funding system. It is this author's argument that the health information system should be part of the on-costs of the insurance system. But even between Scotland and England there are funding differences. In Scotland both hardware, software and training costs are met centrally as a first charge.

How should networks be organised managed and controlled? Any networks should be organised, managed and controlled as above but it raises the fundamental question of how much such patient data should be networked at all outwith the local health care professionals. This is certainly a topic to be discussed in to-morrow's workshop.

4. Case Studies

Many Scottish examples illustrating the above points might be quoted from 1969 to date but only three are included here.

4.1 Woodside Health Centre, Glasgow

1970-72 This was the first major urban health centre in the UK. When it opened it had over 40,000 registered patients and over 30 very independent family doctors who up until then were working out of premises of very variable quality and with mainly non-existant modern records systems.

The family doctors debated and discussed their records systems and obtained a champion to work with them.

Their aims were well defined. They wished simple use of then available main-frame computing to support their indexing of the patients and the filing of their records.

They used a novel but simple Optical Character Reading mainframe system to capture their patient demographic identifiers.

This system was a great success. [1] [2]

4.2 Scottish Cardio-thoracic Surgeons – Surgical Audit

1991-93 This was a nationally funded project to support these surgeons with a commonly agreed surgical clinical audit system.

It had a very complex specification prepared centrally but it did not have wide enough input from all of the surgeons in each of their six geographical centres. The specification was too complex and unrealistic in terms of the then state of the software art.

Under the official rules the cheaper tender won but with hindsight it was quite obvious that both the tenderers underestimated the complexity of the project aims.

The software was based on a Unix platform which was not readily understood by the clinical teams and could not be tailored readily by end users.

To obtain surgeon satisfaction iterative software development became the norm and the supplier could not cope with this financially.

This project was abandoned after an abortive expenditure of around 350,000 Euros although the hardware became re-usable for other work.

4.3 Scottish Primary Care Health Informatics GPASS General Practitioner Administration System for Scotland

There are currently over 4000 Scottish Family doctors and over 80% of their practices use the GPASS system.

This EHCR system has been developed gradually over a period of years. It has had strong democratic management committees. There is a well funded software team. A succession of champions have promoted it over the years. A well developed free education and training programme runs on an on-going basis and within this there are local geographically based co-ordinators who both trouble-shoot and support the educational programme.

GPASS is a success. Its latest Windows' based version has raised the user numbers from under 75% of practices to over 80% [3]

5. Conclusion

Change Management in Health Information and other health applications requires specialised techniques and these must not be ignored.

References

[1] Bryden, J S; Boddy, F A - "Use of optical character recognition equipment in the creation of a patient data file in a large urban health centre" - Journeés d'informatique Medicales, French Government Publication, Toulouse, **1972.**

[2] Boddy, F A; Bryden, J S - "Woodside Health Centre - The Computer Experiment" - Health Bulletin **1972.**

[3] http://www.gpass.demon.co.uk
http://www.show.scot.nhs.uk/gpass/users/
http://www.fays.orknet.co.uk/gpass_user/
http://www.abdn.ac.uk/~gpr117/
http://www.ceppc.org/spice/collecting_data.shtml

Electronic Health Records and Communication for Better Health Care
F. Mennerat (Ed.)
IOS Press, 2002

The Medical Communication and Information System has to be managed by the medical profession

Bertrand Kempf
Honorary Director of informatics, AP-HP, Paris
Phone +33/0-148 78 78 88

Most physicians, politicians and economists do not know that Communication and Information Systems could contribute considerably to improving the quality of our healthcare system, and also to controlling their expenditures.

On the other hand, everybody here knows that the CEHRs (Communicating Electronic Healthcare Records) will help concretely the physicians to have a better understanding of their patients, to help diagnosis process, to improve (qualitatively) and reduce (quantitatively) the tests and therapeutics prescriptions. They will take account of their patients in full knowledge of the facts. So, the result will be dual: quality and efficiency.

Of course, if we want the health professionals to accept the necessary Medical Communication and Information System, and to work correctly and on a long term basis, it has to be as perfect as possible, in its contents, ergonomics, privacy, security etc.

But this is not sufficient. To prevent a failure, ***the system must be conceived, piloted, managed, operated and exploited under the direct authority and responsibility of the medical actors***. That has been my conviction for fifty years, and today, it is my contribution to your working conference.

To be brief and concise, this is what I suggest for France: I propose the creation of "***Regional Agencies for Medical Information***".

The boards and managing teams of these 21 new organisms should be mandated by all the physicians in ambulatory care, by general practitioners, specialists, public and private hospital doctors, and by the other health care professionals. Unions, syndicates, deontological institutions, hospital commissions should be represented, also the patients' associations, and social security.

These bodies should have their own staff, locations, informatics equipment and resources.

They could store, in their electronic safe boxes, the patients' medical records, the CEHRs.

They should have the responsibility and legality for all centralised data uses: for the knowledge and control of professional activities, for epidemiological works, for the data transfer to the pharmaceutical drug industry and to social security, as for medico-vigilance, that means the survey in real time of the apparition of new health risks and accidents.

Besides, these agencies should have the operational responsibility of the telemedicine, of the permanent medical training using networks, of the disposal, via Internet and Intranet, of all information about pathologies, therapeutics etc.

In a few words, that is the political revolution I propose. You could imagine easily, with me, the amazing advantages of the feedback. The obstacles too, which are neither technical or financial.

In France, a very recent law gives new rights to the patients. For instance, a direct access to their own medical records; it organises as well the modes of financial compensation of care risks. Because it creates new obligations for the physicians, it should be fair and wise, in return, to entrust the physicians the operational management of their own information system.

So, altogether, they will commission and supervise the realisation of their own work. So, the power which they deserve should be their own property. Therefore, they will have the power that they deserve.

Let me say something more about the improvement of medical exercise. I am convinced that the physician who has to send to a data bank some information about his patient, knows that he could be judged by his colleagues on the quality of this information. Automatically, it will encourage him strongly, upstream, to be particularly keen about the quality of his medical decision, actions and orders: better medical practice.

As for the control of the health expenses, I rely upon a study which demonstrate that more than one hundred billions French francs are wasted every year in France without any benefit for patients' care. I am sure that the main cause of these useless expenses is the lack of communication, between medical actors, of the CEHRs.

Electronic Health Records and Communication for Better Health Care
F. Mennerat (Ed.)
IOS Press, 2002

Secure communication and co-operation of distributed Electronic Patient Records

Bernd BLOBEL
University Hospital Magdeburg, Leipziger Str. 44, D-39120 Magdeburg, Germany

Abstract. Electronic Health Records (EHR) are moving towards the core application of health information systems. Enabling informational interoperability of shared care environment including EHR, structure and function of components used have to follow open standards and publicly available specifications. This comprises also methods and tools applied. Security services needed have to be an integral part of architecture and operation of the specified and implemented components.
Starting with basic architectural paradigms the Magdeburg Medical Informatics Department was involved in at the early nineties, the secure behaviour of components has been derived. For establishing the required trustworthiness, security models have been introduced and presented in the paper. Beside communication security services based on standardised Public Key Infrastructure (PKI) and security token such as Health Professional Cards (HPC), policy-defined application security services such as authorisation, access control, accountability, etc., of information recorded, stored and processed must be guaranteed. In that context, appropriate resource access decision services have to be established.
As the HARP project result, a component-based EHR architecture has been specified and demonstrated for enforcing fine-grained security services by binding certificates to application components, by the way enforcing policies.

1. Introduction

For establishing efficient and high quality care of patients, comprehensive and accurate information about status and processes directly and indirectly related to patient's health must be provided and managed. Such information concerns medical observation, ward procedures, laboratory results, medical controlling, account management and billing, materials, pharmacy, etc. Therefore, health information systems within healthcare establishments (HCE) converge to Electronic Patient Record (EPR) systems as kernel enabling the view on all the other business processes and building the informational basis for any communication and co-operation within, and between, healthcare establishments (HCE). By that way, inter-organisational virtual electronic healthcare records (EHCR) are built. For providing information and functionality needed, EHCR must be structured and operating appropriately.

2. EHCR Architecture

For a better understanding of the paper's issues, some common definitions regarding the electronic health record (EHR) which includes also aspects beyond the care as patient's being should be introduced.

An EHR is a repository of information about the patient's health available in a computer-readable format. An EHR system at the other hand is a set of components establishing mechanisms to generate, use, store and retrieve an EPR.

Finally, an EHR architecture describes a model of generic properties required for any EPR for providing communicable, comprehensive, useful, effective, and legally binding records, which preserve their integrity over the time independent of platforms and systems as well as of national specialities.

An EHCR has to meet requirements investigated, e.g., in the context of several EHCR projects. Managing objects, an EHCR arises as dynamic process from clinical practice. It performs a complex workflow connected with medical acts. The EHCR is based and supports electronic communication between all parties involved. It documents any diagnostic and therapeutic measures in a standardised structure. Reducing or avoiding redundancy, an EHCR facilitates an optimised unambiguous presentation of medical concepts, preserving the original context and enabling new ones. It reflects chronology and accommodates future developments and views. For managing an EHCR system, the architecture of such distributed and highly complex component system as well as its behaviour (functionality, set of services) must be designed appropriately. The CEN prENV 13606 "EHCR communication" defines in its part 1 an extended component-based EHCR architecture. Such an extended architecture is mandated to meet any requirements through the EHCR's complete lifecycle. According to CEN prENV 13606, an EHCR comprises Root Architectural Components and Original Component Complexes (OCC). The OCC consist of 4 basic components, such as compositions, folders, views, and links. In addition, they may be combined including items, clusters, and headed sections.

Distributed component-based EHCR systems enable the aggregation of those components needed in a specific context. Beside this single model approach, a dual model approach is currently under international development. This model separates the generic object model of the domain and the healthcare speciality-specific or the organisation-specific, department-specific or even person-specific views and restrictions called archetypes. The security-related statements made in this paper are based on the component paradigm used by both general approaches. Depending on the level of abstraction and granularity, they might be expressed in one model or in policy-related archetypes.

Because personal medical data are highly sensitive, communication and co-operation in distributed networking systems must be established in a trustworthy way.

3. Basic Architectural Paradigms

Regarding security with special aspects of the healthcare domain, ethical, legal, social, organisational, and technological issues must be handled. Beside these issues also their management (enforcement) has to be guaranteed. For meeting this challenge, a generic component paradigm has been developed, implemented and tested during the last eight years [1]. Allowing phase transition changing the level of abstraction and/or of granularity, such components enable all the views of ISO/IEC 10746-2 [2]. These views are the enterprise, information, computational, engineering, and technology view at the abstraction level as well as the domain, services, or implementation context regarding the granularity.

If objects require knowledge to be completely useable, reusable, and interoperable on all the different levels mentioned, which can only be provided at the CORBA COSS level, the healthcare vertical facilities need the specification of this knowledge about conditions, relationships, and framework at the business object component architecture level [3]. Therefore, a generic component paradigm was being adopted.

While objects are defined originally as

$$\text{Object} = \quad \text{attributes + operations} \tag{1}$$

the components are characterised by

$$\begin{aligned}\text{Component} = \quad & \text{attributes + operations + structural constraints +} \\ & \text{operational constraints + events + multi-interfaces *} \\ & \text{scenarios + safety + reliability + security + ...}\end{aligned} \tag{2}$$

To make the system requirements, design, and management transparent to the user groups involved, a consistent methodology must be used. Developed and tested within several European projects, such as, eg, ISHTAR [4] and TrustHealth [5], the UML methodology [6] is an appropriate paradigm to deal with the security issues in health information systems like EPR.

4. Security Models

Generic models relevant in the security context are the domain model, the generic security model and the layered security model.

A domain is characterised by components of a system grouped by common organisational, logical, and technical properties. This could be done for common policies (policy domains), for common environments (environment domains), or common technology (technology domains) [7, 8].

A policy describes the legal framework including rules, regulations and ethical aspects, the organisational and administrative framework, functionalities, claims and objectives, the principals (human users, devices, applications, components, objects) involved, agreements, rights, duties, and penalties defined as well as the technological solution implemented for collecting, recording, processing and communicating data in information systems. Because one or more of the policy-defining factors may differ, many policies have to be established in the complex environment of shared care systems. For describing policies, methods such as policy templates or formal policy modelling might be deployed.

Regarding the flexibility in handling properties and policies, the domain is of a generic nature, consisting of sub-domains and building super-domains. The smallest domain is the working place or sometimes even a specific component of a system (e.g., of a server machine). The domain will be extended by chaining sub-domains to super-domains forming a common domain of communication and co-operation, which is characterised by establishing an agreed security policy. Such transaction-concrete policy has to be negotiated between the communicating and co-operating principals, which is also called policy bridging.

For dealing with distributed systems, two security concepts have to be supported: the concept of communication security between two or more principals (e.g., components) and the concept of application security within one component. Communication security services comprise strong mutual authentication and accountability of principals involved, integrity, confidentiality and availability of communicated information as well as some notary's services. As result of the authentication procedure, authorisation for having access to the other principal has to be decided. Application security services concern accountability, authorisation and access control regarding data and functions, integrity, availability, confidentiality of information recorded, processed and stored as well as some notary's services and audit.

5. Roles and Authorisation

Because it is impossible to assign authorisation and access rights within extended domains to any principal specifically, principals are grouped for assigning authorisation and access rights according to the role group members play. Grouping is performed according to defined attributes characterising the group. Such attributes could be qualifications and skills as prerequisites for assigned roles, commonly accepted groups (general professions, legally-defined or regulation-defined groups), etc. For enabling open systems and communication across the border, efforts have been undertaken to harmonise attributes by SDOs (Standard Developing Organisations), e.g., by establishing an international healthcare profession nomenclature [9, 10].

For assigning authorisation and access control to specific principals as group members, attribute certificates must be bound to ID certificates. The Public Key Infrastructure (PKI) needed has been standardised internationally by ISO with the recently approved ISO TDS 17090 "Public Key Infrastructure" [11] and at European scale by CEN/ISSS (Comité Europeéan de Normalisation/Information Society Standardisation System) and ETSI (European Telecommunications Standards Institute) with the European Electronic Signature Standard Initiative (EESSI) [12]. Beside the technical harmonisation, the European Union established also a legal harmonisation for establishing electronic signatures: the EU 99/93/EC "Directive on Electronic Signatures". Contrary to the harmonisation for ID-related certificates, attributes such as specialty, subspecialty and medical disciplines as well as related authorisations (rights and duties) are mostly different. If, e.g., prescriptions are a privilege for Germany's doctors, in Norway this activity is performed by nurses. Therefore, before an agreed terminology and ontology has been introduced, the services (acts) being provided are a better characteristic for defining harmonised roles. Such services are, e.g., observation, physical examination, prescription, nuclear treatment, surgical treatment, anaesthetic preparation, collection of specimen, order, billing.

There are several ways for binding key-related ID certificates to key-less attribute certificates: the monolithic approach, the autonomic approach, and the approach of chained signatures. In the monolithic approach, the attribute certificate is part of the ID certificate. In the autonomic approach, some relevant information in the ID certificate is referred to bind with the attribute certificate. In the binding approach using chained signatures, the ID certification authority's signature is referred to bind with the attribute certificate. The mentioned ISO TDS 17090 fixed the first approach [11].

Considering roles, two specialisation of roles might be distinguished: organisational or structural roles on the one hand and functional roles on the other hand. Organisational roles are established by relationships between entities such as organisations and/or persons. Functional roles are created by acts.

The structure-related role of an HP defines his/her position in the organisational hierarchy of the institution reflecting responsibility and competence of the professional. This schema is a rather static one. With respect to the access control procedures it describes a mandatory model. For this paper out of scope examples of structure-related (organisational) roles of organisation are Naming Authority, Registration Authority, Certification Authority, Physician's Chamber. Examples for structure-related (organisational) roles of healthcare professionals (HCP) in health care systems reflecting decreasing access rights are: medical director, director of clinic, head of the department, senior physician, resident physician, physician, medical assistant, trainee, medical student, head nurse, and nurse.

The function-related role of an HP immediately reflects the position in the healthcare process, i.e., the concrete HCP-patient relationship. It represents a highly dynamic relation, which follows discretionary model approaches. Examples for function-related roles in health care systems reflecting decreasing access rights are: caring doctor (responsible or reliable doctor[1]), member of diagnostic team, member of therapeutic team, consulting doctor, referring doctor, attending doctor, family doctor, attending nurse.

Both roles define the rights and duties of an HP in an Health Care Establishment (HCE). Because HPs fulfil obligations in both the organisational and the functional framework, the resulting access control model combines these two views. According to the codes of conduct, the data protection legislation and the European Data Protection Directive, in most of the democracies the function role dominates the access control model in health information systems. Details are given in [13].

6. Security Use Case

Any EPR security solution must fulfil basic principles for open interoperable systems' design such as conservatism, minimality, simplicity, generality, relevance, flexibility, and scalability. In analysis, design, implementation, and maintenance of systems, the UML methodology is widely used. Adopting the component paradigm, this approach is not only applicable to the systems' IT part.

Modelling the security related basic use cases of component-based information systems, the use cases

- PolicyManagement,
- UserManagement,
- RoleManagement,
- UserAuthentication,
- PatientConsent,
- CommunicationInitialisation,
- InformationRequest,
- AccessControl,
- InformationProvision,
- InformationTransfer, and
- Audit

can be separated [14].

Figure 1 shows one of the basic use case types reflecting the low level granularity use case of access control. Its decision scenario can be refined according to figure 2 which follows the CORBA RAD specification.

[1] In the health care system of several countries (e.g.UK), the family doctor is (or is intended to be, e.g., in Germany) the reliable doctor.

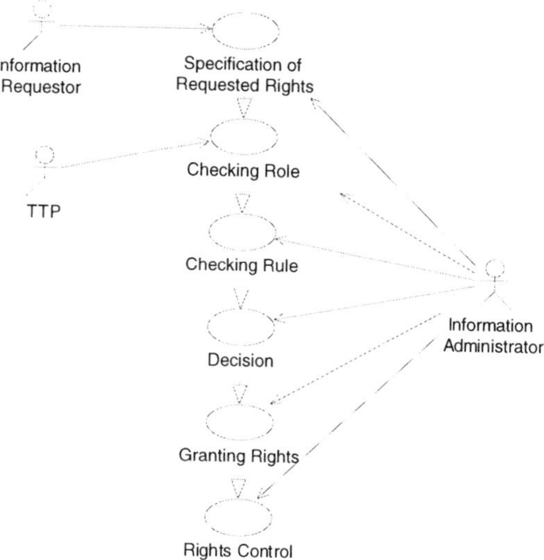

Figure 1. Security-Related Basic Use Case AccessControl

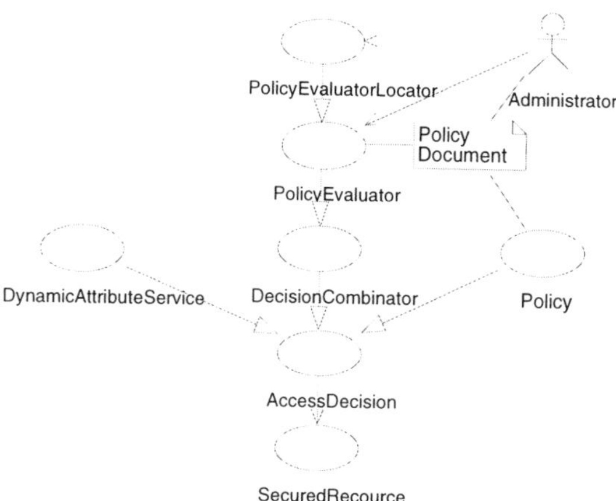

Figure 2. Refined Use Case ResourceAccessDecision

7. Security Infrastructure Enabling Healthcare Networks

The trustworthy environment needed for healthcare communication and co-operation is based on specification and implementation of the aforementioned security services services. Most of these services deploy cryptographic algorithms. For applying asymmetric algorithms such as RSA or elliptic curves, e.g., to provide services for both communication security and application security, such as authentication, accountability, integrity and confidentiality, a security infrastructure has to be established. In Europe, such Public Key Infrastructure (PKI) is based on token for storing the private keys and for processing (signing and verifying) the digital signature mechanism and encoding/decoding as well as on appropriate Trusted Third Party (TTP) services.

At both the European and the German national level, smart cards for health professionals have been standardised as proper token [9, 10]. These Health Professional Card (HPC) standards specify 3 keys for authentication, digital signature and encoding/decoding information or symmetric session key as well as corresponding key-related certificates, but also attribute certificates certifying the card holder's role-defining attributes. For enhancing flexibility in policy and role definitions as well as in role/attribute assignment, especially attribute certificates should be stored and managed on a specific attribute server. Also the legal, organisational and functional infrastructure framework has been specified in Europe as mentioned already.

Supported by several European project's results, the first German demonstrator of an Internet-based secure healthcare network following these standards has been implemented by the Magdeburg Medical Informatics Department. Exploiting experiences about secure communication using strong authentication, encryption, etc. over analogue lines since 1993 or over ISDN lines since 1995, the infrastructure based on HCP and TTP services started its routine use in 1999. This open network aims to facilitate shared care of cancer patients in the region, therefore it is called ONCONET Magdeburg / Saxony-Anhalt. ONCONET enables secure communication of any sensitive multimedia information, but also some application services like secure information retrieval from cancer registry by authorised HP using predefined or free Structured Query Language (SQL) queries. More details about ONCONET can be found in [15].

Regarding the aforementioned application security issues of registries concerning application services (implemented components with their data, operations, restrictions, etc.), following problems could occur. Registries might be organised centrally or decentrally. The former are characterised by separating the site recording information and therefore being responsible for it from the site storing and offering information retrieval. If a registry is centrally organised, the problem of trust whether policy and following authorisation and access rights are correctly enforced occurs. If the registry is decentralised, the management of the entire system requires an adequate architectural solution which isn't in place normally. However, even nowadays Web solutions using component distribution do not support policy enforcement.

For enhancing clinical registry's functionality, specification and implementation of enhanced EHCR interoperability, clinical studies and measures for quality assurance such as quality assurance studies are currently under development. Like the current ONCONET, also these applications have to be trustworthy, interoperable and shall run at the open Internet. They have to use the security infrastructure of HPC and TTP services. Any proprietary architecture shall be avoided.

8. The HARP Cross Security Platform

Real interoperability leads to a closer connection of both communication and application security services. Within the European HARP project funded by the European Commission within the Information Society Technologies (IST) Programme, partners from Greece, Germany, Norway, United Kingdom and The Netherlands specified, developed and implemented enhanced security solutions and TTP services for Internet-based communication and applications [16]. The HARP project's objective is building up entirely secure applications in client-server environments over the Web.

To provide platform independence of solutions in HARP as a real three tiers architecture, the design pattern approach of developing a middleware-like common cross platform called HARP Cross-Security Platform (HCSP) has been used. In HCSP, platform-specific security features have been isolated. Using an abstraction layer, communication in different environment is enabled. According to the component paradigm, an interface definition of a component providing a platform-specific service specifies how a client accesses a service without regard of how that service is implemented. So, the HCSP design isolates and encapsulates the implementation of platform-specific services behind a platform-neutral interface as well as reduces the visible complexity. Only a small portion The solutions concern secure authentication as well as authorisation of principals even not registered before, deploying proper Enhanced TTP (ETTP) services [16]. Especially, it helps to endorse policies by mapping them on processing components. For that reason, HARP components follow the specification of equation (2). Figure 3 demonstrates the HARP ETTP compared with a traditional TTP.

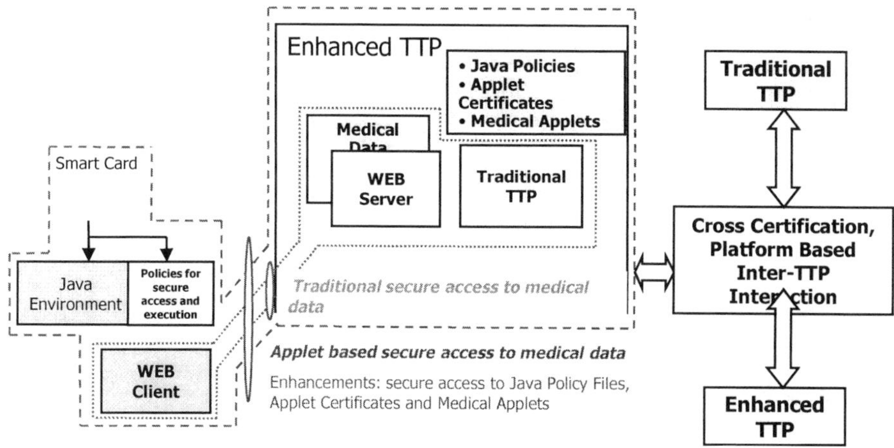

Figure 3. HARP Enhanced TTP vs. Traditional TTP [16]

HARP's generic approach implements several basic principles.

HARP's embedding security into any application to be instantiated over the web-based environment outlined above is based on object oriented programming principles. It is based on Internet technology and protocols solely. The trustworthiness needed has been provided by applying only certified components which are tailored according to the principal's role. In fine-grained steps, it establishes its complete environment required, avoiding any external services possibly compromised. After strong mutual authentication based on smartcards and TTP services, the security infrastructure components are downloaded and installed to be used for implementing the components needed to run the application as well as to transfer data input and output. The SSL protocol deployed to initiate secure sessions is provided by the Java Secure Socket Extension API. The applets and servlets for establishing the local client and the open remote database access facilities communicate using the XML (Extended Markup Language) standard set including XML Digital Signature. Because messages and not single items are signed, the messages are archived separately for accountability reasons meeting the legislation and regulations for health.

Policies are dynamically interpreted and adhered to the components. All components applied at both server and client site are checked twice against the user's role and the appropriate policy: first in context of their selection and provision and second in context of their use and functionality.

Applet security from the execution point of view is provided through the secure downloading of policy files, which determine all access rights in the client terminal.

This has to be seen on top of the very desirable feature that the local, powerful, and versatile code is strictly transient and subject to predefined and securely controlled download procedures. All rights corresponding to predefined roles are subject to personal card identification with remote mapping of identity to roles and thereby to corresponding security policies with specific access rights.

For realising the services and procedures described, an applet consists of the subcomponents GUI and interface controller, smartcard controller, XML signing and XML processing components, communication component applying the Java SSL (Secure Socket Layer) extension, and last but not least the data processing and activity controller. Beside equivalent subcomponents and an attribute certificate repository at the server side, policy repository, policy solver and authorisation manager have been specified and implemented as a "light weight RAD".

After exchanging certificates and establishing the authenticated secure session, servlet security is provided from the execution point of view through listing, selecting and finally executing the components to serve the user properly. By establishing an authenticated session that persists for all service selections, a single-sign-on approach can be realised.

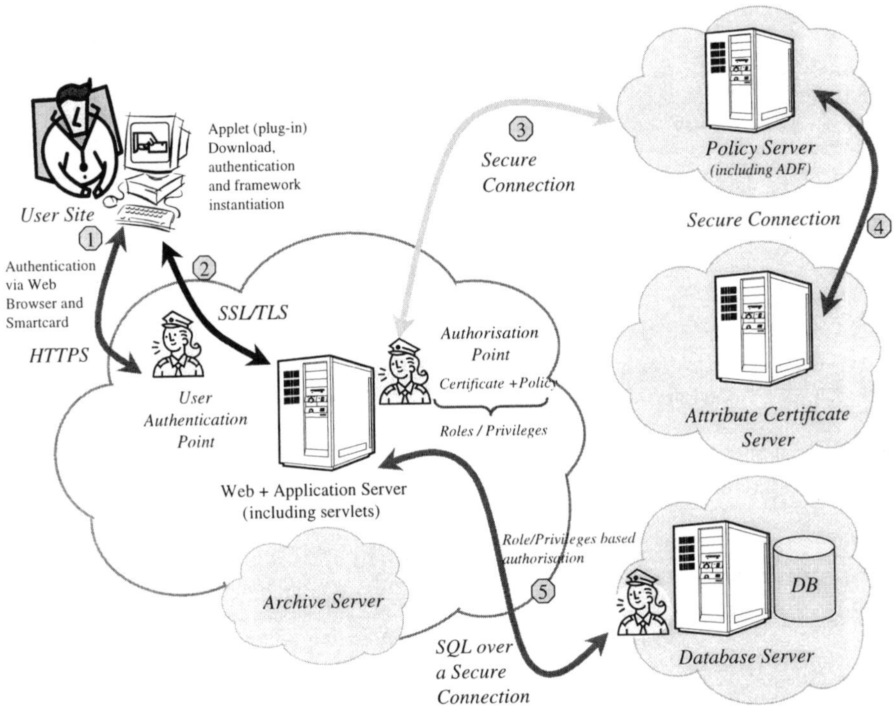

Figure 4. HARP Cross Security Platform [16]

In the server-centric approach, a web-accessible middleware has been chosen based on its support of basic security functionality, e.g., MICO/SSL., Apache Web server with mod_ssl, Apache JServ, and Apache Jakata Tomcat.

Combining the server-centric approach of HCSP, its server-centric approach and the network-centric VPN behaviour, the completely distributed HARP Cross Security Platform can be designed as shown in figure 4.

9. Conclusions

EHCR architecture and subsequently specified and implemented EHCR systems have to comply with comprehensive security solutions solely based on available and emerging standards. Such solutions must be integrated at design and implementation level, involving policy councils, end-users, administrators, developers from the beginning. Communication security services shall be based on PKI, security token and advanced TTP services already established and evaluated at national and international scale.

The European HARP project provides enhanced TTP services and comprehensive development strategies for establishing fine grained application security services. By binding attribute certificates to components appropriate policies can be enforced. These certificates are interpreted at both server and client sides using authorisation services. The HARP Cross Security Platform is solely based on standards including the XML standard set for the establishment of client and server as well as their communication.

Acknowledgement

The author is in debt to the European Commission for funding as well as to the international and national HARP project partners for their support and their kind co-operation.

References

[1] B. Blobel, Application of the Component Paradigm for Analysis and Design of Advanced Health System Architectures. *International Journal of Medical Informatics* **60** (3) (2000) 281-301.
[2] ISO/IEC: Information Technology – Open Distributed Processing – Reference Model: Part 2: Foundations.
[3] OMG, CORBA Specifications. http://www.omg.org
[4] The European ISHTAR Project. http://www.ehto.org/projects/ishtar
[5] The European TrustHealth Project. http://www.ehto.org/projects/trusthealth
[6] H. E. Eriksson, M. Penker, *UML Toolkit*, John Wiley & Sons, Inc., New York, 1998.
[7] B. Blobel, G. Bleumer, A. Müller, K. Louwerse, E. Flikkenschild, F. Ottes, Current Security Issues Faced by Health Care Establishments. ISHTAR Project HC 1028, Deliverable 09 (Final), February 1997; see also B. Barber (Edr.), *Implementing Secure Healthcare Telematics Applications in Europe - ISHTAR*. Studies in Health Technology and Informatics, Vol. 66. IOS Press, Amsterdam, 2001.
[8] OMG: The CORBA Security Specification. Framing-ham: Object Management Group, Inc., 1995, 1997.
[9] CEN TC 251 prENV 13729: Health Informatics - Secure User Identification – Strong Authentication using Microprocessor Cards (SEC-ID/CARDS). Brussels, 1999.
[10] The German HPC Specification for an electronic doctor's license. Version 1.0, July 1999. http://www.hcp-protocol.de
[11] ISO DTS 17090 «Public Key Infrastructure» Part 1 - 3. ISO, 2001.
[12] Council of Europe: 99/93/EC: Directive on Electronic Signatures. Strasbourg, 1999.
[13] B. Blobel, Modelling for Design and Implementation of Secure Health Information Systems. *International Journal of Bio-Medical Computing* **43** (1996) S23-S30.
[14] B. Blobel, F. Roger-France, A Systematic Approach for Analysis and Design of Secure Health Information Systems. *International Journal of Medical Informatics* **62** (3) (2001) 51-78.
[15] B. Blobel, Onconet: A Secure Infrastructure to Improve Cancer Patients' Care. *European Journal of Medical Research* 2000: 5: 360-368.
[16] The HARP Consortium: http://www.ist-harp.org

Electronic Health Records and Communication for Better Health Care
F. Mennerat (Ed.)
IOS Press, 2002

The Protection of Individuals by Protecting Medical Data in EHRs

Barry BARBER
Health Data Protection Ltd,
12 Peterson Court, Worcester Road, WR14 4AA Great Malvern, England

Abstract. The paper discusses the changes in the delivery of Healthcare and the ways in which individuals need to be protected by protecting their Electronic Health Records. A Code of Ethics is needed for health Information Professionals, Data Protection and Security issues need to be taken more seriously. Health Informatics needs to address the issues of safety in the delivery of Healthcare so that it provides solutions to healthcare safety problems rather than increasing the problems to be addressed.

1. The Changing Environment in Healthcare Delivery

The days when one could say to a doctor that "This is between you and me doctor" appear to have gone. The need for the protection of Personal Medical Data is still clearly recognised by the medical and associated healthcare professions. It is recognised in the data protection and other legislation but that protection is not absolute and it does not over-ride all other considerations. From the patients' perspective, the privacy requirements re often context rather than content specific and related to the specific situation of an individual.

The delivery of healthcare has changed by the information explosion and the delivery of care by teams of health Professionals, often operating at different locations. Personal Medical Information is frequently held in centralised Electronic Health records but the globalisation of medicine and the increased use of Telemedicine means that these records and no longer under direct "medical control". No one professional will know everything relevant to the care of a specific individual and hence high quality care requires widespread participation and access to the HER. However, decisions about the disclosure of Personal Medical Information must belong to the patient but they must be informed decisions with the patient being advised that restrictions on disclosure could reduce the ability of the Health Professionals to provide the highest quality of care.

The developments in the area of technology are mainly in the area of local, regional, national and international connectivity. Health Informatics is beginning to be able to deliver the services that were first explored some thirty years ago but with quite inadequate facilities. The opportunities for handling EHRs are dramatically better and it can be expected that these approaches will become universal underpinning of Healthcare and that they will become universally available to Health Professionals for the care of their patients from all locations.

2. Safety or What Happens When It All Goes Wrong?

During the first activities of the EU programme of Advanced Informatics in Medicine [AIM] there was some examination of the next steps and out of these discussions it became clear that safety was a serious issue and the group developed the ideas of Six Safety First Principles for the development of Medical Informatics [1]. This was an interesting development because safety had not appeared to be an issue in medical informatics previously. Curiously, the Healthcare sector is unusual in that it has a serious interest in both security and safety standards. Indeed, the high security counter-measures that arise from risk analysis derive directly from the issues of patient safety. The question derived from work on the security of information systems and the question of "What happens when it all goes wrong?". Some answers to that question were given [2] as the Health Professionals may be mis-led and

- give the wrong treatment
- withhold the right treatment or
- delay any treatment for lack of information.

These actions or inactions may lead to suffering or premature death for individuals or multiple individuals. This may sound far-fetched but there are cases where systems have failed. The most obvious examples are those of the:-

- Therac 25 linear accelerator [3]
- Radiation Treatment Planning Systems
- Alteration of Drug Prescriptions
- Screening Systems
- Loss of Clinical Data
- Loss of Access to Systems

At present there does not exist anything equivalent to the pilots "near miss" reporting systems so that it is often difficult to hard evidence about a security breach but the national press often reports some aspects of these issues when they come to court or when patients are compensated for damages arising from such security breaches.

The health Professional community are becoming more clearly aware of safety issues [4,5,6]. The Harvard Medical Practice study yielded figures as high as 3.7% for the adverse events with half preventable and 14% fatal. The Healthcare system is not as safe as the air transport system but, of course, flying is normally optional while entry into the Healthcare system is not. Health Informatics has potentially much to offer in the endeavour to improve the safety record of the Healthcare sector but it is necessary for it to become part of the solution rather an additional part of the problem..

Clinicians are responsible for the safety of the tools that they use but they cannot check everything. They need to use tools that are "fit for purpose" and designed, developed, maintained and operated to the appropriate standards. However, the systems should be used with common sense and cross-checked where possible in routine use.

3. What Are the Defences for EHRs

The first line of defence has to be the professionalism of all those concerned with the design, development, acquisition, maintenance and use of EHRs. The Health Professionals already have their own Codes of Ethics but at present there is no Code of Ethics for Health Information Professionals [HIPs]. This gap needs to be plugged and the International medical Informatics Association is in process of adopting a suitable Code. Kluge [7] has recently reviewed these issues and outlined the sort of code that is needed and it is hoped that there will be widespread acceptance of the code when it is finally adopted. Exactly as is the case with the other Health Professionals, the law is not enough protection. General ethical principles need to be set in the context of the activities of Health Information Professionals. The EHR is an analogue of the patient and this provides the basis for the ethical basis for the development of a code. It is expected that the code will address the key issues of:-

- Information-privacy & Disposition
- Openness
- Security
- Access
- Legitimate Infringement
- Least Intrudive Alternative
- Accountability

In association with this code there will need to be an established Security Policy to be observed by individual HIPs in their own work as well as a Security policy appropriate to the requirements of Health Care Establishments [HCE] to satisfy their legal obligations. Individual HIPs cannot be responsible for all the security failures of HCEs but they should be aware of them and remedy them where possible.

4. Data Protection Requirements and Standards

The key security requirements for Personal Health Information arise from Article 17 of the Directive [8]. Controllers are required to take technical and organisational measures to protect the data that they are processing, in particular when it is transmitted over a network. In deciding on these security measures they need to have regard to the state of the technology ["state of the art"], the costs of implementing these measures, the risks of the processing and the nature of the data being processed. In healthcare, this is always sensitive or "special category" data. If the Controller does not process the data directly but employs a Processor to do so on his behalf, the Processor must be chosen with sufficient guarantees of security and the Controller must ensure compliance with his security requirements. In addition, there must be a written or equivalent contract and the Processor must only act on the Controller's instructions. CEN TC 251 has developed two standards for the transfer of Personal Health Data outside the EEA [9,10] and these are currently undergoing the CEN Enquiry procedures. There are a number of other CEN TC 251 standards that are relevant to the processing of Personal Health Data. At present the key standards are as follows:-

- ENV 12924 Security Classification & Protection Profiles
- ENV 12251 Password standard
- ENV 12388 Digital Signature Algorithm
- ENV S13608 Parts 1 - 3 Secure Healthcare Communication
- ENV13729 Health informatics - Secure User Identification for Healthcare Strong Authentication using Microprocessor Cards
- ENV 13606 - 3 Electronic Healthcare Record Communication - Part 3: Distribution Rules

Other Data Protection regulations derive from the Council of Europe Convention 108 [11] and the associated recommendation on the Protection of Medical Data [12]. The latter is Healthcare specific and it establishes requirements for the collection and processing of Personal Medical Data, for patient consent, the disclosure of these data, access rights and the correction of erroneous data, security and research uses of these data. It, also, applies to Personal Genetic Data and it sets out requirements on specific issues relating to genetic testing.

5. What Is Meant By Security and Safety?

The traditional definition of security relates to the confidentiality, integrity and availability of data. The property of confidentiality is the assurance that the data are only made accessible to those authorised to have access to those data. The property of the integrity of the data is the assurance that the data are captured correctly and are not maliciously or accidentally, modified during subsequent processing. The property of the availability of data is that the data are available when required for the purposes of the activity. In recent times, the aspect of the accountability has been extracted explicitly from the issue of integrity and it relates to the accountability for any and all aspects of the processing of data so that all actions are identified and capable of being audited as the actions of a specified individual. In Healthcare, the issues of confidentiality have traditionally been taken very seriously although in recent times legal access without patient consent has been accorded in increasing numbers of circumstances. However, the issues of data integrity and availability can be even more serious as patient care can be damaged if Health Professionals believe incorrect information. At the very least the preservation of data integrity requires that measures are taken to:-

- ensure that data are accurately input in to the system
- authenticate the individual who input these data
- ensure that the internal processing preserves that input
- prevent accidental or malicious modification of those data
- ensure accurate presentation of the processed data.

There are a number of standards concerned with the general management if information security:

- ISO 17799 Code of Practice for Information Security Management
- ISO/IEC TR 13335 Guidelines for the Management of IT Security [GMITS]

In addition, there have been a number of European projects concerned with the issues of Healthcare information security and many have been published eg SEISEMD security Guidelines [13], ISHTAR [14], MEDSEC [15] as well as EUROMED-ETS, TrustHealth 1 & 2.

The issue of safety tends to encompass a rather broader field that simply the information processing systems, although it certainly includes the design, development, use and maintenance of such systems. The world standard

For safety-related systems is the IEC 61508 standard [16]. It has been utilised in a number of industries and the healthcare sector can benefit from the experience of other industries as well as developing Guidelines for the utilisation of this standard in Healthcare. CEN has already produced a technical report on the available safety standards and started on this work [17] and this now needs to be completed by the development of the relevant guidelines [18]. Redmill and Rajan [19] have produced a survey of a number of the human factors affecting the utilisation of safety-related systems that are relevant to the current discussions about safety issues in healthcare. The IEC 61508 standard is quite a long and complex one and it consists of the following parts:-

1 General Requirements
2 Requirements for safety-related systems
3 Software vrequirements
4 Definitions and Abbreviations
5 Methods for the determination of safety Integrity Levels
6 Guidelines on the Application of Parts 2 and 3
7 Techniques and Measures.

6. Medical Devices

The medical devices legislation is interesting because there is a raher uncertain boundary between EHRs and medical devices. The definition in the European Directive [20] is as follows:-

"Medical Device means any instrument, apparatus, appliance, material or other article, whether used alone or in combination, including the software necessary for its proper application, intended by the manufacturer to be used for human beings for the purposes of:-

- Diagnosis, prevention, monitoring, treatment or alleviation of disease
- Diagnosis, monitoring, treatment, alleviation of, or compensation for, an injury or handicap
- Investigation, replacement or modification of the anatomy or a physiological process
- Control of conception

And which does not achieve its principal intended action in or on the human body by pharmacological, immunological or metabolic means but which may be assisted in its function by such means."

Maybe Health Information Systems and EHRs will become to be regarded as medical devices at some stage. However, whether or not this approach is taken, there are some important lessons that can be learned from the approach that is taken to the control of medical devices. In the first instance, a defined product is "put on the market" by a person or organisation. In some sense this is a defined, "shrink wrapped", item not merely a box into which a variety of software may be emptied and hence the effects of its use in the market may be, and indeed has to be, monitored for adverse events. When this monitoring reveals inadequacies in the product, it can be recalled and modiified or taken off the market. There is a register of persons who have placed medical devices on the market and there is a classification of medical devices in respect of the risks of its intended use. The Directive established national regulatory bodies to over see the working of the legislation and the manufacturers are required to certify that they have carried out the necessary safety proceedures appropriate to the classification of the device in terms of design, manufacture, testing and instructions for use. The national bodies overseeing this legislation can require information from manufacturers in respect of all aspects of all these issues. Health Information Systems and systems supporting EHRs can benefit from the introduction of some of these approaches to safety even if this legislation does not yet apply to such systems.

7. Conclusion

Following this analysis of progress with the security and safety of EHRs, it appears that we need to establish a suitable Code of Ethics for all Health Information Professionals concerned with the design, development, maintenance and use of EHRs. The Data Protection legislation needs to be taken more seriously and suitable Security Policies put in place and adhered to. Proper standards should be used in all aspects of the design, development, implementation and use of HER and in particular suitable guidelines need to be developed for the use of the IEC 61508 standard in the Healthcare setting. None of this is petty bureaucracy but a protection for the patient in an increasingly complex situation.

References

[1] B Barber et al, The Six Safety First Principles of health Information Systems: A programme of Implementation Parts 1 & 2, pp 608 - 619 in MIE-90, 1990, Springer-Verlag, Berlin, ISBN 0-387-52936-5

[2] B Barber, R Vincent & M Scholes, Worst Case Scenarios: The Legal Consequences, , pp 282 - 288 in HC-92, pub BJHC 1992, ISBN 0-948198-12-5

[3] I Peterson, "Fatal Defect: Chasing Killer Computer Bugs", Vintage Books, New York, 1996, IBN 0-8129-2023-6

[4] B Jarman, The Quality of Care in Hospitals, JRCP Lond, 75 - 91, vol 34, Jan/Feb 2000
Reducing Error: Improving Safety, BMJ issue 7237, 18 March 2001

[5] BMJ, Reducing Error and Improving Safety, Issue 7237, 18 March 2000, collected papers on Healthcare Safety

[6] TA Brennan, et al, Incidence of Adverse Events and Negligence in Hospitalised Patients: results of the Harvard Medical Practice Study, N Engl J Med, 1991, 324, 370-376

[7] E-H Kluge, The Ethics of Electronic Patient Records, Peter Lang, 2001, ISBN 0-8204-5259-9

[8] Directive, 95/46/EC, of the European Parliament and the Council "On the Protection of Individuals with regard to the Processing of Personal Data and on the Free Movement of such Data", 24 October 1995, OJEC 281/31 - 50

[9] Draft TC 251 ENV, Guidance on Handling Personal Health Data in International Applications in the Context of the EU Data Protection Directive, out for CEN Enquiry, 2001

[10] Draft TC 251 ENV, International Transfer of Personal Health Data Covered by the EU Data Protection Directive: High Level Security Policy, out for CEN Enquiry, 2001

[11] Council of Europe Convention 108, For the Protection of Individuals with regard to Automatic Processing of Personal Data, 1981

[12] Council of Europe Recommendation "On the Protection of Medical Data", R(97)5, 1997

[13] SEISMED Consortium, Data Security for Health Care, Studies in Health Technology and Informatics vols 31 – 33, IOS Press, Amsterdam 1996
vol I Management Guidelines ISBN 90 5199 264 5
vol II Technical Guidelines ISBN 90 5199 265 3
vol III User Guidelines, ISBN 90 5199 266 1

[14] ISHTAR Consortium, Implementing Secure Healthcare Telematics Applications in Europe, Studies in Health Technology and Informatics vol 66, IOS Press, Amsterdam 2001, ISBN 90 5199 489 3

[15] MEDSEC Consortium, Security Standards for Health Care Information Systems, IOS Press, Amsterdam 2002, in press

[16] International Electrotechnical Commission, Functional Safety of Electrical/ Electronic/ Programmable Electronic Safety-Related Systems, IEC 61508, May 2000
Council Directive, 93/42/EEC "Concerning Medical Devices", 14 June 1993, OJEC 169/1-43

[17] CEN/TC251/N99-001, Report on Safety & Security related Software Quality Standards for Healthcare [SSQS], 5 February 1999, CR 13694

[18] B Barber, F-A Allaert & E-H Kluge, Info-Vigilance or Safety in Health Information Systems, MEDINFO 2001, pp1229-1233, IOS Press, Amsterdam 2000

[19] F Redmill and J Rajan, Human Factors in Safety-Critical Systems, Butterworth-heinemann, Oxford, 1997

[20] Directive of the Council 93/42/EEC of 14 June 1993 "Concerning Medical Devices", OJEC 12/7/93, L169/1 - 43

Electronic Health Records and Communication for Better Health Care
F. Mennerat (Ed.)
IOS Press, 2002

Electronic Health Care Records in Europe: confidentiality issues from an American perspective

Alexandru I. PETRISOR[1], MSPH; Julia M. CLOSE[2], BA
[1] *Department of Environmental Health Sciences, Norman J. Arnold School of Public Health, University of South Carolina, 800 Sumter Street, Columbia, SC 29208, USA*
[2] *Department of Government and International Studies, College of Liberal Arts, University of South Carolina, Columbia, SC 29208, USA*

Abstract. The confidentiality and security issues related to the European Electronic Health Care Records have been approached in the United States as well. This paper synthesizes several solutions and comments on these issues from the legal viewpoint in the United States, as well as some preoccupations of the academic world to improve and standardize the quality of the security and confidentiality of data from studies involving human subjects.

1. Introduction

The EUROREC 2001 Work Conference, organized in Aix-en-Provence, France, raised several questions related to issues concerning the European Electronic Health Care Records. The particular area of interest presented in this intervention is related to confidentiality and security of information. We will be presenting some solutions implemented in the United States, in the academic world, particularly in the Norman J. Arnold School of Public Health at the University of South Carolina, and the legal frame governing the implementation of other solutions by health agents, and some reactions and suggestions provided by a panel of discussants from the Norman J. Arnold School of Public Health.

2. The Academic World

In the European vision, security is a combination of availability (prevention of unauthorized withholding), confidentiality (prevention of unauthorized disclosure), and integrity (prevention of unauthorized modification). It involves attributes of software that bear on its ability to prevent unauthorized access, whether accidental or deliberate, to programs and data [2].

In the United States, according to the Federal Policy for the Protection of Human Subjects (Basic Department of Health and Human Services Policy for Protection of Human Research Subjects), information must be presented to enable persons to voluntarily decide whether or not to participate as a research subject. It is a fundamental mechanism to ensure respect for persons through provision of thoughtful consent for a voluntary act. The regulations insist that the subjects be told the extent to which their personally identifiable private information will be held in confidence. For example, some studies require disclosure of information to other parties. Some studies inherently are in need of a Certificate of Confidentiality, which protects the investigator from involuntary release of the names or other identifying characteristics of research subjects. The Institutional Review Board will determine the level of adequate requirements for confidentiality in light of its mandate to ensure minimization of risk and determination that the residual risks warrant involvement of subjects [4].

In the light of these procedural guidelines, any research involving human subjects in the Norman J. Arnold School of Public Health, disregarding the manner of conducting the study, must received a prior approval of the Human Subject Ethics Committee. The application represents the base for assuring confidentiality, through the following two items [1]:

(a) "Would the type of data you are collecting from each subject possibly be construed in an invasion of privacy?"
(b) How will subject's privacy be protected? What are the procedures for safeguarding each subject's rights with respect to the following: safety and security of the individual, privacy and confidentiality (including protection and anonymity of data), and embarrassment, discomfort, or harassment?

3. The Legal Frame

The US legal frame governing issues related to confidentiality and security of individual data, including the health care data, is represented mainly by two legislative pieces: The Freedom of Information Act (FOIA), and the Privacy Act.

The Freedom of information Act was passed by the US Congress in 1966 and amended in 1974. It is based on Madison and Hamilton's arguments that openness in government will help people in making the choices necessary to a democracy, therefore people need to be informed. According to FOIA, any member of the public may obtain the records of the agencies of the federal government (agencies, offices and departments of the executive branch of the federal government, such as the National Security Council, federal government-controlled corporations, such as the US Postal Service or Amtrak, or independent federal regulatory agencies, such as the Federal Trade Commission, Environmental Protection Agency, or Federal Communications Commission).

FOIA applies only to agencies of the federal government, however every state has laws guaranteeing citizens access to the records of state agencies. Records that can be obtained with FOIA vary. People have requested information on health and safety reports on silicone breast implants from the Food and Drug Administration, records on the assassination of Kennedy from the FBI and CIA.

FOIA allows the access to two types of information: structure and functions of the agencies: records related to taxes, public health, consumer product safety, labour relations, national defence, and environmental issues, and record that the government has about people (themselves): records only about oneself under the Privacy Act of 1974 [3].

The Privacy Act of 1974, which became effective on September 27, 1975, can generally be characterized as an omnibus "code of fair information practices" which attempts to regulate the collection, maintenance, use, and dissemination of personal information by federal government agencies. Broadly stated, the purpose of the Privacy Act is to balance the government's need to maintain information about individuals with the rights of individuals to be protected against unwarranted invasions of their privacy stemming from federal agencies' collection, maintenance, use, and disclosure of personal information about them. It was also concerned with potential abuses presented by the government's increasing use of computers to store and retrieve personal data by means of a universal identifier, such as an individual's social security number. The Act focuses on four basic policy objectives:

(a) Restrict disclosure of personally identifiable records maintained by agencies.
(b) Grant individuals increased rights of access to agency records maintained on themselves.
(c) Grant individuals the right to seek amendment of agency records maintained on them upon a showing that the records are not accurate, relevant, timely or complete.
(d) Establish a code of "fair information practices" which requires agencies to comply with statutory norms for collection, maintenance, and dissemination of records.

Like the Freedom of Information Act, the Privacy Act applies only to a federal "agency", thus, state, local government agencies and private entities are not subject to the Act. Privacy Act rights are personal to the individual who is the subject of the record and cannot be asserted derivatively by others. However, the parent of any minor, or the legal guardian of an incompetent, may act on behalf of that individual, noting "there is no absolute right of a parent to have access to a record about a child absent a court order or consent". The records regulated by the Privacy Act include, without limiting to, information about education, financial transactions, medical history, and criminal or employment history. To qualify as a "record," the information must identify an individual [5].

4. The Panel's Reaction

A mini-conference organized in the Norman J. Arnold School of Public Health at the University of South Carolina was meant to present some ideas of the EUROREC '01 Conference, focussing on issues related to data security and confidentiality. The participants were international students and they made several interesting remarks:

(a) Some student from Canada suggested the increased importance of a unique identifier to be used as a key to accessing individual health care records. The health care providers in Canada use magnetic cards, similar to the solutions presented at EUROREC '01 by the representatives of Germany and The Netherlands. One of the problems is that this card can store a limited amount of information and not the entire record. As a result, it is necessary to identify the minimum information to be stored on a card.
(b) Even though the exchange of health care records is not generalized in India, there is a special system used by radiologists to submit a radiological picture in order to request a second opinion. Referred as PACS (Picture Archive Communication Systems), the system was adopted in some other countries as well.

References

[1] Coker AL, Sanderson M. EPID 741: Epidemiologic methods I. Course materials. University of South Carolina, 1999
[2] Telemedicine glossary. Glossary of standards, concepts, technologies and users. Unit B1: Applications relating to health. 3rd Edition. 2001 working document. April 2001. DG-INFSO B1, Version 3.10
[3] The Website of American Civil Liberties Union- http://www.aclu.org. 2001.
[4] The Website of the Office for Human Research Protections (Division of the United States Department of Health and Human Services)- http://ohrp.osophs.dhhs.gov. 2001
[5] The Website of the United States Department of Justice- http://www.usdoj.gov. 2001

Electronic Health Records and Communication for Better Health Care
F. Mennerat (Ed.)
IOS Press, 2002

Information Architecture for a Federated Health Record Server

Kalra D [1], Lloyd D [1], Austin T [1], O'Connor A [1], Patterson D [2], Ingram D [1]
[1] *University College London, CHIME, Holborn Union Building, Highgate Hill, London, N19 3UA*
[2] *The Whittington Hospital, Highgate Hill, London N19 5NF*
Correspondence to: d.kalra@chime.ucl.ac.uk

Abstract. This paper describes the information models that have been used to implement a federated health record server and to deploy it in a live clinical setting. The authors, working at the Centre for Health Informatics and Multiprofessional Education (University College London), have built up over a decade of experience within Europe on the requirements and information models that are needed to underpin comprehensive multi-professional electronic health records. This work has involved collaboration with a wide range of health care and informatics organisations and partners in the healthcare computing industry across Europe though the EU Health Telematics projects GEHR, Synapses, EHCR-SupA, SynEx and Medicate. The resulting architecture models have fed into recent European standardisation work in this area, such as CEN TC/251 ENV 13606. UCL has implemented a federated health record server based on these models which is now running in the Department of Cardiovascular Medicine at the Whittington Hospital in North London. The information models described in this paper reflect a refinement based on this implementation experience.

1. Requirements

The very extensive investigations of user and enterprise requirements that have taken place over ten years have sought to capture the diversity and specialisation across primary, secondary and tertiary care, between professions and across countries. These requirements identify the basic information that must be accommodated within an EHCR[a] architecture to:

- capture faithfully the original meaning intended by the author of a record entry or set of entries;
- provide a framework appropriate to the needs of professionals and enterprises to analyse and interpret EHCRs on an individual or population basis;
- incorporate the necessary medico-legal constructs to support the safe and relevant communication of EHCR entries between professionals working on the same or different sites.

---

[a] The Terms Electronic **Healthcare** Record (EHCR) and Federated **Healthcare** Record (FHCR) have been used by many projects and publications over the past decade and are used here when referring to historic work. The preferred adoption of the term Federated **Health** Record (FHR) in this paper reflects a slightly wider scope to include the recording of aspects of a patient's health that might not result in health care services being provided.

A detailed review of requirements for this domain was published by the GEHR project [1, 2, 3, 4], and this set of requirements informed the subsequent work of CEN ENV 12265 [5] and the Synapses project [6]. The EHCR-SupA project recently consolidated European and international published requirements into a single project deliverable [7]. This publication has been used as the starting point of a new ISO Work Item on EHCR Requirements.

2. Representing Contextual Information

The work of GEHR and Synapses has drawn attention to the essential nature of contextual information captured alongside the individual clinical entries at the time of recording. Although several other projects have each developed their own EHCR information architectures, they share the objective of formalising a set of contexts that may be associated with any health record entry[b].

The term "context" has been widely used by different projects and organisations to describe certain aspects of the inter-relationships between parts of a set of record entries or to describe the constituent parts of an individual entry. Each group appears to have identified a specific data set for context, so that, when the work of EHCR architecture, medical knowledge, and terminology groups is compared, several different kinds of contexts emerge. In practice most of these need to be represented within an EHCR, while a few are more applicable to a medical knowledge service interfacing with a population of patient records.

Table 1 below summarises the overall set of contexts that the authors believe need to be mapped to classes and attributes within an EHCR architecture.

Table 1: The range of contexts that may be associated with health record entries

Compositional Context
• Record entry names to provide a label for each data value
• Compounding hierarchies of clinical concepts to express complex concepts
• Grouping hierarchies for sets of clinical concepts with common headings, to:
  • preserve the way in which entries were originally organised by the author
  • identify the way in which the clinical concepts relate to the health care activities and processes surrounding the patient

Data Value Context • Formal representations for all data types, including text, quantities, time, persons and multi-media • Names of term sets, versions and registering agencies • Natural language used in a recording • Accuracy, precision and units for quantities • Normal ranges

[b] A health record entry is considered in this paper to be a quantum of information that is entered into a record, usually constituting a single fact, observation or statement.

Qualifier Context
• Presence / absence • Certainty • Severity • Site and laterality • Prevailing clinical circumstances (e.g. standing, fasting) • Justification, clinical reasoning • General comments • Knowledge reference (e.g. a journal reference)
Ethical and Legal Context
• Authorship and duty of care responsibilities • Subject of care • Dates and times of healthcare actions and of their recording • Version control • Access rights • Emphasis • Preservation of meaning on transferring the record to another site
Care Process Context

Links and pointers:
• to other parts of the record, e.g.
  • cause and effect
  • request and result
  • process (act) status (e.g. a test that is requested and subsequently cancelled)
• to a defined problem
• to an episode of care
• to a stage in a protocol
• to a decision support system

3. Information Architecture

The Synapses approach to distributed health records utilised the methodology of database federation to a standard and comprehensive schema, the Federated Healthcare Record (FHCR) information architecture, mediated and managed through a set of middleware services [8, 9].

In building on the Synapses work, the challenge being addressed by UCL in the design of the federated health record (FHR) information architecture is to provide a formal representation of the generic characteristics applicable to any potential health record entry arising from feeder systems or through clinical applications, now or in the future. In practice, this challenge can best be addressed through a pair of interrelated information models rather than through a single model.

1. The FHR Reference Model, which represents the global characteristics of health record entries, how they are aggregated, and the general set of context information attributes described as requirements in Table 1. This model corresponds conceptually to the EHCR architecture of GEHR [10], the Synapses federation schema (the SynOM) [11] and to the information model of ENV13606-1 [12]. It is intended to be applicable to any health domain, in any potential organisational setting. It also reflects the stable characteristics of an electronic health record, and is embedded in the federated record server at a program code level.

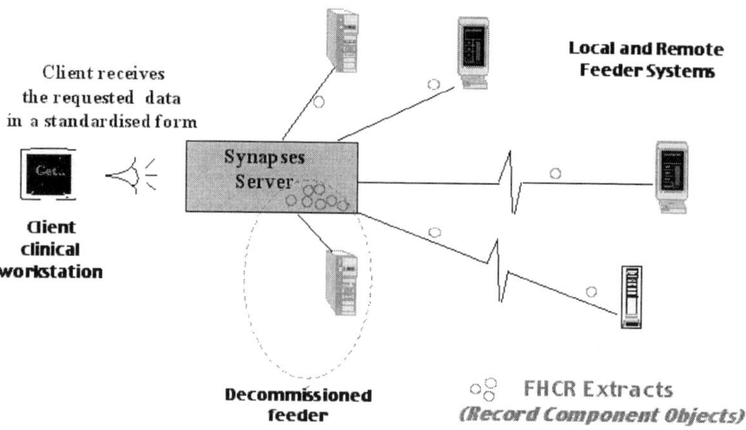

Figure 1: Distributed access to record components within a Synapses federation

2. The FHR Archetype Model, which extends (and effectively constrains) the Reference Model for particular domains or organisations by specifying particular record entry names, data-types and aggregations of these. This model is used to map the specific data schemata of feeder systems and clinical applications. Such schemata (known as Archetypes) will be subject to frequent change as clinical practice and information systems evolve. This model corresponds conceptually to the Synapses Object Dictionary [13, 11] and to the Archetype concept of the Good Electronic Health Record project [14]. This part of the information architecture is deliberately implemented in a way that facilitates and audits changes to the definition of clinical Archetypes over time within an FHR Archetype Object Dictionary component.

These two information models are described in the next two sections of this paper.

4. FHR Reference Model

The UCL Federated Health Record Reference Model (FHR-RM) defines a set of classes and attributes that represent the clinical context and medico-legal status of health record entries as a hierarchical set of Record Components. The goal for this model, in contrast to the Archetype Object Dictionary, is to represent the generic and domain-independent characteristics of Record Components.

The UCL FHR-RM is drawn below showing its class inheritance hierarchy (in red), and its aggregation (containment) hierarchy. The diagram conventions are based on the UML notation. The attributes have been omitted from the overall diagram below, and are defined later in this section.

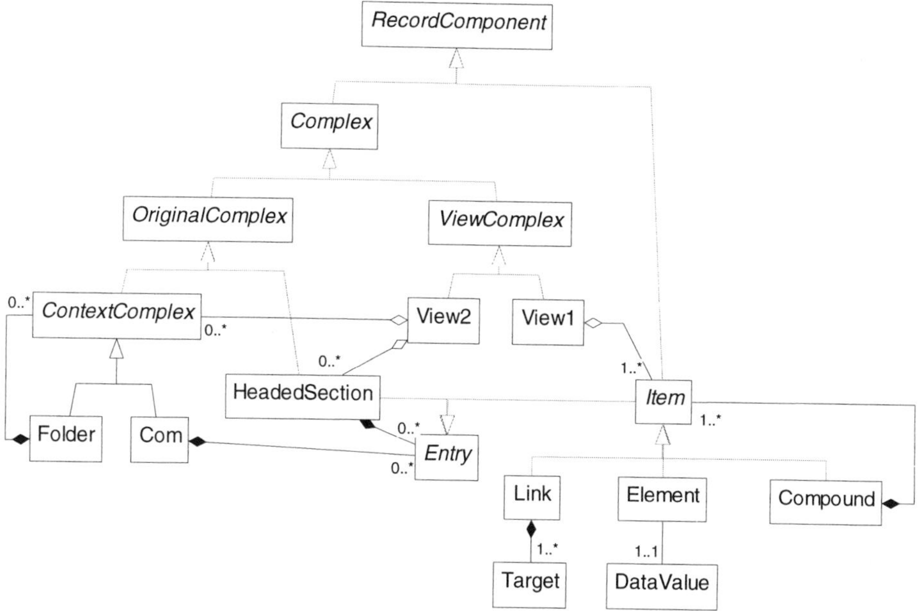

Figure 2: Class Inheritance and Aggregation within the FHR-RM

4.1 Description of the principal FHR-RM Classes

RecordComponent

RecordComponent is the abstract base class for Complex and Item. It defines the common attributes applicable to all of the major classes of the FHR-RM for:

- Record authorship, ownership and duty of care responsibilities
- Subject of care
- Dates and times of health care actions and of their recording
- Version control
- Access rights
- Emphasis and presentation

The complete set of attributes and their data types is presented later in this section. The FHR-RM distinguishes between the aggregation necessary to convey compound clinical concepts and the aggregation within a record that provides a way of grouping observations that relate to the health care activities performed. An example of the former would be *blood pressure*, which is a compound concept composed of *systolic* and *diastolic* values. An example of the latter would be the grouping together of observations under a general heading of *Physical Examination*.

The Complex and Item constructs respectively represent these two broad categories of aggregation.

Complex

In the FHR-RM, Complex is the common abstract super-class for the grouping of observations that relate to the health care activities performed. Two broad categories of Complex are reflected in the FHR-RM through two abstract sub-classes.

1. OriginalComplex: this set of classes represents the original organisational structure (grouping) of sets of record entries, as defined by the author(s) of those entries; it provides the medico-legal representation of the underlying information.
2. ViewComplex: this set of classes provide the means by which alternative groupings and sub-sets of the original information may be organised and preserved as permanent views in a patient's record, unlike those generic views provided in an ad hoc way by a client system.

OriginalComplex

Three concrete classes of OriginalComplex are defined in the FHR-RM, to provide for the nested aggregation of original groupings for record entries.

Folder

Folders define the highest-levels of organisation within health records. They will often be used to group large sets of record entries within departments or sites, over periods of time, or to demarcate a prolonged illness and its treatment. Examples of Folders include an episode of care, an inpatient stay, or one stage of a disease process. Folders can contain other Folders, and/or Coms.

Com

A medico-legal set of record entries required by the author to be kept together (to preserve meaning) when information is physically moved or copied to another persistent store. This is to ensure that all persistent EHR stores comprise whole Coms. This explicitly includes caches and cache mechanisms. The Com also defines the medico-legal cohort for the inclusion of new entries within an EHR: any new EHR entry (even if stored on a local feeder) must be a whole Com. Coms cannot contain other Coms or Folders. Examples include:

- the data entered at one date and time by one author (similar to a GEHR Transaction);
- the information gathered through the use of a protocol or template;
- a serialised set of readings taken over time but contributing to one examination;
- the definition of structures corresponding to electronic documents.

HeadedSection

This class is intended for grouping observations under headings *within* a Com. It therefore provides for the fine granularity grouping and labelling of record entries with names that relate the clinical concepts to the health care activities and processes surrounding the patient. Examples of HeadedSection names include presenting history, symptoms, investigations, treatment, drug prescription, needs, or plan. HeadedSections may contain other HeadedSections and/or Items. They cannot contain Coms or Folders.

ViewComplex

Two concrete classes of ViewComplex are defined in the FHR-RM, to provide for two differing mechanisms by which views may be generated.

View1

The View1 provides a means for grouping entries within Coms, at a similar hierarchical level in a record to the HeadedSection. However, the data within a View1 is derived through the use of a predefined query procedure i.e. a View1 comprises a query that generates a set of entries dynamically at the time of a client request. The mechanism by which search criteria can be defined in a generic, durable and portable manner within the View1 class is presently being developed.

View2

The View2 provides a static view of original information, through a set of references to the original entries or to groups of entries (i.e. Items, HeadedSections and/or Coms). It therefore provides a mechanism by which information within one Com may logically appear inside another Com, since the originals of these cannot be nested. This class cannot include object references to other instances of View2, to avoid recursive loops of such references.

Item

This abstract class provides an aggregation construct for clinical concepts that are composed of one or more individual named clinical values (e.g. *pulse, blood pressure, drug dose, heart sounds*). These entries may be aggregated within a hierarchy to represent complex clinical concepts, but such a composition is distinct from the record structure grouping hierarchy provided by the Complex classes. This class also provides a means by which point-to-point linkage or linkage nets within a single FHR can be represented. The Item class hierarchy is described later in this section.

4.2 The Attributes of the RecordComponent Class

The tables below list the attributes of the RecordComponent class. These are inherited throughout the FHR-RM class hierarchy and may acquire instance values at any level of a hierarchy of record entries. Some of these attributes have been defined as mandatory, and must be incorporated within any FHCR in order to comply with this specification. If mandatory information is not present in the underlying feeder system data then a null attribute value must be included within the Record Component object. Other attributes, marked as optional, have been included to meet published requirements or on the basis of implementation and deployment experience. The attribute data types are all of a base type; complex attribute data types have deliberately been avoided to ease implementation and the processability of federated records. The cardinality of all Mandatory attributes is 1, and that of Optional attributes is 0 or 1.

Subject of care

RecordComponent attribute	Mandatory Optional	Description of intended use	Type
SynPatUID	Mandatory	This is the "Subject of Care" attribute and will identify the patient about whom the record component provides information.	STRING
SubjectOf Information	Optional	This will identify the person about whom the information in a record component relates if not the subject of care e.g. if the information is about a family member, such as the patient's father or mother. PERMITTED VALUES: {patient, relative, foetus, mother, donor, personalcontact, otherperson, device} DEFAULT = "patient".	STRING

Note: the values for SubjectOfInformation are taken from ENV13606-2 (Domain Termlist)

Record authorship, ownership and duty of care responsibilities

FHR-RM attribute	Mandatory Optional	Description of intended use	Type
RecordingHealth CareAgent	Mandatory	The healthcare agent responsible for physically including this record component into the patient's source record.	STRING
Responsible HealthCareAgent	Optional	The healthcare agent responsible for effecting the care and for authoring this record component.	STRING
LegallyResponsible HealthCareAgent	Mandatory	The healthcare agent with senior clinical responsibility for the patient at the point of care documented by this record component e.g. Consultant in charge.	STRING
Information Provider	Optional	The person providing healthcare information if not the subject of care (e.g. a family member, friend, another clinician, an electronic device).	STRING

Note 1: information passed to the record server is deemed to be from authenticated sources. Digital signatures are not considered to be part of the FHR information model, but might be stored within an EHR server on an enterprise-specific basis.

Note 2: although countersignature is sometimes required for health record entries, these are usually handled at an application level and do not necessarily form part of the FHR. In cases where more than one actioning healthcare agent needs to be recorded the UCL team have so far proposed that two from the available set of healthcare agent attributes above should be used, such as the RecordingHealthcareAgent and the ResponsibleHealthcareAgent.

Dates, times, locations of health care actions and of their recording

FHR-RM attribute	Mandatory Optional	Description of intended use	Type
RecordingDateTime	Mandatory	The date and time this record component was included in the patient's source record (NOT the date and time it was brought into the federation).	DATETIME
HealthcareActivityBegin Time	Optional	The date and time of the health care activity to which this recording relates (this may differ from the RecordingDateTime if a delay occurred before a record could be authored e.g. a home visit at night).	DATETIME
HealthcareActivityEnd Time	Optional		DATETIME
ObservationBegin Time	Optional	The date and time (or intervals) of any health or care acts which occurred in the past but are being recorded at the present e.g. an operation performed several years ago.	DATETIME
ObservationEnd Time	Optional		DATETIME
HealthcareActivity Location	Optional	The enterprise, department or other location at which the patient is receiving the care documented in this entry (for audit, management, financial or access rights purposes).	STRING
AcquistionTimeDate	Optional	The date/time at which this Record Component was added to a Federated Record if its origin was elsewhere e.g. if received as a message from another record system; this attribute is necessary because the RecordingDateTime would represent when the original entry was recorded, not when it was received into the federated health record.	DATETIME

Locale	Optional	To document the time zone and geographical location of the recording clinical system, for example permitting international interpretation of other dates and times recorded.	STRING

Note 1 : the UCL implementation of Healthcare Activity and Observation attributes (using the Java Calendar class) permits the recording of begin or end times to be specified to an arbitrary granularity, permitting an author, for example, to record that observation occurred between 1960 and 1965.

Version control

FHR-RM attribute	Mandatory Optional	Description of intended use	Type
RevisedVersion	Optional	A reference to the version of this Record Component that replaces this version, if it has been revised (referenced via its RC_UID).	STRING
RevisedBy	Optional	A backward reference to the Record Component that this version has replaced, if it has been revised (referenced via its RC_UID).	STRING
Authorisation Status	Mandatory	PERMITTED VALUES: {unattested, attested, obsolete, revision}.	STRING

Access rights

FHR-RM attribute	Mandatory Optional	Description of intended use	TYPE
AccessAmend Rights	Mandatory	PERMITTED VALUES: {admin, audit, clinical, team, profession, hcp} This set of values reflects an ordered set of sensitivity levels. The anticipated default in most EHR systems will be "clinical" i.e. the record component is accessible to all staff involved in the clinical care of the patient. This attribute is used to differentiate sensitivity levels *within* a single FHR, and are supplementary to any restrictions on overall access to each patient's FHR as a whole.	INTEGER

Note: this attribute permits a sensitivity level to be assigned to Record Components at any level of granularity, as part of a broader approach to access control summarised later in this paper.

Emphasis and presentation

FHR-RM attribute	Mandatory Optional	Description of intended use	Type
Emphasis	Optional	At present this attribute is limited to a Boolean. If set to true the information in this record component was emphasised by the original author.	INTEGER

Note: there is some debate about the importance of representing more detailed aspects of presentation within the FHR. The view taken by the authors is that the specification of presentation characteristics is not necessary nor feasible for all entry instances within the records of individual patients. Where enterprises wish to retain a medico-legal reference to information display characteristics used for a given time period by certain applications, for example through a pointer to an XML Stylesheet, these ought to be retained by each enterprise or by the developers of clinical applications.

Class identifiers

FHR-RM attribute	Mandatory Optional	Description of intended use	Type
Name	Mandatory	This attribute preserves the actual name of the record component used in the original source record; this may be identical to the corresponding Archetype name, but might not be in the case of synonyms.	STRING
RC_UID	Mandatory	An internal reference identifier for each record component, provided by the FHR server.	STRING
SynObjectUID	Mandatory	The unique identifier of the Archetype that provides the template for this set of record components (Note: the Name attribute may not always be identical to the Archetype name).	STRING
ParentRC	Optional	The primary information context, i.e. it is a reference to the record component at the next higher level in a record structure.	STRING
EHCRSource	Optional	The unique identifier of the feeder system contributing this record component to the federated health record; this is important for medico-legal reasons, including the ability to link all parts of the FHR to relevant Data Controllers.	STRING

Other Attributes

FHR-RM attribute	Mandatory Optional	Description of intended use	Type
AuthorsComment	Optional	A free-text comment associated with the record component as a whole (not primarily with its value), intended for use by the author; it might be used by a revisor to explain the rationale for the revision.	STRING
RcuLink	Optional	The RC_UID(s) of other record component(s) in the FHR linked by the author (e.g. to relate an allergic rash to a previous drug prescription). Note: these other components must already be in the record, and therefore the references will be to past or accompanying present entries.	STRING
RcuLinkBack	Optional	This reference represents the reciprocal of the above link, from an historic target record component to the source: it will therefore point forwards in time. Some EHR systems may not permit the retrospective editing of record components to insert this attribute.	STRING

Note: The RcuLink and RcuLinkBack sttributes have been implemented using the Java Vector class to permit multiple targets to be specified. The RCU link attributes overlap in function with the Link class described below. This is deliberate to reflect the varying way in which internal links are represented by different feeder systems at present.

Item

The Item abstract class hierarchy provides a means to represent compound and elemental clinical concepts, using the concrete classes Compound and Element respectively. A set of context description attributes is associated with the Item objects, which are largely derived from the CEN EHR Domain Termlist standard ENV 13606-2. Other attributes such as Justification and ProtocolRef permit both a human and a software reference to the rationale behind a clinical entry, including the specification of a protocol or step in a protocol that was used during that part of clinical care. The Item class also inherits the attributes defined in the RecordComponent class, with the option to override the value of any of these at a local level.

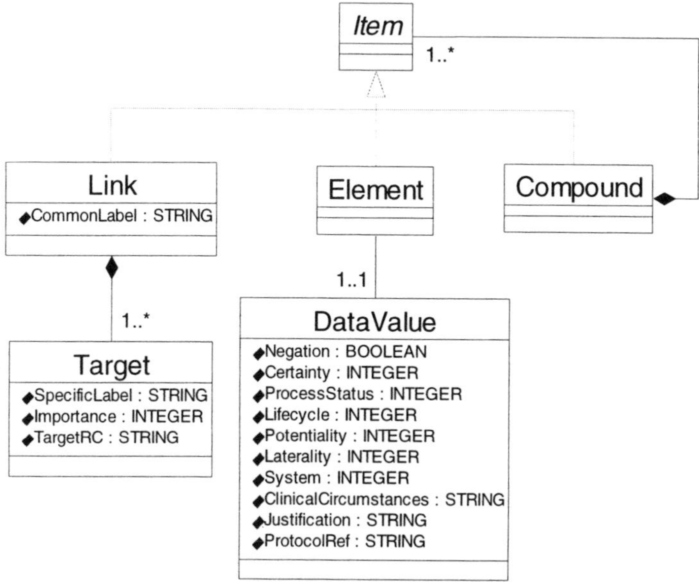

Figure 3: Item Class Hierarchy

An important aspect of the FHR-RM, including the Element, is the binding of a Name attribute (acting as a label) to each content value, providing the individual quantities, dates, images or clinical terms with a primary context in any given record entry.

The Compound class provides an aggregation construct for clinical concepts that are composed of one or more individual named clinical values (e.g. *pulse, blood pressure, drug dose, heart sounds*). These entries may be aggregated within a hierarchy to represent complex clinical concepts, but such a composition is distinct from the record structure grouping hierarchy provided by the RecordItemComplex classes such as the HeadedSection.

An additional child class of RecordItem is Link. This class provides a means by which point-to-point linkage or linkage nets within a single EHR can be represented. From an aggregation perspective, Links behave as Elements: they are leaf nodes in an FHR object hierarchy.

Content Classes

The Element supports a range of data types for the DataValue that may be assigned to any element entry. These generic classes are a distillation of the original foundation work of GEHR, EHCR-SupA, and CEN/TC 251 ENV 13606.

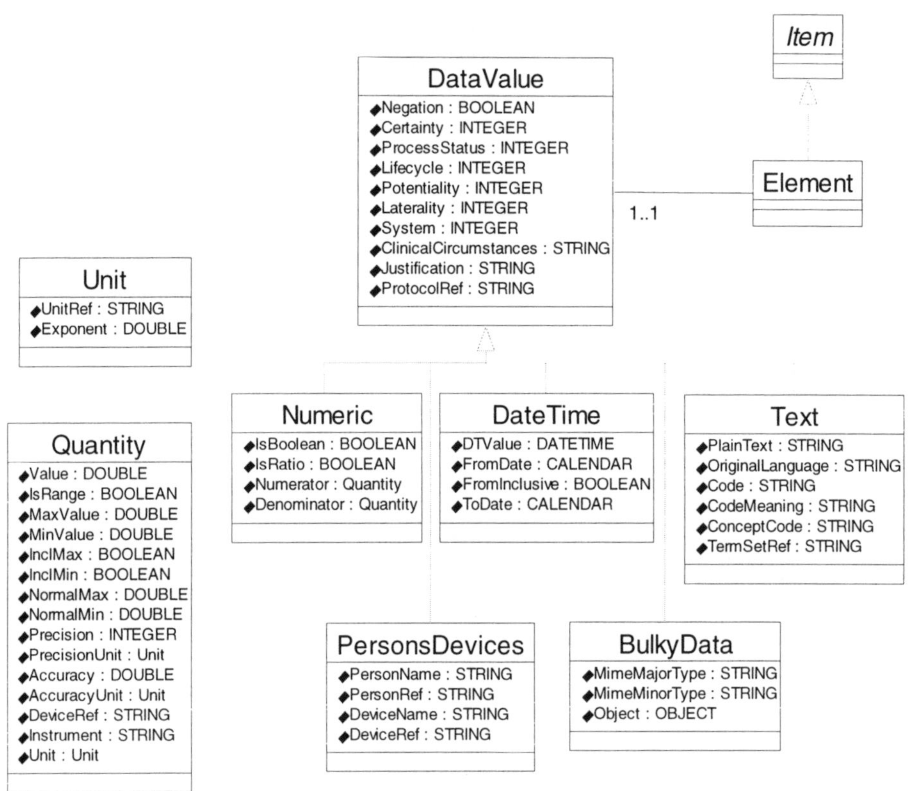

Figure 4: Object model of Element content

Separate dictionaries for units and for referencing terminology systems are under development. The model for persons and devices above will reference the richer information objects in the Persons Directory Service (see below), which will later also include a register of devices. The name strings are also included in the PersonsDevices class for medico-legal safety, to ensure that these attributes of a record component's content can be interpreted even if that Directory Service is somehow unavailable.

It should be noted that ENV 13606-4 defines a set of specific content models for commonly used objects such as drug prescriptions. The UCL FHR-RM deliberately does not define specific record objects of this nature: they are instead capable of being defined in and implemented through the Archetype Object Dictionary. This approach attempts to separate the most stable aspects of a health record model (through the FHR-RM) from those where local variation or evolution over time are most likely to occur (via the Archetype Object Dictionary).

5. FHR Archetype Object Dictionary

The classes and attributes of the Reference Model, described in the previous section, are deliberately defined at a high level of abstraction to provide an information model that can be applied to any potential health record entry. However, the individual feeder systems providing data to the FHR server are likely to be highly specific to the local requirements of individual sites, to specialities and to groups of professionals.

The Archetype Object Dictionary provides the formalism by which the specific clinical data sets and aggregates normally found in health records and in contemporary feeder systems can be defined. Archetype entries utilise the FHR-RM classes as basic building blocks, using the Name attribute of each class instance to generate specific clinical hierarchies that can be directly mapped to feeder system data schemata and can be the target of a client request.

The Archetypes can be mapped onto the data representations used in each individual feeder system through a set of access methods. These might be defined jointly by the developers of each feeder system and the developers of the FHR server at each installation, or might be derived from published interface specifications. The references to the access methods are logically integrated within the Archetype Object Dictionary during the "sign-up process" by which each feeder system is connected to the federation. In a "live" federation, a request by a client application or middleware service for a set of Record Components will result in the invocation of the relevant method(s) by the FHR service in order to retrieve the necessary health care record data from a feeder system.

Other features of the Archetype Object Dictionary are the mapping of Archetypes to clinical concept tags, and the inclusion of validation criteria that might be used to verify the instantiation of a Record Component's candidate data value. These are shown diagrammatically below.

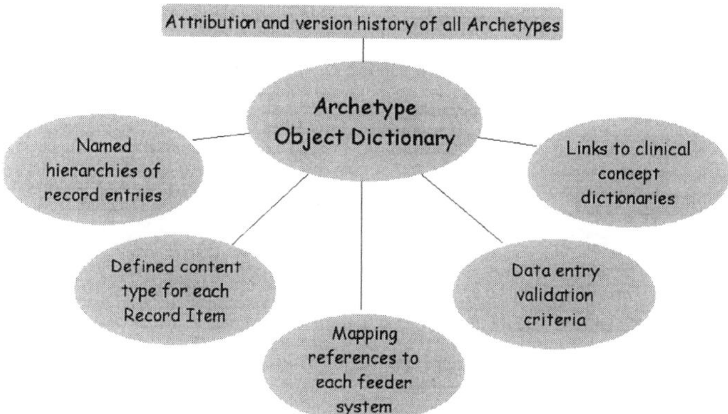

Figure 5: Functional sub-components of the Archetype Object Dictionary

The Archetype Object Dictionary Client component is described in a later section of this paper on Middleware Services.

5.1 Object Model of the Archetype Object Dictionary

The formal object model of the Archetype Object Dictionary is closely related to the FHR Reference Model. It extends the RecordComponent class of the FHR-RM through the addition of one compound attribute that is used to represent the information about the creation, versioning and use of each library definition, and supports the mapping of that definition to a set of medical knowledge concept tags.

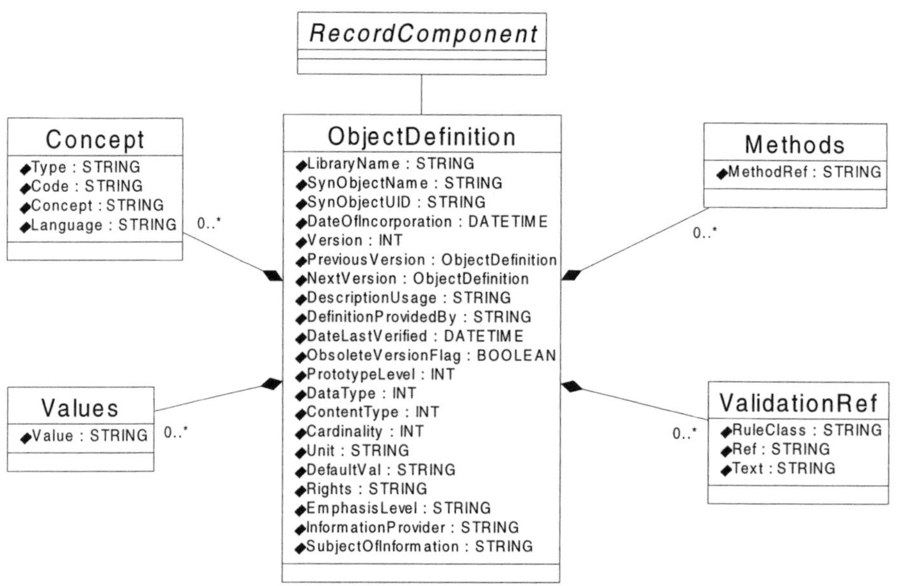

Figure 6: Information Model of the Archetype Object Dictionary

ObjectDefinition Class

The ObjectDefinition class contains the attributes relevant to managing the library entries associated with each Archetype. This includes the formal definition, author identification and version of any local or national standardised data sets within the Dictionary. In addition, some descriptive text (a definition or explanation) may be provided to clarify the intended clinical use of the object. It will also be necessary to store information about changes that occur to Archetypes over time; this might mean recording if this particular object is the current definition, and the identification of its predecessors and/or successors. The individual attributes of ObjectDefinition are described below.

ObjectDefinition attribute	Mandatory Optional	Description of intended use	Type
LibraryName	Mandatory	Archetypes are authored within libraries to permit traceability and the managed distribution of these within multi-agency domains.	STRING
SynObjectName	Mandatory	This is the standard preferred name by which the Archetype is known.	STRING
SynObjectUID	Mandatory	This UID is used to uniquely identify this Archetype within Record Components.	STRING
DateOfIncorporation	Mandatory	When the Archetype was authored in this Library.	DATE
Version	Mandatory	The version number.	INT

PreviousVersion	Optional	A reference to the previous version if this is a revision.	ObjectDefiniton
NextVersion	Optional	A reference to the successor version if this Archetype has been revised.	ObjectDefiniton
DescriptionUsage	Optional	A textual description of how this Archetype was intended to be used for record entries, intended as guidance for those mapping feeder systems or clinical applications.	STRING
DefinitionProvidedBy	Mandatory	The reference source guiding this Archetype definition, such as a clinical guideline.	STRING
DateLastVerified	Mandatory	When the reference source was last checked to confirm this Archetype is still valid.	DATETIME
ObsoleteVersionFlag	Optional	To permit Archetypes to be marked as obsolete even if a revision has not been authored.	STRING
PrototypeLevel	Mandatory	This attribute permits selective sharing of parts of an Archetype library to others. PERMITTED VALUES: {0-2} (2=PRIVATE, 1=PRIVATE_SHARABLE, 0=PUBLIC).	INT
DataType	Mandatory	The FHR-RM class to which this Archetype applies. Permitted Values: {0-7} (0=Folder, 1=Com, 2=HeadedSection, 3=Compound, 4=Element, 5=Link, 6=View1, 7=View2).	INT
ContentType	Mandatory	Specifying the Data Value type for Archetypes whose DataType is Element. Permitted Values: {0-5} (0=No_Content, 1=Text, 2=Numeric, 3=Date_Time, 4=Persons_Devices, 5=Bulky).	INT
Cardinality	Mandatory	Indicating the number of instances of this Archetype that may be created within any one instance of its parent e.g. 1 to many.	STRING
Unit	Optional	Specifying the unit of recording for Archetypes whose DataType is Element.	STRING
DefaultVal	Optional	Providing a default value on instantiation for Archetypes whose DataType is Element.	STRING
Rights	Optional	Permitted values for these Record Component attributes may be specified in the Archetype definition, for example in the case of a Family History Archetype to indicate that the SubjectOfInformation may not be the patient.	STRING
EmphasisLevel	Optional		STRING
InformationProvider	Optional		STRING
SubjectOfInformation	Optional		STRING

Values Class

This class permits the author of the Archetype to specify a fixed possible value list for Archetypes whose DataType is Element.

MethodRef Class

This class stores a set of method references that may be used to identify feeder system data relating to this Archetype.

Concept Class

This class enables a client application to reference an Archetype through the use of a locally-defined label, an abbreviated name or a language translation of it. It will also enable an application to identify the set of available objects that correspond to a clinical subject heading. This class is a place-holder for the methodology by which Archetype definitions can be appropriately linked to, for example, GALEN ontology or terminology services.

Concept attribute	Mandatory Optional	Description of intended use	Type
Type	Optional	The classification system or ontology from which the code has been derived.	STRING
Code	Optional	A code referencing the clinical concept within that classification system or ontology.	STRING
Concept	Optional	A rubric for that code, included for safety and to permit searches to utilise this class of information if that classification system or ontology is not available as a live look-up service.	STRING
Language	Optional	The natural language used for the rubric.	STRING

ValidationRef Class

This class, which is still undergoing evaluation, is a place-holder for the expression of rules regarding the validation of instance values for element objects, or the interdependence of values on other components of an Item or Complex. These rules would be used primarily during data entry rather than retrieval. For example, an entry value may be drawn from a pick-list or reference database (such as *drug name*), it may be subject to upper and lower limits (such as *height*), or its value may be restricted by other values in the record (such as the patient's age or gender).

This class contains a set of rules that must be evaluated against any candidate value for an Element conforming to this Archetype. A string text message can be returned to the clinical application if a condition is met. This provides a useful means of providing messages back to end users:

- if the value they have offered is not permitted;
- if they need to re-affirm the value (e.g. it is a rather unusual value, but not impossible;
- if the value is accepted but some further action advice needs to be communicated back to the user.

The three situations map to three sub-types of rule, reflected in three values for the RuleClass attribute: REJECT, CONFIRM, ACCEPT.

If more than one rule has been defined for an Archetype, the provisional intention for the service implementing this class is to evaluate rules in the order:

1. REJECT
2. CONFIRM
3. ACCEPT

This class is a place-holder for the methodology by which Archetype definitions can be appropriately linked to electronic guidelines and to other decision support services.

ValidationRef attribute	Mandatory Optional	Description of intended use	Type
RuleClass	Optional	Action to be performed if the rule condition is met. PERMITTED VALUES: {0-2} (0=ACCEPT, 1= CONFIRM, 2= REJECT}	INT
Ref	Optional	The rule string to be evaluated against a candidate value for an Element of that Archetype.	STRING
Text	Optional	A string to be returned by the Federated Health Record server to the calling application if this rule is met.	STRING

6. Middleware Services

The federated health record is derived through a set of services that support access to distributed sources of health records. The FHR Server provides a set of middleware services that enable a requesting service (e.g. a healthcare professional using a client clinical application, or another middleware service such as a decision support agent) to access electronic health record information from a diversity of repository servers (*feeder systems*). These feeder systems may hold clinical data in a variety of different structures, which may range from rigorous electronic health record architectures to quite simple table structures such as those found in departmental systems. The feeder systems may be on-site at an institution or connected remotely through telecommunications services.

The FHR implementation at UCL provides the means by which Record Components (aggregate sets of entries forming part of a patient's federated health record) can be retrieved, added or revised according to a schema defined in the Archetype Object Dictionary. These actions take place in accordance with the user's role-based privilege and the sensitivity of the Record Components involved, and are registered in an access audit trail.

The components outlined here are believed to constitute one of the first live implementations of a generic record server that provide proof-of-concept validation of many constructs in the current CEN EHCR standard. Recent work at UCL has resulted in considerable refinements to the Reference Model on the basis of practical experience, including some simplifications, which might helpfully inform the pending first review of ENV13606 by CEN Working Group 1.

The North London demonstrator is utilising the following UCL FHR component services:

Federated Health Record services: a scalable run-time FHR environment supporting distributed access to record components from new and legacy feeder systems.

Archetype Object Dictionary Client and services: a means of facilitating feeder system sign-up and of navigating a federation environment. It enables clinicians or engineers to define and export the data sets mapping to individual feeder systems, and to relate these to the schema requirements of clinical applications accessing the record server.

Persons Directory services: storing a core demographic database to search for and authenticate staff users of the system and to anchor patient identification and connection to the patient's federated health record.

Expert Advisory (Decision Support) services: for anticoagulation management, to calculate the patient's next treatment regimen and next monitoring interval.

Web-based applications: to provide end-user clinical views and functions.

6.1 Component engineering approach

The FHR Reference Model has been implemented as a set of Java™ classes (and an XML DTD) that provides a reference model for:

- the federated record persistent repository
- the Archetype Object Dictionary
- feeder system mapping
- client server communications

All of the main components are written in Java. The federated access to distributed clinical databases is managed through a set of directory services accessed via the Java Naming and Directory Interface (JNDI). The components are deployed within a middleware environment managed through Novell Directory Services and JINI™, an open standard service-integration technology. The services are presently deployed on a Windows™ NT server (to suit local hospital requirements) and a second deployment using Linux™ has been tested. IPv6 web server and servlet runner applications are required for the 6WINIT project (see below) and will be deployed on the Linux™ version.

As well as accessing distributed feeder systems, the UCL FHR services incorporate a principal record database, using ObjectStore™ (from Object Design Inc.), that can be used as a local cache and provides a robust repository for data originating from feeder systems that are to be decommissioned. This object oriented database stores record components in a form native to the federation architecture. An Oracle version of the record server has also been developed and will also be tested in live use late in 2001.

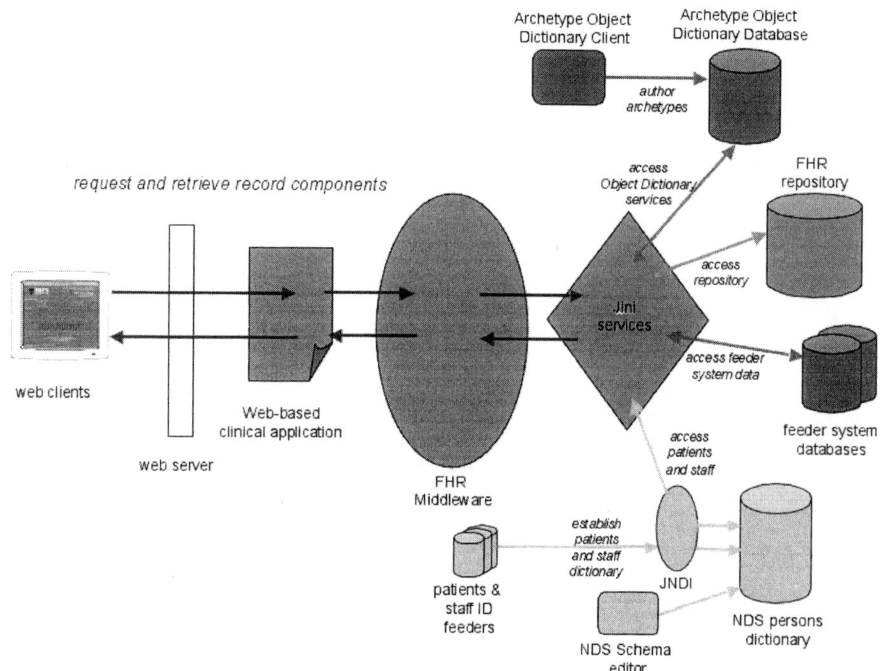

Figure 7: FHR components handling the run-time request for and retrieval of patient records

New web-based clinical applications have been written, using Java servlets, to provide end user access to the patient records held within the FHR server. The web servlet scripts extract single or multiple instances of patient record objects from the FHR repository and map the output object attributes to cells within HTML tables. At present these applications exclusively use http for client-server communication.

Some additional middleware components have been authored specifically for use in the management of anticoagulation therapy. A previous decision support methodology (i.e. the algorithm and tables for warfarin control) has been re-engineered using Java. This service is now provided through specific agents called from a dedicated client and these return data to this client.

6.2 Archetype Object Dictionary Client

The UCL Archetype Object Dictionary Client (ODC) component:

- provides an authoring tool for Archetypes in terms of their constituent compound clinical concepts;
- includes the formal definition, author identification and version of any local or national standardised data sets within the Dictionary;
- incorporates pointers to access methods which can extract data held on feeder systems to which the FHR services are connected;
- ensures adequate version control and maintenance procedures to accommodate revisions of Archetypes over time.

The Archetype Object Dictionary Client component has been written entirely using Java Foundation classes and Swing, allowing true cross-platform deployment. It utilises an object database PSE Pro, from Object Design Inc., which is also a Java application and is similarly capable of installation on any platform that supports a Java Virtual Machine. The licence for PSE Pro permits the distribution of run-time versions alongside the Archetype Object Dictionary application, removing the need to purchase any additional third-party software. The ODC permits the structure of the record object definitions to be captured in a way that the user originally intended for maximum performance and flexibility.

The core features of the ODC are listed below.

ODC Class Hierarchy
ODC Archetype Properties
Creating New Archetype Entries
Cardinality on Instantiation
Validation Criteria
Data Retrieval Methods
Copying and Pasting Archetypes in the Hierarchy
Publicising Archetypes
Deleting an Archetype
Marking an Archetype Obsolete
Revising an Archetype Definition
Reviewing the Version History
Tracking Archetypes having Multiple Parents
Exporting the Database
Saving the Database
Help about screen

Future work will enable synonyms for clinical object names to be identified and linked to preferred terms, and offer a multi-lingual set of clinical object names. Data entry validation criteria may also be incorporated, and their linkage to run-time protocol components is being explored.

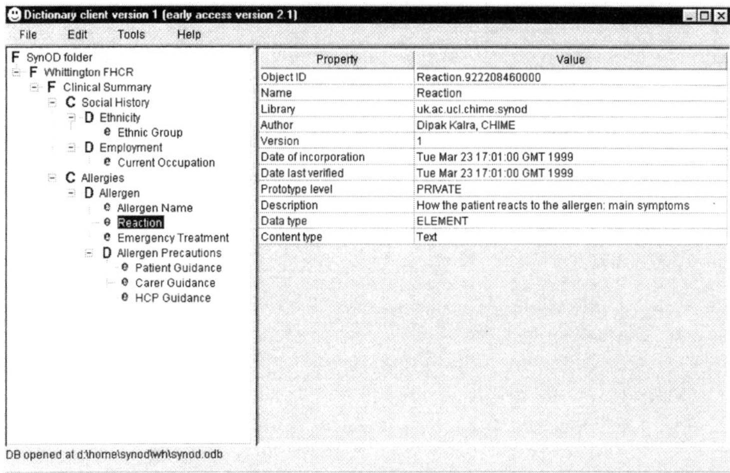

Figure 8: Example screen from the Archetype Object Dictionary Client

6.3 FHR Persons Directory Service

The Persons Directory Service is a component providing information on the identification of patients, healthcare professionals and other staff to the other FHR services. It provides a repository of person names and other demographic information, together with their access rights status, that can be used to identify persons within an FHR or to authenticate access rights to a given set of record components.

The Persons Directory provides a means of registering staff and patients within a consistent repository as part of the FHR. This model has been proposed, and implemented as the Persons Directory Service, in order to provide a means of searching for patients, confirming the correct patient has been chosen, and providing a basic demographic data-set as part of each patient's federated health record. In many situations where an FHR server is deployed there is likely also to be a regional or national directory of patients and also of healthcare agents, which would replace the service described here. The overall engineering approach to the FHR middleware would permit the replacement of the Persons Directory Service with a local alternative quite easily.

The information model builds on the early work of GEHR and Synapses, which has been refined by the EHCR-SupA project. The models proposed here by UCL are a simplified but consistent representation of the Healthcare Agent subsystem defined in CEN/TC 251 ENV 13606 (EHCR Communication). This model is deliberately not intended to mimic a full patient demographic server such as a hospital PAS.

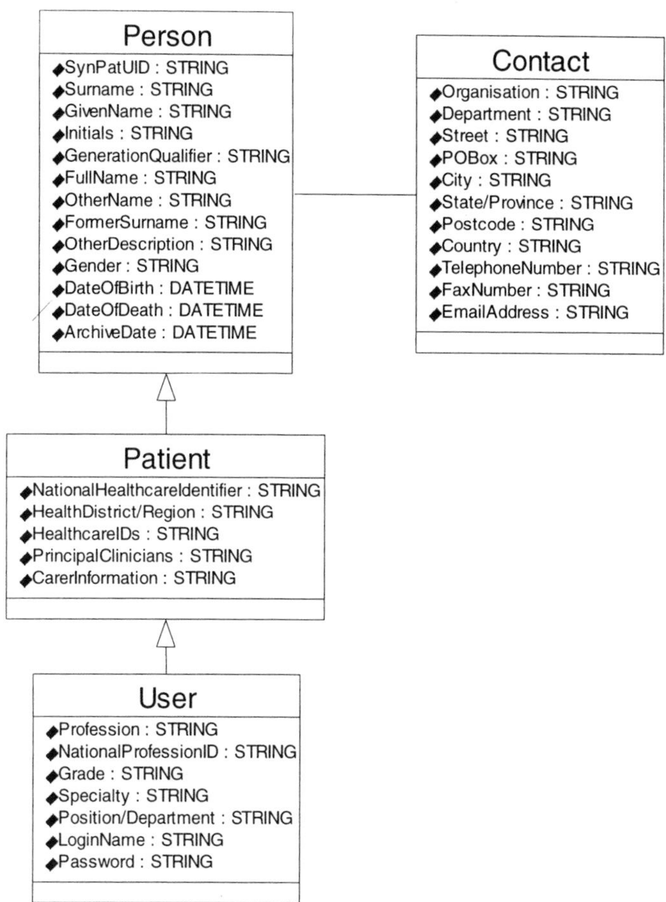

Figure 9: Information Model of the FHR Persons Directory

The data repository uses and extends Novell NDS objects and its metadirectory, and is accessed via Java Naming and Directory Interface (JNDI) APIs. This entails some configuring of the NDS tree and its class models to optimise it as an object repository for patient and staff identification. For deployment purposes, Novell eDirectory has been used as the product to provide and manage the NDS services.

A Software and Devices Directory is also being developed using NDS, and is intended to provide a registry of all electronic sources of FHR information (such as monitoring devices and decision support software) that might be referenced within a patient's record.

6.4 Access Control

A combination of internal services is used to deliver an overall access control framework governing access to FHR information, reflecting enterprise policies by:

- determining user profiles from available authentication and certification services;
- limiting patient searching within organisational contexts;
- limiting access to sub-categories of the record based on roles e.g. a department or speciality.

Specific structured parts of each patient's FHR can record individual patient consent to:

- map a user's role-based privilege to the sensitivity of individual record components;
- permit access to sub-categories of the record based on roles e.g. for research or teaching;
- exclude named persons from adopting certain roles for accessing individual patient records.

These services are in the process of being implemented and tested, and will be published later.

7. North London Demonstrator Setting

The UCL FHR components have so far been implemented along with two clinical applications: one in cardiology (anticoagulant therapy management) and one in respiratory medicine (asthma home monitoring). The anticoagulant application is now live, and new applications to capture basic medical summaries and for the management of chest pain clinics and are being designed for deployment during the 6WINIT project lifetime. The asthma home monitoring application is restricted to a research context and is not as yet envisaged as a live clinical service.

7.1 Anticoagulant application

This application provides a set of HTML web clients to enable the management of anticoagulation therapy by clinical staff (or patients) trained to monitor this. The overall application includes forms to deal with requests for and the display of existing data, and also with data entry. The system incorporates drug dosing decision support and recommends monitoring intervals between blood tests. It has been written to replace a legacy application, and is the first live clinical application to test the FHR server. This application is being used daily by staff at the Whittington Hospital, running clinics with up to 110 patients per day. It will shortly be accessed from outside the hospital by a community pharmacist, and it is hoped to include other pharmacists, GPs and patients as users within the next 12 months. Only some of the actual FHR objects and attribute values are shown on user screens, to meet the needs of the users who run the anticoagulation clinics at the Whittington.

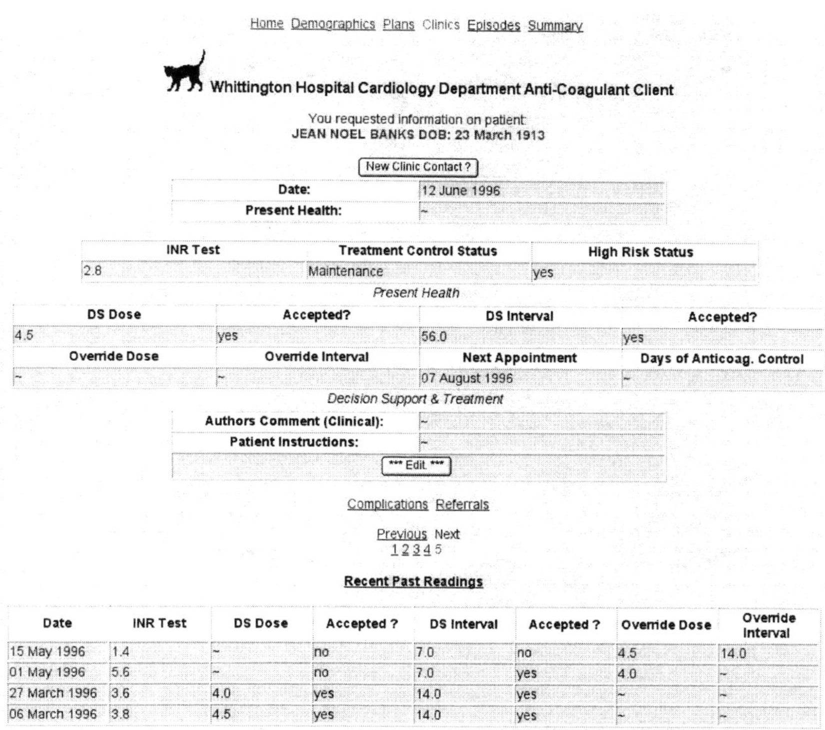

Figure 10: Anticoagulant Client - viewing a clinic contact

7.2 The 6WINIT Project

The IPv6 Wireless internet INITiative (6WINIT) project is a European IST Framework V initiative involving major European telecom companies, equipment manufacturers, solutions/software providers, research laboratories and end-user hospitals. Its objectives are to validate the introduction of the new mobile wireless Internet in Europe - based on a combination of the new Internet Protocol version 6 (IPv6) and the new wireless protocols (GPRS and UMTS/3GPP). The UCL north London demonstrator, based at the Whittington Hospital, is one of the three clinical sites. Work in progress is expected to demonstrate applications using wireless and IPv6 Internet services to access FHR services during 2002.

7.3 Chest Pain Management

A new application is being written to provide clinicians with access to the record of patients having non-acute chest pain (i.e. possible heart disease) symptoms. The primary clinical application will be hosted on the same FHR server as the anticoagulant system, and share the same core middleware services. The intention is for this application to be accessed from workstations in the Whittington Hospital and from selected GP practices.

7.4 Mobile views

Two views of a patient's medical summary will be created, one for emergency care and one for patients who wish to view their own record. For this we hope to utilise 6WINIT mobile networks and PDAs supplied through consortium partners. The emergency view is expected to be a helpful demonstration of secure mobile use of the 6WINIT networks, and is a high-profile strategic goal of the UK Department of Health.

7.5 NHS ERDIP Demonstration

The UCL record server components have been selected by South West Devon ERDIP for the development of a cardiovascular EHR connecting local hospitals and GPs. This work will replicate and extend the Whittington implementation of the record server to suit the requirements of a regional network of collaborating hospitals and general practices.

7.6 Further developments

Further developments planned for the medium term include collaborative work with General Electric/Marquette to incorporate investigation reports (in particular, bio-signals) within the federated record. This integration will explore new facets of live feeder system federation and distributed access to multimedia data.

8. Conclusion

UCL is in the process of establishing an international foundation (*open*EHR), co-ordinated by UCL and with specific collaborating centres in Australasia and the US [15]. This will operate as a non-profit body to foster high quality electronic health records amongst the purchaser, vendor and user communities. The generic components of the UCL federated health record server described here will next year be offered as Open Source products through the *open*EHR Foundation.

The experience gained to date in the design, implementation and deployment of a generic federation health record server has revealed many issues that still need to be explored and empirically tested before any claim could be made to have met the challenge of delivering ubiquitous and appropriate access to health information. The work described in this paper should be seen as steps on a journey towards that vision, hopefully with future opportunities to partner a number of organisations internationally in the same way that we have valued so far.

References

[1] Ingram D, Southgate L, Kalra D, Griffith S, and Heard S. The GEHR Requirements for Clinical Comprehensiveness.. The Good European Health Record Project, Deliverable No. 4. European Commission, 1992.
Available from http://www.chime.ucl.ac.uk/HealthI/GEHR/EUCEN/del4.pdf

[2] Ingram D, Hap B, Lloyd D, Grubb P et al. GEHR Requirements for Portability. The Good European Health Record Project, Deliverable No. 5. AIM Office 1992.
Available from http://www.chime.ucl.ac.uk/HealthI/GEHR/EUCEN/del5.pdf

[3] Ingram D, Lloyd D, Baille O, Grubb P et al. GEHR Requirements for Communication Capacity. The Good European Health Record Project, Deliverable No. 6. AIM Office 1992.
Available from http://www.chime.ucl.ac.uk/HealthI/GEHR/EUCEN/del6.pdf

[4] Ingram D. The Good European Health Record. In: Health in the New Communications Age. Laires, Laderia, Christensen, Eds. pp66-74. IOS Press, 1995.

[5] Hurlen P (ed.). ENV 12265: Electronic Healthcare Record Architecture. CEN TC/251 PT 1-011. 1995. Brussels.

[6] Grimson J, Grimson W, Berry D, Kalra D, Toussaint P and Weier O. A CORBA-based integration of distributed electronic healthcare records using the Synapses approach. Special Issue of IEEE Transactions on Information Technology in Biomedicine on Emerging Health Telematics Applications In Europe, Vol 2, No 3; 124-138. 1998.

[7] Dixon R, Grubb P, Lloyd D, Kalra D. Consolidated List of Requirements. EHCR-SupA Project Deliverable 1.4, May 2000.
Available from http://www.chime.ucl.ac.uk/HealthI/EHCR-SupA/del1-4v1_3.PDF

[8] Grimson J et al. Synapses - Federated Healthcare Record Server, Procs. Of MIE 96, Copenhagen, August 1996, J Brender et al (Eds), IOS Press, 695-699.

[9] Grimson W, Groth T (Eds). The Synapses User Requirements and Functional Specification (Part B). The Synapses Project. Deliverable USER 1.1.1b. EU Telematics Application Programme Office 1996.

[10] Lloyd D, Kalra D, Beale T, Heard S, Maskens A, Dixon R, Ellis J, Camplin D, Grubb P, Ingram D. The GEHR Architecture. The Good European Health Record Project, Deliverable No. 6. AIM Office 1995.
Available from http://www.chime.ucl.ac.uk/HealthI/GEHR/EUCEN/del19.pdf

[11] Kalra D (Ed). ODP Specification of Synapses - Part 3: Information Viewpoint. The Synapses Project. Available from http://www.cs.tcd.ie/synapses/public/html/projectdeliverables.html

[12] Kay S, Marley T (Eds). ENV13606 Electronic Health Record Communication - Part 1: Electronic Health Record Architecture. CEN TC/251 PT 1-026. 1999. Brussels.

[13] Kalra D (Ed). The Syapses Object Model and Object Dictionary. The Synapses Project. Deliverable USER 1.3.2. EU Telematics Application Programme Office 1997.

[14] Beale T. The GEHR Archetype System. The Good Electronic Health Record. Aug 2000. Available from http://www.gehr.org/technical/archetypes/gehr_archetypes.html

[15] See http://www.openehr.org

Electronic Health Records and Communication for Better Health Care
F. Mennerat (Ed.)
IOS Press, 2002

Standards Supporting Interoperability and EHCR Communication – A CEN TC251 Perspective

Tom Marley
University of Salford, United Kingdom

Abstract. This paper has been submitted by Tom Marley. Tom was a member of the project team which produced ENV13606 Part 1: and acted as liaison to the Part 4 project team. Tom is currently writing up the document on General Purpose Information Components.

1. Why the CEN TC251 Focus?

There are currently three standards organisations that are producing standards in health informatics in the international arena: CEN TC251, Health Level 7 and ISO TC215.

- CEN TC251 produces standards for the European market and has traditionally focussed attention on communication between organisations rather than within organisations. This inter-organisational communication presents more of a challenge than the intra-organisational communication which can often be resolved locally using commercially available tools such as datagates. CEN TC251 has recently produced its pre-standard ENV13606 which deals with EHCR communication and is currently developing a further multi-part standard on General Purpose Information Components which will complement this work.

- Health Level 7 (HL7) has focussed its attention on intra-organisational communication using messages. Over the past few years HL7 has been developing its revolutionary version 3 messages based upon a strict message development framework, an underlying Reference Information Model (RIM) and a message development toolset. However, two aspects of this work should be noted in particular:
  a. the HL7 RIM is not a model of healthcare or of the EHR; it provides a set of templates which are used when describing activities, materials, persons, observations, etc.
  b. the focus of the messages that are being developed is still mainly concerned with intra-organisational communication, and in particular messaging between hospital departmental systems for administration, orders and reports.

  A new HL7 Special Interest Group has been set up for EHR matters led by David Markwell from the UK and is using ENV606 as its starting point.

- ISO TC215 is more recently formed but does not have the structure or commercial support to do other than to take input from other standards bodies in order to promote and harmonise existing work to produce fully international products.

2. Which standards are we considering here?

The most relevant CEN TC251 standards work for consideration are:

a. CEN ENV13606 (1999) - HealthHealth Informatics - Electronic healthcare record communication

b. the current work of CEN Project Team 41: General Purpose Information Components.

A discussion on these two topics are the subjects of the remainder of this paper.

3. CEN ENV13606 Health Informatics - Electronic healthcare record communication

This prestandard, produced in 1999 is in 4 parts:
- Part 1: Extended Architecture
- Part 2: Domain Termlist
- Part 3: Distribution Rules
- Part 4: Messages for exchange of information

The prestandard has been implemented and validated in a number of countries and steps are being taken to revise and update the work to a full EN (European Standard).

Due to restrictions of space this paper concentrates upon Part 1: the Extended Architecture which was based upon, and replaced, the previous CEN ENV12265 entitled 'electronic healthcare record architecture'. ENV12265 was the first ECHR standard and not only spawned 13606 but also led to implementations and work under the Advanced Informatics in Medicine banner. The most notable of these outputs were GEHR (Good European Healthcare Record) and Synapses.

It should be noted that the emphasis of ENV13606 is healthcare record communication and does not attempt to set standards for how systems should organise healthcare records internally. When one looks at the products of 13606 it should be kept in mind that the parts do not represent identical views of the healthcare record. In particular, the differences between parts 1 and 4 may be summarised as:

- Part 1: provides a logical view of healthcare record architecture when communicated, where communication is considered as:
  - communication across space. This includes inter-organisational communication
  - communication across time. This covers aspects of referring to historical data and also covers archiving
  - communication across responsibility. For example, communication between nursing and clinician responsibilities.

- Part 4: provided an implementable specification for the design of messages used for the purpose of sending the healthcare record in whole or in part between computer systems. These messages were validated within a GP to GP communication domain.

3.1 Architectural Principles

Within 13606 Electronic Healthcare Record Architecture is defines as:

A set of principles governing the logical structure and behaviour of electronic healthcare records that enables safe communication of the healthcare record as a whole or of any selected part(s) of the record

Note here that the architecture described in Part 1 of the standard is a 'logical structure, not an implementation structure. This means, for example, that if an architectural principle states that all communicated record components are to be attributed to their source, this does not mean that the item of data communicated must carry this attribution, only that the source of the information must be accessible and unambiguous.

The most important of the architectural principles of 13606 was inherited from 12265 and relates to the **Original Information Context** within the healthcare record. Conformance to this architectural principle ensures that the clinical information as entered into the electronic healthcare record by one or more healthcare agents remains safely intact and unambiguous (i.e. nothing is inadvertently or deliberately lost or added, irrespective of why, when, who, where, and how it is communicated). The original context will include:

- which subject of care the information relates to
- the date and time the information originated
- the source of the information
- the date and time the information was entered into this healthcare record
- who was responsible for this entry

In addition it may be important to communicate information about the context under which the information was collected and possibly whether the information has connections or links with other information within the healthcare record.

3.2 Architectural Components

There are a number of architectural components which may be considered as 'containers' and which allow other components (the content) to be grouped and provided with some contextual information, etc. These 'container' components are:

Table 1: Record container type components

ComponentType	Description	May contain
The 'EHCR root'	The EHCR record for the patient (as a whole)	Folders Compositions
Folder	Used for large groupings of record components. In some cases all of the patient EHCR originating from a single healthcare provider may be contained in a single folder	Folders (sub-folder) Compositions
Composition	In GEHR this would be called a *transaction*' and in other places a *contribution*. The composition is intended a container for record components relating to : - one time and place of care delivery - a single session of recording, or - a single document	Headed Sections Data Clusters Data Items Also other compositions but only where these are references or included compositions that originated elsewhere
Headed Section	Record component representing a sub-division within a composition, the content of which have	Headed Sections Data Clusters

ComponentType	Description	May contain
	a common theme or are derived through the same healthcare process. For example: examination findings, family history, current medication	Data Items
Data Cluster	Record component used to aggregate data items and/or other clusters to represent a compound concept. For example: blood pressure, results of a battery of laboratory investigations, treatment schedule consisting of several individually specified preparations or dosages	Data Clusters Data Items

Apart from these 'container' record components there are two other components that we need to mention, the Data Item and the Link Item.

Non-container type record components

Data Item	Single unit of data that in a certain context is considered indivisible.
Link Item	Record component that provides a means of associating two other instances of architectural component and specifying the relationship between them.

3.3 Representation of complex data

It was found during the UK NHS validations of ENV13606 that certain types of clinical information were not easily represented using the standard without the creation of complex data items. Moreover, the Data Cluster was often used to group data items in ways which were inappropriate and which were not underpinned by clear definitions of the types of relationships between their constituent parts. To some extent these effects can be mitigated as in GEHR by careful use of headings, which help to provide better understanding for humans. However, the use of a better heading facility, which GEHR certainly does present, does not suffice when it comes to increasing machine processability. For this we have moved to the process of describing common reusable concepts for which we can provide with rules, semantics and vocabularies. These are being explored and standardised by CEN in its General Purpose Information Components initiative, and by GEHR (Australian version) in its Archetypes.

4. CEN Project Team 41. General Purpose Information Components

As pointed out above, there is a need to identify and standardise our descriptions of common information components for the purpose of communication. Thus, for example, there are many instances where it is necessary to communicate a drug regimen, e.g. in a prescription message, a dispensing message, in a referral letter, as a part of a discharge summary, etc. Once we identify this common need we can look at all of the varieties of drug regimen and either define a single GPIC (with sufficient optionality to allow for differences in the regimen descriptions, or by defining different regimen GPICs for particular purposes.

This process has resulted in a wide range of such GPICs, which in turn may be combined in carefully controlled ways so as to be able to build up more complex GPIC structures.

4.1 GPIC Example – Analysable Object

In the CEN GPIC document. an analysable object is defined as information about something derived from or to be derived from a living subject of care or a physical location as part of a dignostic or laboratory investigation. Examples of analysable objects that were considered are:

- An X-ray image, a series of X-ray images, part of an X-ray image. The image may exist in a digitised form or as a film
- An electrocardiograph (ECG) monitor tracing or a twelve lead ECG
- An organ removed during surgery or post-mortem, a biopsy, a particular slide containing a section taken from a biopsy
- A view observed through an endoscope, an observation during an echocardiographic examination
- A sample of meat taken from a food shop

The figure below illustrates how the GPIC is modelled, although it does not show information about the attribute description, cardinalities nor the underlying vocabularies.

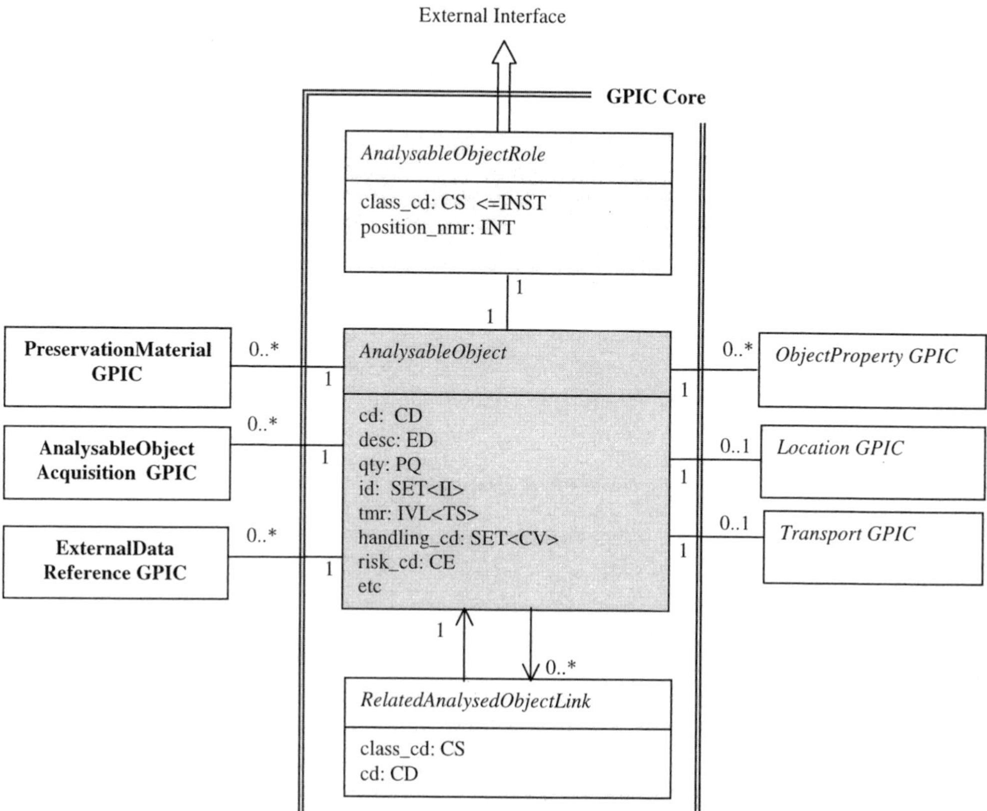

Figure 1. **An Example General Purpose Information Component**

The blue box indicates the core of the GPIC and all provisions as regards attributes and associations described within this boundary must be observed if conformance is to be achieved. The figure also indicates the optional relationships between this core and the extended GPIC. These extensions are all to other GPICs and are optional. It must be stressed that in interfacing with the central GPIC, the context of the satellite GPIC is constrained, which in turn may cause constraints to the vocabularies and attribute values that are utilised within these satellite GPICs.

5. Conclusion

ENV13606 is in need of updating taking into account the findings of the validations and of the implementations that have taken place. In addition it is proposed that the EHCR standard utilises reusable components being developed by CEN in PT 41 and by GEHR (Australia) in its Archetypes.

Electronic Health Records and Communication
for Better Health Care
F. Mennerat (Ed.)
IOS Press, 2002

Unified EHR Standards - Is convergence possible?

Thomas BEALE
Deep Thought Informatics, Mooloolah, Qld 4553, Australia
thomas@deepthought.com.au

Abstract. This paper examines the current state of the art in standards for the electronic health record (EHR) and messaging, and proposes a theoretical design basis for the EHR which is formal yet flexible, and which takes into account many of the difficulties experienced in the past. Recommendations are given for how convergence of EHR specifications might occur, in order to achieve a unified standard suitable for all clinical and cultural contexts.

1 Introduction

The level of activity in standardisation of health information has probably never been greater than at the present time. The difficulties of the domain of clinical medicine, particularly the size, complexity and rate of change of information concepts, have meant that progress in the past has been slow, and the primary goal of widespread, interoperable health information systems has generally not been realised. However, recent advances in information modelling techniques, interoperability technologies, and the formal understanding of the domain seem to point to the possibility of truly interoperable systems in the future.

Principal players in the standards arena include the standards committees ISO/TC 215, CEN TC/251 [4], the HL7 Organisation [11], OMG Health Domain Task Force (HDTF; previously Corbamed) [16], a number of terminology standards groups such as SNOMED [22] and Galen [7], guidelines standards projects such as GLIF [8] and ProForma [18], and long-running EHR standards-oriented projects like SynEx ("Synergy on the Extranet") [12] and GEHR (Australia) [9]. Although work produced by these various groups is sometimes seen as competitive, this impression is not technically or politically justified. Most of the current standards developments are aimed at meeting different technical requirements, and are in some cases located in significantly different cultures of clinical medicine, such as typified by the more social models of Europe and the private payor models of the US.

The possibility of globally harmonised standard(s) for health information systems is seen as attractive by most clinicians, software vendors, health providers, and organisations such as insurers and national health departments, since it would mean that software solutions would be reusable, systems would be interoperable, and personal health data would be widely comprehensible. Achieving harmonisation among the various standards is requires each group to attain an understanding of the domain broad enough to include the situations or requirements being addressed by other groups, and then searching for common technical definitions.

This paper attempts to characterise two of the main standards paradigms, namely 'messaging' and 'EHR' in terms of their scopes and purposes, and goes on to provide a summary of design principles for an EHR standard. The ideas presented here are the basis of current work in the non-profit *open*EHR Foundation, CEN and GEHR, and draw heavily upon work in HL7. It is hoped that they will prove useful in standards development both in the messaging and EHR arenas.

2 Approaches to Interoperability

In the current standards environment, two paradigms of health information standards development are apparent. The first, exemplified by the HL7 and EDIFACT standards, is usually known as 'messaging', and is agnostic as to the contents and behaviour of systems. The other approach, exemplified by the CEN 13606 standards, Corbamed standards, and the Good Electronic Health Record (GEHR) is a systems-oriented approach, and consists of identifying the characteristics of information and behaviour found in (or available from) various systems, particularly EHR systems. Significant confusion has existed in the industry about the relative merits of each approach. Both are valid but have different applicability and scope, as discussed below.

2.1 Historical Context

Historically, message standards such as the HL7 version 2.x specifications and EDIFACT described the semantics of information in terms of message structures. There are two reasons for having done so.

Standardised receiver interface: receiver systems, typically health record systems, clinical applications etc, need to be able to receive data (lab results, etc) from disparate source systems. For this to be technically and economically feasible, the structure, content and semantics of received messages needs to be standardised, allowing the receiver system to treat all messages in a uniform way.

Standardised source system message model: many source systems are based on relatively simple, in-house information models, or information models which may be disciplined but concern only the information stored at the source (such as lab test data or images, which may be only a fraction of the total information of interest for a patient). A standardised message specification is one way of enforcing discipline on the information emitted by disparate source systems, without having to say anything about how they work internally. It also serves as a software specification for the maintainers of the source systems.

Source systems, and in most cases to date, receiver systems such as hospital health record systems, are often not based on standardised information models, and consequently, message specifications are a natural way to deal with the requirement of communicating health information, without having to say anything further about how participating system functions internally. This has been the historical approach of organisations like HL7, and has proven itself in actual use.

In more recent times, the advent of information systems based on standards (even if only the *de facto* standard of a common vendor), as well as generic interoperability mechanisms such as CORBA, COM, SOAP, and the platform-independent XML data representation standard has meant that information can be transferred between systems without a message-level specification. Accordingly, current EHR interoperability standards do not mention protocols or messages as such; likewise version 3 of HL7's standard is oriented towards semantic content descriptions of messages rather than the mechanics of sending byte streams between computers. The main points of comparison between the two approaches are the purpose, scope and applicability to particular systems.

2.2 Domain Scope and Purpose

One of the obvious differences between messages and health records is that messages sent between systems may relate to numerous things not of interest to the health record, for example:

- billing;
- patient administration;
- operational (i.e. low-level) information about orders, materials, or demographic entities.

The main reason for this in a standard such as HL7 is that messages are specified for all possible system interactions, according to use cases describing communication exchanges. Such interactions may or may not involve the EHR system, and may include numerous messages between other systems. The HL7 version 3 standard defines a reference model designed to accommodate all such exchanges, and consequently includes a selection of semantics from all major systems in its scope. EHR standards on the other hand describe either the semantics of information in health record systems (GEHR), or what can be emitted by one (CEN ENV 13606), and do not describe the contents of messages due to general use case-based interactions. Standards for other systems are similar, such as the DICOM [5] imaging standards, and various standards for guidelines and decision support, e.g. ProForma [18], Asbru [1] and GLIF [8].

2.3 Level of Clinical Abstraction

Health records differ from messages in another crucial aspect: they are *accumulators of clinical-level health information*. Messages deal with clinical and other information at an *operational* level. Models describing messages do not describe a time-based accumulator of information, but rather discrete packets of information as sent at distinct points in time between cooperating systems, due to exchanges described by particular use cases.

As an example, consider the notion of an "order for treatment" such as a prescription. The clinician's view of an order is that of a stateful process, where the treatment goes through various states, such as: "proposed", "ordered", "executing", "completed" (with exception states as needed). New information relating to each state is successively incorporated into the record as events in the real world unfold. The level of abstraction of the information is at the clinical level, that is to say, at a level of detail required for the patient care process.

By contrast, in the messaging world, it is argued in HL7 version 3, Unified Service Action Model section [11] that the various phases of an order should not be treated as states in the HL7 reference model, but as distinct message types. When one considers the dynamics and purpose of messages, this argument is justifiable, since there will be separate (possibly numerous, repeated) messages at each phase of treatment, between a number of systems. The state machine paradigm is therefore inappropriate. The design of message content is based on consideration of use cases in which each message appears rather than a full informational representation of the treatment process.

In general, we can say that:

- Messages are discrete packets of information designed to transmit a quantum of information between two systems at a point in time, rather than descriptions of processes or things evolving in time.
- The type of information in messages is operational, and is primarily for consumption by computer systems, whereas the information in the health record is primarily destined for human carers, and omits most of the operational detail, which is of no interest to clinicians.

2.4 Messages versus EHR Extracts

Another point of comparison is between the type of communications between peer EHR systems and between non-EHR systems. According to CEN ENV 13606 and GEHR, peer EHR systems communicate logically using something called an "EHR extract", which is not the same as the kind of messages used when one of the systems is a non-EHR system. An EHR extract is a selection of items from the total EHR, and of the same form and level of abstraction, and is intended for integration into the same patient's EHR at a destination system.

The contents of an EHR extract are generally significantly larger than the typical message, and consist of numerous items of information (e.g. a family history, current medications, therapeutic precautions, entire chains of entries for a problem); the model of access control will be different as well. EHR extracts are more likely to be sent between providers, whereas many messages are likely to be between systems inside the same provider organisation.

One could in fact think of the specification of the semantics of EHR extracts, along with the use cases in which they are transmitted, as being a small 'messaging standard' for EHR transmission.

2.5 System-of-Systems versus Single Model

Reference models for the EHR are typically formulated as one of a family of models, each representing a major service in a distributed health computing environment, such as terminology, demographics, decision support, imaging, guidelines, billing and so on. The 'system-of-systems' approach supports open computing environments, but brings with it the challenge of synchronising the standards.

The messaging approach of HL7 uses a single reference model, in the form of the HL7 version 3 Reference Information Model (RIM) to describe all possible messages, and therefore includes elements of the semantics of all services. The challenge here is making a single model fit the needs of all possible communications between systems, including systems which have their own well-defined models of information such as imaging, guidelines, and the EHR.

However, neither the approach used by GEHR (the same approach could be used with the CEN standards) nor that of HL7 is so simple. In fact, both have a second level of models which provide the domain-level definitions of information inside and flowing between systems. The meaning of the reference model in HL7 is that of a 'language of communication', while in GEHR and CEN, it is a 'language of representation'. A challenge for the single model approach is to show how significantly different systems can communicate using one language.

2.6 Methodology

The two levels of models found in HL7 and GEHR are best understood by a comparison of the methodologies for developing the second layer of formal domain concept models. The archetype methodology used in GEHR, and under consideration by CEN for forthcoming versions of the ENV 13606 standards is described in section 3.2 below.

The HL7 version 3 methodology might best be described as 'sub-schema-ing'. Instead of archetypes, the HL7 approach uses R-MIMs (restricted message information models), and CMETs (common message element types) based on the HL7 Reference

Information Model (RIM). Each R-MIM is a specialised schema, or model in its own right, of a family of related messages, and is derived from the RIM by:

- removal of classes and attributes not relevant to the particular message being defined;
- cloning of classes to provide compositional replication;
- addition of some constraints.

The result is that each R-MIM is like a small RIM, with its own class names and namespace. R-MIMs are expressed using a diagrammatic language, authored using the Microsoft Visio tool. R-MIMs are further refined to produce Hierarchical Message Definitions (HMDs), which are effectively templates for messages. CMETs are templates for re-usable subparts of messages which are likely to occur in more than one message. Figure 1 illustrates the refinement methodology.

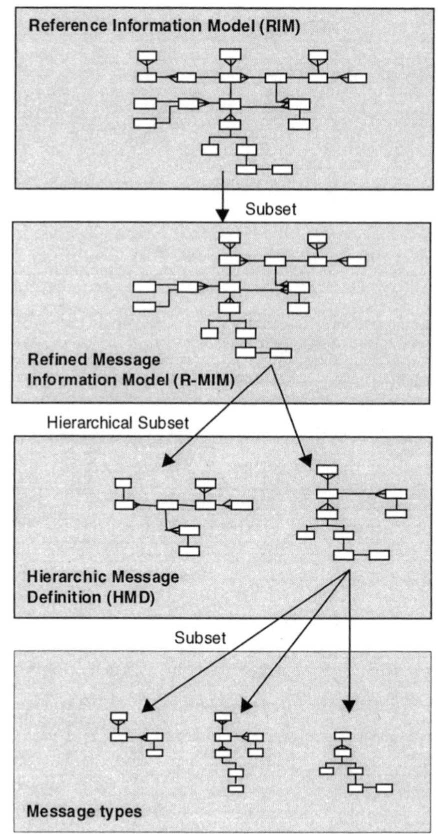

Figure 1 HL7 version 3 Refinement Methodology

The differences between this approach and the archetype approach include the following:

- In HL7, the reference model (the RIM) is only an informative definition of the language of R-MIMs, rather than being a model of information instances. To find out what model data are instances of requires the particular HMD and CMETs to be available.

- Message data items are not instances of RIM classes in the object-oriented sense, but of the classes found in HMDs and CMETs.
- Each new R-MIM (and its HMDs and CMETs) causes new class definitions to be created.
- Since each type in an R-MIM is a pseudo-subtype of a RIM type (+/- attribute modifications), links from the R-MIM classes to the generating RIM classes are also needed, if general RIM-based validation capability is required.
- According to HL7 experts, R-MIMs are not currently intended to be directly comprehensible by domain experts without special training.

2.7 Summary

Table 1 summarises the differences between EHR and messaging standards approaches. The important lesson from this comparison is that EHR and messaging standards satisfy different requirements. The important distinction is one of purpose, between 'models of messages between systems due to dynamic interactions' and 'models of information in/available from systems'.

Table 1 Comparison of Message and EHR Standards

	Message Standard	EHR Standard
Purpose	Define contents of messages according to use cases of system interaction.	Define semantics of patient health record information.
Domain Scope	Clinical, demographic, billing, administration, etc.	Clinical.
Users	Operational computer systems	Humans: clinicians, the patient, epidemiologists, researchers, statisticians. Computer Systems: decision support, guidelines, etc.
Level of Abstraction	Operational – highly detailed	Clinical – the level required by clinicians
Communication	Small, numerous messages.	Usually large EHR extracts.
Reference Model	Single model for all systems.	Model per service.
Methodology	Messages based on refinement sub-schemas of reference model.	Data are instances of reference model, structured by archetypes.

3 Design Principles for the EHR

The design principles described here result from a long history of development work in the GEHR (Australia) project, drawing upon work from CEN TC/251, HL7 version 3, the original European GEHR project [10], and numerous other sources.

We commence by defining what we mean by the term 'EHR', followed by a short description of the 'archetype' design paradigm, which is central to formulating standards for 'future-proof' information systems. The abstract structure for an EHR standard based on this is outlined. Following this, the basis for an EHR reference model is described. Of the numerous sources of design principles available, two primary sources which provide the main structure of the model are discussed, namely, a system of ontologies for the clinical domain, and a context theory of information acquisition.

3.1 What is the EHR?

There are significantly different understandings of the term "EHR" in various parts of the world. An "official" definition which accurately describes our idea of the EHR is that of the Australian Electronic Health Records Taskforce [15]:

An electronic longitudinal collection of personal health information usually based on the individual, entered or accepted by health care providers, which can be distributed over a number of sites or aggregated at a particular source. The information is organised primarily to support continuing, efficient, and quality health care. The record is under the control of the consumer and is stored and transmitted securely.

Some other statements which we can make about the EHR as understood here include the following:

- The EHR is *patient-centred*, and ideally includes information relevant to all kinds of carers, including allied health, emergency services as well as patients themselves. This is in contrast to provider-centred or purely episodic records.
- The EHR contains observations (what has occurred), opinions (decisions about what should occur), and care plans (what should occur).
- The level of abstraction of the EHR is *generalist*, that is to say, specialised information such as images, guidelines or decision support algorithms are not typically part of the EHR *per se*; rather interfaces (discussed below) exist to standards for other, specialised systems.
- The EHR is a *sink* of diagnostic and other test data.
- The EHR is a *source* of clinical information for human carers, decision support, research purposes, governments, statistical bureaux, and other entities.
- The EHR is a long-term *accumulator of information* about what has happened to or for the patient.

In summary, the EHR is a history of all clinical thoughts, observations and decisions about the care of a subject, and as such, it exhibits a kind of 'clinical integrity', meaning that no matter what part of if it is viewed, a complete clinical story is available.

3.2 Design Paradigm

The archetype approach, described by Beale [3] is a two-level approach to modelling, aimed at building 'future-proof' information systems which are capable of processing formal models of domain-level concepts called *archetypes*, in order to structure information during creation and modification. Software and databases are built solely on the basis of the reference model, which is small (less than 100 classes) and defines domain-generic information concepts. An allied model, the *archetype model*, defines a constraint language. Archetypes are formally instances of this model, and each archetype simultaneously defines a domain concept, such as "blood pressure" or "biochemistry results", and the constraints for validating every item of data comprising an instance of the concept. Archetypes are used at run-time during content creation or during batch input to validate all data going into the EHR. Archetypes also provide a 'street-map' for existing data, enabling some classes of querying to be very efficient.

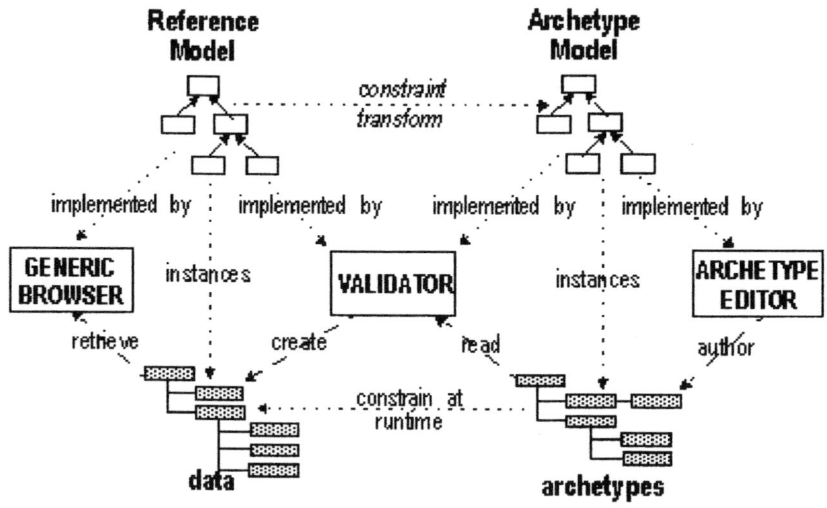

Figure 2 Archetype Software Meta-architecture

Figure 2 illustrates the relationships between the models and types of software. The latter are as follows:

- *Domain Model Editor*: a GUI application for creating new domain concept definitions, based on the constraint model;
- *Validator*: any component which creates or manipulates valid data using archetypes. This is based on the reference and archetype model classes;
- *Browser*: a generic browser can be built, based solely on the reference model, although a smarter browser can be built using the archetype model as well (when viewed in an appropriate GUI).

Almost all applications in a real system are instances of the 'validator' component; that is, they have the property of being able to manipulate data in the presence of the constraints expressed by domain models.

The constraint transform relationship between the reference and the archetype models is a new kind of formal relationship between models, and is not typically treated in the object-oriented literature. However, it is not technically difficult to devise such a relationship, and it has been implemented in the GEHR (Australia) [9] and SynEx [12] projects.

The most important property of systems based on this scheme is that instance data (shown at the bottom left) are not only technically conformant to the reference model (as per the usual object-oriented class/instance relation), but are also conformant to one or more archetype instance (bottom right). That is, they are both *valid reference model instances, and logical instances of domain models*. Further, the variability expressed in archetype constraints enables more than one data instance to be identified as instances of the same domain model. Other properties include:

- term coordinations are formed by *meanings* concatenated along paths;
- constraints are expressed on structure, names, and values;
- the archetype as a whole constitutes a formal model of a domain concept easily understandable by a domain expert.

The importance of a two-level modelling approach such as the archetype approach for EHR standards cannot be understated: it is the key to building systems flexible enough to work in completely different contexts, to enabling knowledge-level interoperability, and to ensuring non-obsolescence.

3.3 Structure of an EHR Standard

A standard for the EHR should be defined as part of a family of standards which collectively represent the major services in a distributed health computing environment, including terminology, demographics, and inferencing systems. This 'system-of-systems' approach described by Maier [13] means the EHR standard does not have to try to be everything, but can rely on other standards to provide the services it requires. It also allows standards to be layered, and released incrementally, making the overall standards process much more manageable than it would be with a monolithic approach (Messerschmitt and Syzperspki [14]). A notional health information systems environment is illustrated in Figure 3.

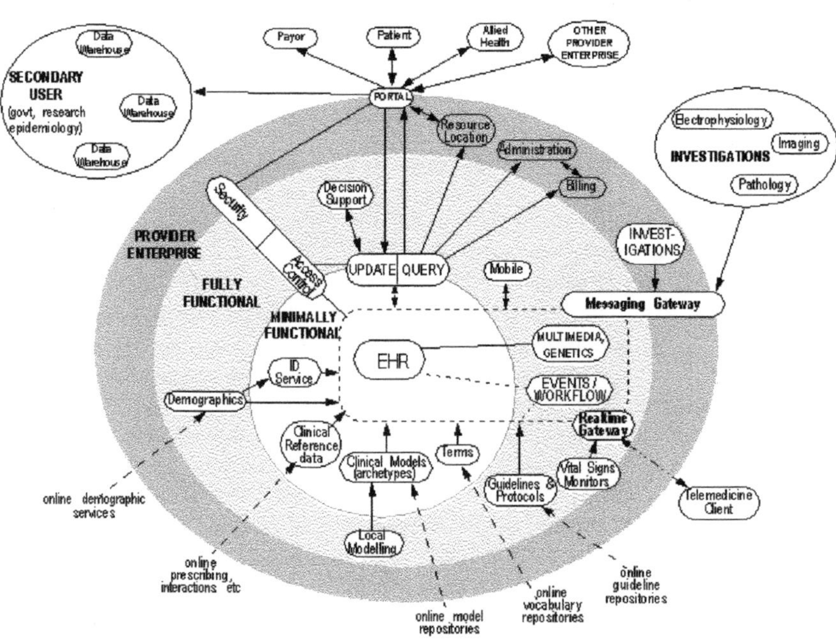

Figure 3 System-of-systems Health Information Environment

What is the vertical structure of each standard in a system-of-systems? We know that in almost all cases, each system is a confluence of the following artefacts:

- software based on a reference model (i.e. an object model);
- formally expressed (i.e. computable) knowledge patterns, models or templates;
- actual data.

We can therefore say that the standard for each service will consist of a reference model level, and a knowledge level (or in fact many levels, as shown in the section below on ontologies).

In the end, it is the form of data we want to standardise, to make it interoperable, and also tractable for computation. This is done by standardising models of data, which requires standardisation of the reference model, the model of knowledge patterns, and knowledge patterns themselves. With the archetype approach, the standard will consist of a reference model, an archetype model, and knowledge expressed a repository of archetypes, terms or other definitions.

3.4 Interface Between Standards

In the system-of-systems approach, most standards have interfaces to other standards, meaning that their respective models have to be compatible. EHR standards have important interfaces to standards for terminology, demographics, inferencing systems, and diagnostic data sources, such as imaging, at both the reference model and knowledge levels. Here we will describe some general principles of interfaces at the reference model level, and the interface with terminology at the knowledge level.

3.4.1 Interfaces at the Reference Model Level

The problem of relationships between reference models is mostly understood by software engineers as a question of what goes in the object model (i.e. class model) for each standard, and in particular, how to represent common concepts in compatible ways in related standards. The most basic principle we can state is that there should be only one model in which any given concept has its primary, or most sophisticated definition.

All other models in a system of standards which need to use a concept primarily defined in a particular standard are obliged to map to it somehow. There are three broad strategies for doing this: *reference*, *encapsulation*, and *summarisation*. In the first case where a system can assume the presence of other systems, its reference model need only include a reference version of the concept modelled primarily in other reference models. For example, the model of coded terms and relationships in Galen [7] and SNOMED [22] servers may be quite sophisticated, but the model of 'coded term' in the EHR and other reference models need only contain the attributes *code* and *terminology identification*. Similarly, the EHR reference model should model demographic entities simply as identifiers which can be decoded in a demographic server.

Now, while this principle is theoretically true, there are some complications. Firstly, the need for interoperability imposes itself on all systems: if data is sent from one service, such as the EHR service, to a location where other services (e.g. terminology and demographics) are not available, the received information will not be completely intelligible. This is the general case in the world today, even for EHRs sent between hospitals or hospitals and GP sites, and does not seem likely to change because of the difficulties in establishing large trusted domains. We can therefore say that models of concepts primarily defined in other standards may need to be augmented in order to make instances intelligible outside the original computing environment. For example, while the strict model of 'coded term' in the EHR reference model would include only the code and the identifier of the terminology, to make EHR data interoperable, the term *expansion* should also be included, since not all recipients might have access to the same terminologies.

The next complication is due to two related needs: the need for *summarised data*, and the need for *uniform access*. Consider that almost all 'after-the-fact' people or systems using the EHR mostly want access only to specific sections of data which are found in their full glory in specialised systems. One example is in imaging: most users of EHR data after the actual treatment event for which images were created are only interested in the particular images regarded as diagnostic by the specialist; these are typically much smaller than the complete sequences taken during scanning sessions, and which may continue to reside on an image database somewhere. Electrophysiology results follow the same usage pattern. In a similar fashion, after-the-fact guidelines users are likely to be interested only in the key characteristics of guidelines which may have been executed for a patient, such as the goal, the final status, and other clinically interesting facts, such as drugs administered and total time taken. In all cases, users are interested only in summary versions of the original data.

The second aspect of after-the-fact EHR use is that most users (again, both human and machine) would prefer to be able to go to the EHR service only, and obtain everything they need, rather than having to interrogate each specialist system looking for the particular items they need. In other words, it is preferable to have summarised versions of specialised data available via a uniform interface of the EHR service.

There are two strategies for achieving summarised, locally available data in a given system. One is to *encapsulate* relevant pieces, along with sufficient meta-data to allow users and other applications to know what to do with them (e.g. launch a certain image viewer); the other is to include a simplified version of the information transparently. The first requires the addition of an encapsulation concept to the reference model, and is most likely to be used with bulky diagnostic data. The second may require additional modelling, or more likely, the use of archetypes to structure existing primitives to represent the desired information, and is more likely to be used to include a simple version of a guideline that was executed for a patient.

3.4.2 Interfaces at the Knowledge Level

Although interfaces exist between the EHR and various other standards at the knowledge level, we will discuss here arguably the most important: the interface with terminology. The interface between models for the EHR and for terminology has been at the forefront of debate in health informatics for some years, and with good reason. Rector [20] provides an excellent analysis of why terminology is so difficult, and brings up many issues, some of which are touched upon here.

At the simplest technical level, terminologies are used for two purposes in the EHR:

- As *names* of items which form the semantic context structures of data values. Many clinicians think of terms in this role as 'labels', as in "family history" or "blood pressure" corresponding to questions asked or tests performed.
- As *data values*, for values expressed textually. In this role, a limited set of term, such as genders, pain levels, blood types etc forms the value *range* for the datum. Clinicians often think of terms in this role as 'answers' to questions or 'results' of tests.

Rector [19] characterises the problem of the interface of EHR and terminologies in terms of the notion of *encapsulation* - the amount and form of information in a terminological entity – and the choice between *pre-coordinated* and *post-coordinated* terms. The latter in particular is a serious problem because there are many concepts which are composites of more basic concepts, and the inclusion in a terminology in "pre-coordinated" form would vastly increase the size of the terminology, making it impossible to manage.

Another problem has to do with the *volatility* of combined concepts. While the combination "left ear 1000 Hz hearing threshold" might be typical in audiology test results used in Australia in 2001, there is nothing to say that such tests won't be restructured in the future, based on different frequencies, or even a completely different arrangement of the data, rendering the old combined term obsolete. Likewise, there is no guarantee of applicability in other health systems. Clearly, it would be dangerous to include such volatile concepts in terminologies which are intended as widely usable repositories of reliable domain definitions.

Pre-coordination leads to volatile terminologies of astronomical size, *only a fraction of whose terms might ever be used* in practice. It is therefore not a realistic or desirable option. The other alternative, *ad hoc* post-coordination maintains little or no control over the terms generated - the number of which is infinite, and creates serious problems for standardised use of terms and interoperability.

Real solutions to the problem become possible once it is seen that the choices are not limited just to pre-coordinated terminological entities or *ad hoc* post-coordination at the point of use. There is clearly a need for domain concept models of *information in-use*; models which describe particular coordinations of terms as used in a particular context, such as a certain pathology test or heading structure for physical examinations. Such models can be implemented using a mechanism such as archetypes. Other implementations exist, such as the *fils-guides* (guide paths) of the Odyssée [2] product. The 'categorial' structures described in CEN ENV 13606-2 were a precursor to these solutions.

The use of formal domain concept models provides a place for *standardised post-coordination of terms*, according to actual uses. This solves the problem on a number of levels. If the archetype or similar approach is used, post-coordinated terms are not defined in limbo, but as part of a whole archetype representing a self-standing concept such as "biochemistry results". This means that sensible groups of post-coordinated terms ('paths' in archetypes) are created and identified together by analysing whole, often well-understood concepts logically. Further, archetypes contain constraints not just on term use but on structure and values, so they constitute a nice encapsulation of all that needs to be said about a given concept, not just statements about naming. There are further advantages:

- archetypes are self-contained, easily manageable, and can be made obsolete or superseded as appropriate;
- actual post-coordinated terms are *constrained* at the point of use (say in the EHR or a guidelines engine) through the runtime use of archetypes;
- archetypes can be specialised to meet the needs of a particular environment while fulfilling the constraints of the parent archetype to guarantee interoperability.

If archetypes are standardised, the problem of each instance of a particular concept in disparate EHR data being slightly different depending on software, users, and other contextual factors goes away. The result is that EHR content is interoperable at the level of domain knowledge concepts, not just standardised data items.

Based on the use of archetypes, we can also state some guidelines for developing terminologies, and for the kinds of terms expected by an EHR architecture, as follows.

- Terminologies should limit themselves to *non-volatile reference concepts*, making their development and management much more tractable, and improving their quality. The job of terminologies should be seen as providing a "level 0" ontology (see below), which supports higher-level ontologies expressed in terms of archetypes or other formal models.
- They can and *should include relationships* between elements, in order to express meaningful networks of concepts describing things in the real world, and allowing queries to be posed. The only rule is that the relationships express non-volatile facts.
- They *should not include pre-coordinated terms*, except where the combination is universally accepted and used, and there are is a clear 'convenience' argument. Atomic source terms should continue to exist in the terminology, allowing systems using archetypes or templates to create other coordinations based on the same atomic terms.

– Terminologies which are to be used to provide base terms for archetypes or other domain concept models (i.e. names of things), have to be designed using a *description* rather than a *classification* mentality, i.e. describing in more or less detail the thing under investigation.

3.5 Ontologies for the EHR

The discussion so far provides some general precepts for building a reference model for an EHR standard. In order to elucidate the actual structure of such a model, we need to explore the domain of clinical information in some detail. A common approach is to try to classify knowledge structures of the domain into *ontologies*, or 'languages of knowledge'. In practical terms this means identifying the different kinds of information in the domain, and deducing the major ontological levels which exist. Table 2 shows a set of ontologies which have been devised by the GEHR (Australia) project, and which correspond strongly to the reference models used in the CEN ENV 13606 standards, as well as numerous implementation efforts. Each ontology corresponds to a level of knowledge used in the domain, beginning with 'principles', or what most clinical professionals see as accepted facts. Level 1 corresponds to structures of information which occur due to particular use cases, such as observations, pathology tests or other investigations. Level 2 contains organising concepts, which describe how clinicians organise gathered information into a sensible documentary form. Levels 3 and 4 describe the compositional constructs of 'transaction', 'folder' and 'EHR', while level 5 describes concepts relating to the transmission of EHR information.

Table 2 Ontologies for the Clinical Domain

Level	Meaning	Expression	Examples
0 - principles	Vocabulary and quantitative semantics of domain, facts true for all instances and all use contexts	Semantic terminology networks, quantitative models.	• textbooks • SNOMED-CT, Galen • statements about quantitative data
1 – descriptive	The smallest self-contained descriptions of distinct phenomena: concepts which describe observation, analysis or prescription of something in the real world.	Compositions of level 0 concepts	• blood pressure • body part measurement • medication order • adverse reaction • history of specific family member • structures implied in LOINC lab codes
2 – organising	Structural information concepts whose purpose is to organise information according to norms of practice, in the same way as headings in a paper document.	Hierarchical structures containing level 1 concepts.	• problem / SOAP headers • alcohol and tobacco use headings • family history headings • referral headings • heading structures for physical examination

3 – unit of work	Unit of information capture, committal, review, modification and communication.	Compositions of level 2 concepts	• transaction, e.g. family history, current medications, problem list, patient contact
4 - accumulation	Concepts relating to collections of information over the long term	Collections of level 3 concepts	• folders, e.g. persistent, event, demographic transactions, etc • EHR
5 - communication	Concepts relating to the packaging of information for the purpose of sharing.	Extracts or packages derived from level 4 information	• document • EHR extract

The utility of a multi-level ontology is twofold. At the reference model level, each ontology provides a 'root class'. In the *open*EHR model, level 0 provides the concept of 'Data value' or 'Data item'. Level 1 provides the concept 'Entry', level 2 'Organiser', level 3 'Transaction', and level 4 'Ehr'. Level 5 provides the class 'Ehr_extract'.

At the knowledge level, the ontologies provide the key for finding and formulating archetypes. Level 0 is primarily expressed as terminologies and quantitative models, while the other levels can be expressed using various levels of archetypes. An archetype for the concept "blood pressure" would thus be one of many in the level 1 ontology, and one for the well known "problem/SOAP" heading structure would be a model of Organisers at level 2.

In summary, ontologies lead to the beginnings of a reference model, as shown in Figure 4.

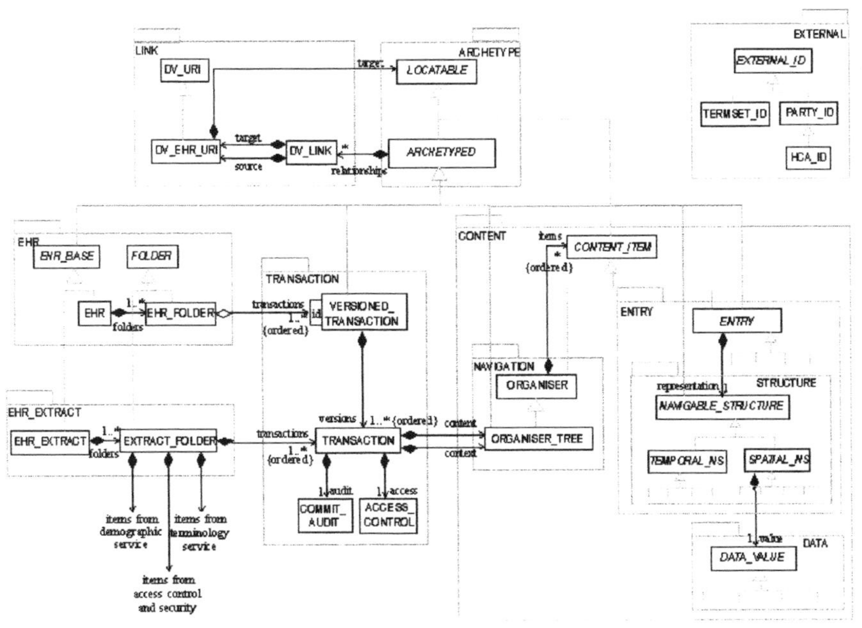

Figure 4 A Proposed *open*EHR Reference Model

3.6 The Context Basis of the EHR

In order to discover the detailed classes and attributes of the reference model, an investigation into the acquisition of clinical information is required. Specifically: what information is gathered, and what contextual information is recorded with it to guarantee that it remains valid. An initial look at the information acquisition process reveals some obvious contexts, including:

- the context of *gathering information*, such as performing an observation or thinking of a diagnosis;
- the context of *clinical activity* in which information gathering occurred, such as a patient visit or a pathology test; and
- the context of a *user interacting with the computer system* containing the EHR.

Experience has shown that, hidden within these 'visible' contexts are a number of sub-contexts, all of which become clear by considering examples in which they differ. The problem of identifying and characterising contexts has been approached here by starting at the reductionist level of 'data values' - what it is carers are ultimately interested in, if they are to make decisions and perform actions. The analysis described in the following sections reveals a number of levels of context, each contained within the next, which are visualised in Figure 5.

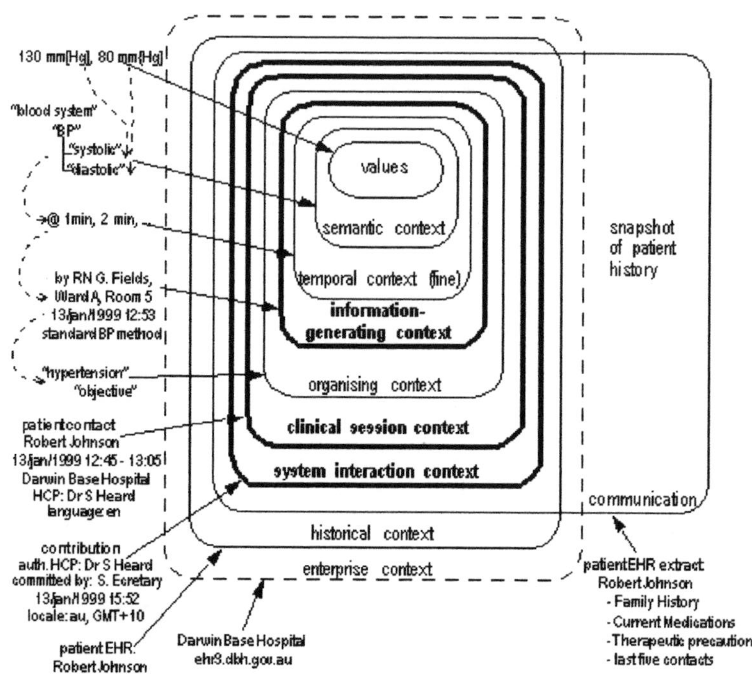

Figure 5 Context Model for the EHR

3.6.1 Values

At the core, clinical information consists of atomic values expressing either an idea (e.g. a diagnosis) or something in the real world (e.g. a clinical datum, a demographic entity). Values are expressed as text, coded terms, quantities, dates, times and so on.

3.6.2 Semantic context

Values are given semantic meaning within contextual knowledge structures which locate the values *with respect to the human subject of the statements* made in the information-gathering context. (The subject of the statements is not be recorded in the semantic context, but in the information-gathering context, since all statements, including repetitions in time, are about the same subject.)

It is important to realise that the subject of statements might not be the subject of the record, but a related person, the family, or an organ donor. Examples include the heart rate of the foetus found during the antenatal examination of the mother; and the result of an HIV status undertaken on an organ donor but recorded in the record of the person having an organ transplant.

Things measured on the patient's body are contextualised by their location, typically expressed hierarchically. Thus, for example, the value "110 mm[Hg]" is meaningful in the context of "blood pressure/systolic". Here the subject of the statements is the patient.

Other semantic structures may be anatomical, such as "renal system / kidney, left". Typically only enough structure is given to avoid ambiguity; thus, clinicians would only realistically use "kidney, left", however, there may well be value in fully locating all values with full paths in the EHR, since it might make some categories of queries much easier to satisfy.

Values for such things as tests on biological materials such as blood or urine are similarly located within semantic structures - typically lists or tables - which describe a breakdown of the characteristics of the material along compositional, chemical or other lines (e.g. ability to culture, genetic etc). In this case, the subject of the statements is the person from which the biological sample has been taken. This may not always be the subject of the record, as in the case of blood tests for a prospective organ donor.

3.6.3 Temporal Situation (fine-grained)

Values within semantic structures must be situated on a real-world timeline, showing when they were true. For most observations in a primary care context, there is only a single time-point. For time-series data typically found in hospitals, the structural pattern (but not usually the exact values) is repeated in time.

3.6.4 Information-Gathering Situation (fine-grained)

The fine-grained real-world situation in which the information is gathered or created constitutes a context which needs to be documented in order to describe the quality of the information. Information-gathering might be carried out by different parties in different situations. Examples include: the subject of the record in their own home by taking a measurement of their own weight or blood sugar; a GP in the surgery performing an auscultation; a pathologist testing blood; a radiologist scanning a patient.

Information is also created whenever a subjective statement is made, such as a diagnosis or opinion from the clinician, or whenever the patient recounts their experience of a problem. Clinicians also create knowledge whenever they decide upon a course of therapy, care plan or other prescription for the patient.

In all cases, this context is characterised by the creation of a single, meaningful item of knowledge, documented by a number of attributes, such as where it occurred, who was the knowledge gatherer, who was the subject, how the knowledge was arrived at, and why it was obtained or created. Numerous distinct information-gathering contexts could exist within the one clinical activity context (e.g. the measuring of blood pressure, auscultation of chest, inspection of throat are three information-gathering contexts within one GP visit).

As already noted, the subject of the knowledge gathered in this context, i.e. the subject of all statements made, is sometimes not the subject of the record, but a foetus, a donor, a family member, or someone unrelated.

3.6.5 Organising Context

Clinical information is not just added to the EHR in an unorganised way; it is arranged by its author into navigational structures, using hierarchical ‘heading’ structures and potentially alternative ‘views’. In this context, organisational models of clinical practice (such as “problem/SOAP headings”), narrative enquiry (e.g. question structures such as “history of presenting complaint”) or classification are applied based on accepted practice norms. Practitioners in different situations (e.g. intensive care versus primary care), or from different medical cultures may well record the same observations (e.g. patient temperature) under entirely different heading structures. The organising context thus corresponds to the ‘logic of practice’, whether it be investigation, reporting or planning.

3.6.6 Clinical Activity Context (coarse-grained)

Information is gathered or created and then organised and committed to an EHR system during and because of a clinical activity. This may be a patient contact with a GP or specialist in a hospital, with a social worker, or it may be a pathology test session during which a test order is completed by a technician. Within any given clinical activity, numerous information-gathering situations may exist, each described by their relevant context attributes; the information from each of these situations may be contextualised under different organising contexts.

The clinical activity is characterised by a clinician, a subject, which is usually the patient, and takes place at a health care facility at a particular time.

Clinical activities normally take place in a longer term care plan or situation. Rossi-Mori [21] suggests that a motivation for the activity should be identified. He raises the examples such as “check-up”, “palliative care” or “revascularisation”. How specific or general the description of motivation needs to be remains to be seen.

3.6.7 System Interaction Context

The information gathered during a clinical activity is committed to the health record system, itself an important context. The person who enters the data (i.e. actually uses the EHR software) is identified (and is often not the treating clinician), along with the particular system, the time and reason for committal, and any other information which may be relevant. Locale information of language used by the system, time-zone and is also required if the record is ever likely to be transmitted elsewhere, or absorb extracts from elsewhere.

The design of the units in which information is committed is crucially important, since they constitute the quantum of information update in the EHR system. Committal units must make sense in their own right, or in other words, exhibit *clinical integrity*. Committal units may also be considered as ‘documents’ in some systems. In GEHR and *open*EHR, committed units are ‘transactions’.

3.6.8 History Context

The EHR is an accumulator of committed changes, and as such is the long term temporal context for health information. It is no coincidence that health records are also known as 'patient histories'. The history context is characterised by the patient for whom the record is compiled.

3.6.9 Communication Context

This context describes the situation in which health record information is communicated between systems, and is characterised by the identities of the source and destination systems, the requesting and receiving and authorising clinicians, and when the exchange occurs.

3.6.10 Enterprise Context

The context of the health care provider in which clinical activities take place and EHR systems are found is characterised by the identification and location of the provider, and possibly other details, such as the provider internet domain.

3.6.11 Context Attribute Model

Table 3 lists the context-related attributes found by a detailed study into the contexts described above. The set of contexts relates strongly to the ontological levels described earlier, and provides a more detailed breakdown. Each set of attributes is used as the basis for formal attribute definitions in the root class for each level in the reference model.

3.7 Other Design Factors

Putting together a complete reference model for the EHR requires consideration of a number of other aspects of health information which have proved difficult in the past, including:

- uncertainty in subjective information;
- approximate, or fuzzy values, particularly in dates and times;
- flavours of null, i.e. the meaning of empty data items;
- how to correctly model negation of terms;
- where domain entities such as 'Person', 'Address' and so on should be modelled;
- the problem of incompatible terminologies used in the same record;
- the non-availability of terminologies for some users;
- the need for an indelible record which still allows logical modification;
- the effect of implementation formalisms such as programming languages, XML and databases.

Initial solutions for most of these problems have been described by various authors (including authors of both current CEN and HL7 standards), and constitute a significant part of the current challenge for EHR standardisation and software development.

Table 3 Context Attributes for the EHR Reference Model

Context	Meaning	Attributes
Value	Quantitative and qualitative data values. Qualitative values are often coded terms.	• [data values] • data interpretation [1]
Semantic	Semantic context of values, with respect to subject of statements.	• logical structure (e.g. list, table, tree) formed with coded or plain text names [1]
Temporal (fine-grained)	Occurrences of structured data in real world time, as measured or observed	• reference time [0..1] • time offset of each event [1]
Information gathering	Real world context of making an observation or thinking of something: the who / how / when / where / why of the information gathering situation.	• human subject of statements (relative to subject of record) [1] • location of information gathering [1] • identity of information gatherer [1] • how information was gathered [0..1] • confidence [0..1] • normal/abnormal [0..1]
Organising	Structural knowledge model in which gathered information is organised by clinician	• hierarchy of headings [1]
Clinical activity (coarse-grained)	Real-world clinical context in which activities occur, e.g. patient visit, pathology lab test.	• human subject of clinical activity [1] • identity of healthcare facility [1] • identity of clinician [1] • start time [0..1] • end time [0..1] • reason, i.e. motivation for clinical activity [1] • principal language of interaction [1]
System interaction	System context of contribution committed to EHR.	• identity of person committing to EHR [1] • identity of clinician legally responsible for committal [1] • time of commit to EHR [1] • identity of EHR system [1] • language of recording [1] • locale details [0..1]
Historical	Patient EHR	• identity of patient [1]
Communication	Context of system/system communication of EHR extracts.	• identity of originating system [1] • identity of target system [1] • identity of requesting clinician at target [1] • identity of authorising clinician at origin [1] • reason for transfer [1]
Enterprise	Context of provider enterprise in which system exists, and clinical activities take place	• identity of enterprise [1] • internet domain of enterprise [0..1]

4 Strategies for EHR Standards Convergence

Convergence of existing specifications for the EHR into a universal standard hinges more on common acceptance of the underlying systems and design paradigms, and theories of information gathering, than alignment of technical aspects such as data types or class names. Nevertheless, it is the latter which is required if a common formal definition for the EHR is to be agreed and standardised. Clearly, the primary quality of a universal standard must be 'flexibility'; that is, within its formal definition, it must allow for the multiplicity of actual health record structures and semantics found in different clinical contexts, languages and cultures. Some of the core areas which require agreement if convergence is to be a serious possibility include:

- the technical requirements of the EHR;
- the use of a two-level design paradigm such as the archetype methodology;
- the general concept of a system-of-systems environment;
- the form of the standard, i.e. type and number of models and other specifications;
- the approach for mapping to implementation technologies;
- a common theory of ontologies and context, supporting development of a universal reference model;
- a common approach to terminology use;
- a core set of archetypes or other standardised domain models for major clinical areas such as general practice, basic pathology, and the major hospital-based uses of the EHR;
- a common set of data types;
- continual implementation-based testing.

Participation by all standards bodies and other interested parties is to be encouraged. The key to success is recognition of a diversity of opinions, whilst at the same time defining and following a common technical vision underpinned by good theory and proven by implementation work.

References

[1] Asbru / The Asgaard Project. See http://smi-web.stanford.edu/projects/asgaard/

[2] P Ameline, Odyssee Project. See http://www.nautilus-info.com/odyssee.htm.

[3] T Beale, Archetypes. See http://www.deepthought.com.au/it/archetypes.html.

[4] CEN TC/251. See http://www.centc251.org.

[5] CEN/ TC 251 Health Informatics Technical Committee. ENV 13606-2 - Electronic healthcare record communication - Part 2: Domain term list.

[6] Digital Imaging ad Communications in Medicine (DICOM). http://medical.nema.org/dicom.html.

[7] Galen. See http://www.openGalen.org.

[8] Guideline Interchange Format (GLIF). See http://www.glif.org/.

[9] Good Electronic Health Record (GEHR). See http://www.gehr.org.

[10] Good European Health Record (GEHR). See http://www.chime.ucl.ac.uk/HealthI/GEHR/Deliverables.htm.

[11] HL7 International. See http://www.hl7.org

[12] Dipak Kalra et al. Software Components developed by UCL for the SynEx Project & London Demonstrator Site. UCL, 2001. See http://www.chime.ucl.ac.uk/HealthI/SynEx/.

[13] M Maier, Architecting Principles for Systems-of-Systems. Technical Report, University of Alabama in Huntsville. 2000. See http://www.infoed.com/Open/PAPERS/systems.htm

[14] D G Messerschmitt, C Syzperspki , Industrial and Economic Properties of Software: technology, processes and value. University of California Berkeley Computer Science Division Technical Report. UCB/CSD-01-1130. 2001

[15] National Health Records Task Force, Australia. The Health Information Network for Australia. July 2000. See http://www.health.gov.au/healthonline/connect.htm.

[16] OMG Health Domain Taskforce (HDTF). See http://www.omg.org.

[17] *open*EHR Proposals. See http://www.gehr.org/openEHR/.

[18] ProForma language for decision support. http://www.acl.icnet.uk/lab/proforma.html.

[19] A L Rector, The Interface between Information, Terminology and Inference Models. MEDINFO 2001 proceedings. IOS press, Amsterdam.

[20] A L Rector, Clinical Terminology: Why Is It So Hard? Yearbook of Medical Informatics 2001.

[21] A Rossi-Mori, F Consorti, Assembling clinical information. Note sent to HL7 EHR-SIG discussion list, 2001-04-19.

[22] Systematized Nomenclature for Medicine (SNOMED). See http://www.snomed.org/.

Electronic Health Records and Communication for Better Health Care
F. Mennerat (Ed.)
IOS Press, 2002

Standards in Electronic Health Care Records: the EADG/BACH paradigm

Alain Maskens, M.D., Ph.D.
avenue Lambeau 62
B - 1200 Brussels

When it first started to be used in real practice, the electronic healthcare record system I helped create and develop from 1985[1], almost immediately induced a high level of frustration amongst the initial users. Why? Mainly because they rapidly felt prisoners of the somewhat rigid structures and contents pre-imposed in the various sections of the record. Even the initial practice for whom these specific screens had been designed rapidly identified the need to modify them. The diversity of situations actually found in real life, and even the variability of needs over time for one same patient, made flexibility and adaptability of the record contents and structures an important requirement

Initially, every aspect of the record structure was in fact solidly wired within the source code and underlying data store structure. Therefore, any change required by the users forced us to enter modifications in the source code and recompile it. As soon as we realised that the requests for modifications were becoming frequent, we were forced to rapidly mover towards a different paradigm. We adopted a flexible data storage architecture, and we separated the medical record *templates* ('sections', 'data sets' ...) from the code and kept them into separate files, which we could more easily adapt without modifying the source code.

But eventually, we had to design tools such that the users themselves could create and modify their own templates, in a totally independent manner. This tool was first developed in 1988[2]. With such a tool, for instance, users could themselves create data sets that were specific for particular medical situations, such as a common GP consultation, an ante-natal clinic, a diabetes follow-up examination, etc.

With time, further developments were made in two directions. On the one hand, users were offered constantly more potential to customize their records and their data entry tools. They were provided with tools to create their own lists of preferred contents for the medical items. Or they could select specific data types to be used with given items. Or they could create computation formulae to be applied with relevant items (e.g. BMI, predicted delivery date, ..). Or, they could selected from several display options for a particular item.

The other development was a natural extension of the previous steps: once users were capable of creating their own medical view of the record, their wish was to be able of sharing it with others. Since all customisation data (e.g. the specification of the templates) were stored in separate files, it was rather simple to offer our users ways to copy such files to other users. We then saw expert users take on an active role in the development of specific medical record environments which they started sharing with colleagues working in the same specialty, organisation, country.

---

[1] *HEALTHone*, from Health Data Management Partners s.a., Brussels (www.hdmp.com)

[2] "*Heditor*". The main contributor to the development of Heditor has bee Mr. J. Geboers.

But it is only the way instances of records wore populated with relevant data which was customisable. All data entered into the records according to these templates were in fact represented using a common data architecture which always corresponded to the same, single model. The components used to create templates (e.g. medical items and their attributes) did very precisely correspond to those used to structure the healthcare records themselves. As a result, records created with our system under whatever form of customisation remained fully compatible with the underlying common architecture. Thus, EHCRs created by one particular user with one particular set of customised templates and other specialised features, could easily be transferred, read, and analysed by any other user of our system, whatever his or her own type of customisation.

It is my practical experience that this approach has worked extremely well, with today several thousand users of our system in different countries and healthcare settings all creating highly customised healthcare record instances which do however all build upon a common data architecture model.

This story has limits: it is only the users of our system which share this deep compatibility and exchangeability of their data. But what it tells is that

1) Healthcare professionals are willing to accept standardisation at the data architecture level, provided they retain the freedom to use this in a highly flexible way. They need to adapt to their specialty, and within in, to the numerous specific situations which may occur. In addition, not all medical schools or institutions share the same views about the way to organise the provision of care, to manage particular diseases, or to represent their domain in the healthcare record.
2) It also tells us that the real experts in designing these 'domain' views are not the software developers, but healthcare professionals themselves.

Let me propose here a comparison. A software house could be compared to a manufacturer of music instruments. The music instrument will be specified so as to be capable of producing specific sounds, based on the (standard) specification of the scale, and different other peculiarities of the sound, such as its harmonics. But the manufacturer is not at all an expert in playing the music instrument. That is where you need the musicians, who will play an almost infinite variety of melodies with this single instrument. Some musicians then may acquire a special competency in creating tunes of a high quality: they are the composers. And composers will create tunes, and propagate these by expressing them using music scores. The latter are based on a representation model consistent with the same standard definitions of the scale and notes (musical components) as those used to build the instruments. What we see here is that we have three categories of functions: the manufacturers, the composers, and the players. This principle allows for the diversity we witness today in the world of music. When however the score is part of the instrument (as is the case, for instance, in the barrel organ or barrel piano), then variety is killed.

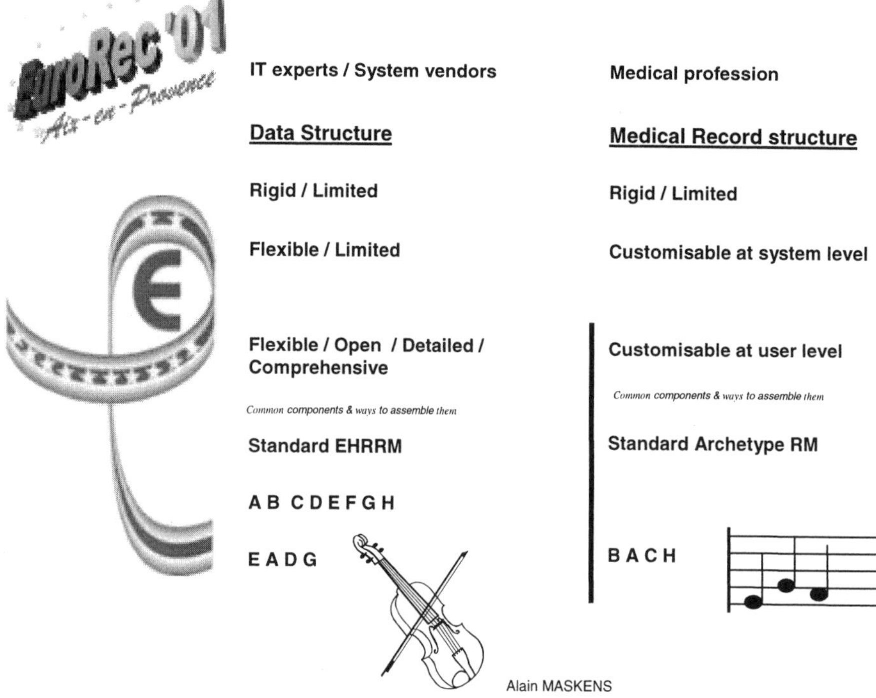

But it can only work because of the consistency of the underlying standard models. The components of the data model (the scale and notes: A B C D E F G) are used in the instruments (e.g. the corresponding strings in a violin: EADG), and are also the basis of the reference model of the system used for expressing the tunes (the score).

The score of course corresponds to what we have called here above 'templates'. It is a concept which has been progressively emerging from several directions. Perhaps one of the precursors of this concept can be found in the way the *Zentralinstitut für die kassenärztliche Versorgung* in Germany developed its healthcare message formats: it used the combination of a rather simple, flexible, common data model, completed by a number of different specifications well adapted for different aspects of the healthcare domain: administrative data ("ADT"), clinical data ("BDT"), laboratory data ("LDT"), or even complex situations such as diabetes follow up[3]. The work of CHIC[4], one of the early European cooperative projects in healthcare informatics, in which François Mennerat was a contributor, was amongst the first attempts to recommend a number of data sets to be used in general practice. SYNAPSES[5], a more recent European project, also identified the need to specify specialised 'clinical objects' and establish a 'clinical object dictionary' as a key constituent of a middleware capable of federating records from various sources.

---

[3] www.zi-koeln.de

[4] DE CLERCQ E, The CHIC concepts : towards standardised GP electronic healthcare records, PROREC NEWS, june 1997,

[5] www.chime.ucl.ac.uk/HealthI/SYNAPSES

The recent work of the GEHR foundation on archetypes[6], presented at this conference, is a further and important effort in this direction. The suggestion is clearly made to separate, in future versions of the EHCR standards, the data architecture of the record on one side (standard *electronic healthcare record* reference model), from the corresponding representation of templates or archetypes, on the other side (standard *archetype* reference model). I do personally support this suggestion, as it would bring at the standards level the benefits we have experienced in the context of our own proprietary developments.

[6] www.deepthought.com.au/it/archetypes.html

Electronic Health Records and Communication for Better Health Care
F. Mennerat (Ed.)
IOS Press, 2002

Sharing clinical information. Principles and task-oriented solutions

Angelo Rossi Mori (1, 2), Fabrizio Consorti (2, 3), Fabrizio L. Ricci (1, 2)
(1) Consiglio Nazionale delle Ricerche, Roma, Italy (2) PROREC Italia
(3) Istituto IV Clinica Chirurgica, Università La Sapienza, Roma, Italy

Abstract. Increasing cooperation among health professionals — within and across organizations — require a suitable sharing of clinical information from heterogeneous (electronic) documentation. Information originates from healthcare activities and may be organized within record systems in relation to health issues, episodes of care, episodes of illness, etc. Implementation of record systems depends on tasks and attitudes within each particular healthcare environment, that determine (i) the balance among functions of the record system, e.g. supporting human memory and decision making, supporting workflow management, recording circumstances about stored data, (ii) the particular organization of a record, (iii) the details of clinical statements that should be explicit or understood.

In this paper we present a set of features of record systems and of their context that affect sharing of clinical information.

1. Introduction

Rationalisation of healthcare provision — supported by the information and communication technologies — relies on multiple uses of the same clinical information, both for several tasks of an user and for co-operation among health professionals [12, 13].

The evolution of organisational models towards continuity of care, including intense co-operation between hospitals and primary care, brings together highly heterogeneous Electronic Patient Record (EPR) systems. The organisation of clinical information within applications is determined by diverse users' perspectives, hampering direct reuse of data.

We recently analysed various EPR systems — from different healthcare environments in various European countries — and the approaches of several European Projects [1]. We described 5 kinds of attitudes towards organisation of clinical information within the record:

1. pure chronological list;
2. interpretative attitude in record systems oriented towards health issues;
3. workflow-oriented attitude, focussing on interactions and passage of responsibilities among professionals;
4. episode-oriented attitude, focussing on the process of care in one location;
5. process-oriented attitude, including and generalizing the above ones.

Each attitude responds to the requirements of a particular healthcare organisation and results in a different typology of record systems. We generalise here our previous results, by producing a schema to explain different perspectives on record systems and to justify the consequences on record organisation. Furthermore, we consider the possible modalities to share clinical information among professionals, from the usage of a server to handle notifications about changes in the life cycle of care processes, to federated health record.

2. An unified schema on healthcare situations and related documents

We present a schema (fig. 1) to show the relations among (i) the activities on a subject of care, (ii) the healthcare situations that are the context for these activities, and (iii) the related documentation, i.e. the possible levels of aggregation of documents into various kinds of record systems. The schema is then organised in three vertical zones.

With respect to similar schemata (e.g. in [22]), here the basic principle is that each record system refers either to a situation of care provision or to a period of life of the patient.

The schema is explained in the rest of the present paragraph.

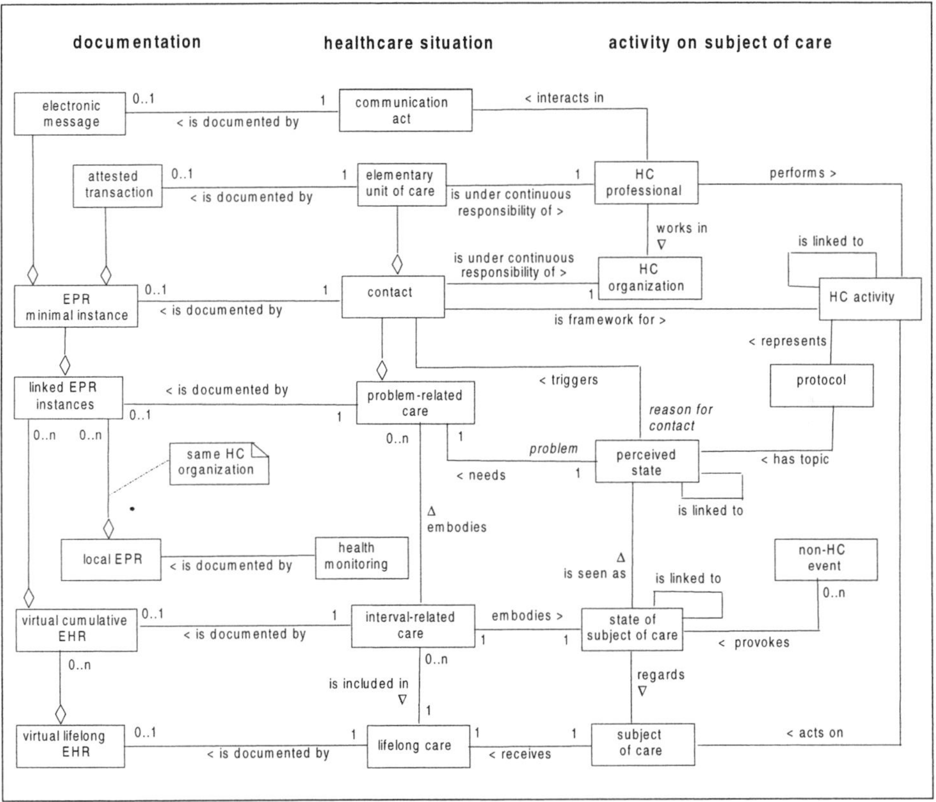

fig. 1 High-level model of healthcare activities, healthcare situations and related documentation (only items relevant for discussion are considered; a diamond represents "part-of"; roles are in italics)

2.1. The right zone: the activities on a subject of care

On the right zone we represented the activities performed by a "healthcare professional" (or a point of service) according to an implicit or explicit "protocol", to face a "perceived state" of a "subject of care" (a person or a group). A "state of subject of care" can be any actual illness or a state of risk, that may be seen as a "perceived state", either by the subject of care or by the healthcare professionals. In turn, the perceived state may assume either the role of "reason for contact" (when it triggers a "contact"), or the role of a "problem" (if used to organise data collection, decisions and thus "problem-related care").

2.2. *The middle zone: the healthcare situations*

In the middle zone we represent a set of healthcare situations [21, part 2] that may be considered as the context for activities on one side, and thus as the focus for documentation on the other side. The situations show an increasing complexity, from the top to the bottom of the schema:

- at the top, there are (i) the minimal unit of care under the continuous responsibility of the same healthcare professional, i.e. an "elementary unit of care" documented by an "attested transaction" and (ii) the minimal act of communication, i.e. the "communication act" documented by an "electronic message";
- in the middle zone, the situations are determined by
  - a contact with a single healthcare organization ("contact"),
  - any single problem or health issue ("problem-related care"),
  - all the problems and contacts with a single healthcare organization or an individual GP ("health monitoring"),
  - all the problems considered during a particular interval, determined by a particular state of the subject of care, e.g. a patient's illness ("interval-related care");
- at the bottom, there is a class for the entire life of the subject of care ("lifelong care").

Note that for a general practitioner, the "elementary unit of care" and the "contact" coincide roughly with an encounter.

The class of *episode of illness* was avoided in our schema, because it may correspond to various "states of subject of care", according to user's interpretations. In fact, apart co-presence of diseases, different recurrences of the *same* disease can be related in different ways to the idea of "episode of illness", e.g.:

- in asthma, the same disease is manifested by recurrent attacks,
- in ulcer, recurrences of new episodes can appear in the same facilitating environment, i.e. as a unique problem of *recurrent ulcers*,
- in pneumonia, completely independent episodes can occur in the same patient,
- in diabetes, a set of complications can be seen as episodes of the same chronic problem,
- in genetic diseases, a latent state can trigger a late episode.

We assume that in our schema we provided the primitives to express the different definitions, as well to deal with care between recurrences and controls. A detailed solution to these issues goes beyond our goals.

Analogously, we also avoided to represent an *episode of care*, because it can be defined in various ways by different perspectives. According to the point of view of the different professionals involved in the care provision and/or of the managers of facilities, it could correspond to a contact, to the care provided for a specific problem, to the care provided for a principal problem AND certain secondary (related and unrelated) problems, including complications. In the ideal case of shared care, episodes involve a set of coherent activities by different organisations, to face a *unique* problem, with local sub-problems. In our schema, this is represented by a unique (ideal) situation of "problem-related care", documented by a "linked EPR instances", i.e. a folder (implemented with an appropriate mechanism) containing documents from many contacts within the various organisations. Non co-ordinated healthcare organisations will have local objectives (not integrated into a common objective) and thus they will see different unrelated problems. They will thus originate independent episodes of "problem-related care" from the same illness, with different time intervals.

2.3. The left zone: the documentation (EPR and EHR)

On the left zone, the basic documents (electronic messages and attested transactions) are *in principle* organised into more and more complex folders, i.e. the documentation is organised according to the healthcare situations represented in the middle column.

Documentation may envisage future actions (orders, intents, plans), register patient's awareness and decisions (consent, attitudes), provide descriptions, or just notify the occurrence of an event.

The basic descriptive documents arising from activities are:

1. diagnostic reports, e.g. reports describing what has been measured by a device, or observed in an image;
2. activity reports, e.g. the description of what has been done during a performed activity, as in surgical procedures (note that there are also mixed procedures, e.g. PTC colangiography, producing an integrated diagnostic & activity report);
3. attested syntheses / summaries of what has been seen and done, from previous documents. A synthesis can be made either by the sender of a message (e.g. discharge letter) or by the receiver (e.g. a note into the journal about relevant clinical information extracted from the received message, that may be also put into the folder as a blob).

The notifications refer to various kinds of events, such as transfer of responsibilities (care mandates), opening and closing of health issues, changes in the life cycle of procedures.

Symptoms, signs and lab results usually may appear in a record system either as items included into more complex documents (i.e. together with interpretations and recommendations) or as sequences of self-consistent statements.

The local collection of basic documents is called here "Electronic Patient Record" (EPR), whereas the view including many EPR located in different systems is called "Electronic Health Record" (EHR) [10, 11, 21].

Note that "*integration*" of clinical information into an EHR may be accomplished at various degrees, i.e. actual *implementation* of a record system can be achieved in multiple ways:

- by creating a real synthetic new EPR with most relevant clinical information;
- by updating an individual EPR using clinical information from external sources, either by automatic extraction or through an attested synthesis;
- by collecting selections of clinical information from different sources into the same datawarehouse;
- by including just links to original EPRs;

In the absence of any integration, i.e. if EPRs are actually produced in the diverse facilities, but no effort is made to link them each other by transfer or pointing, an user is obliged to attempt to locate EPRs each time when a real need arises, perhaps with the assistance of the patient or paper-based documents.

We will analyse the implications of these solutions in the rest of this paper.

3. Documenting healthcare situations: need for adequate homogeneity

If a computer application needs to process in a uniform way either generic or detailed clinical information from different sources, an adequate coherence in the organisation of the documentation is needed. We refer to our schema (fig. 1) to characterise a few relevant situations and the related documentation (table 1).

Documents assigned to the same situation require a suitable level of homogeneity, according to the processing tasks to be performed at that particular level of organisation.

Note that homogeneity does not imply that the individual documents must be actually resident on the same physical support and that they are managed by the same application.

Table 1. Description of healthcare situations and related documentation

elementary unit of care	It is the minimal unit that is under the continuous responsibility of one HC professional, e.g. a visit of a general practitioner (i.e. an encounter), an interactive telecommunication with the patient, a discussion/review of documents. It is documented by an "attested transaction", i.e. the minimal self-consistent significant unit in a EPR, signed by one professional
contact	A contact is the set of units of care that are under the continuous responsibility of the same healthcare organization, as an hospital stay (for a general practitioner — when considered as a HC organization — a contact coincides with an elementary unit of care). It is documented by a "EPR minimal instance", i.e. the minimal folder (including also copies of sent and received messages) that can be considered as patient record.
problem-related care	Problem-related care may consist of one or more contacts for the same (main) problem or health issue, perhaps faced by many cooperating organizations. It may require the linkage of multiple EPR instances, one for each contact. Many situations — *as seen by a professional* in relation to a preventive activity or an illness — can have the *role* of problem. An illness may be seen as many coexisting problems.
interval-related care	An illness-related interval goes from onset of illness to complete recovery or stable outcome (i.e. after convalescence without further care). The care situation in this interval includes the patient's process of illness and the care related to a principal problem (and to many possible secondary problems). An illness-related situation without care (and no documentation) is possible, as well as care without illness (e.g. prevention). The cumulative folder is any integration of the EPRs for care related to each problem , plus a possible synthetic repository.
health monitoring	A local record is maintained by an HC organization that is in charge of the person's health (e.g. GP record, diabetic folder, occupational risk folder, data collection for follow-up of preterm newborns, elderly care record). In particular, a "GP record" contains (virtually or physically) all the documents generated during the encounters, and perhaps copies of messages and links to other records.
lifelong care	It is a virtual EHR (i.e. a theoretical union of all the records generated during all the episodes of care in any healthcare organization) related to the whole existence of the subject of care (the patient's life, or the materno-fetal unit, or a couple for genetics)

4. Attitudes about organisation of record systems

In the introduction we mentioned 5 attitudes about organization of records. In §2.1 we presented a schema (fig.1) where a set of situations of growing complexity was related to folders of increasing size. In this paragraph we describe the influence of the attitudes about organization of records on the implementation of actual record systems, according to the users' needs in particular environments. In fact, different environments (e.g. GP vs. hospital ward) typically focus on different healthcare situations and thus on different kinds of documentation. We don't consider here paper-based records, electronic scanning of paper-based record, or free-text (word-processor) records.

All the attitudes show a different balancing of clinical and organisational issues and different levels of complexity in representing and reconstructing clinical statements. The different healthcare situations behind each typology set the reference intervals for interpretation of fuzzy time expressions in section headings and in data elements. For example, the words "presenting", "present", "current", "past" (applied to symptoms, complaints, drugs) have a certain amount of ambiguity: they could apply to a medium-long term illness, or to an individual episode of its recurrence, or to the contact, or to a set of contacts for the same problem. The same applies to the idea of "history".

With a precise model in mind —and perhaps in future with a more clear vocabulary— a solution of most of the ambiguities should be at reach, allowing a correct computer-based processing.

4.1. Time-oriented attitude

The minimal structure in the corresponding record systems is a chronological list.

Every attested transaction has at least an explicit "date of registration". Possibly the attested transaction should be organized in elementary entries, where each entry should be associated to a precisely represented "date of event".

Therefore a pure chronological log of unstructured notes for each elementary unit of care can always be present (or derived) in computer-based record systems, e.g. as the clinical journal and the sequence of transactions of a GP.

This kind of record system has no predefined semantic structure, no section headings nor names of data elements that contribute to the interpretation of the individual record items. Each entry must be very close to a complete clinical statement, i.e. all non-obvious details should be explicit in the short form, e.g.:

– "1994 / family history of - diabetes mellitus - confirmed"

Applications in this typology may not be able to handle relations among entries, even if they can be obvious to a human reader.

In absence of widely accepted compositional terminological systems, the clauses are expressed in free text, and/or in a particular (set of) coding schemes supporting all the fragments of the clinical statements (i.e. including status terms about actual subject of information, uncertainty, etc.). Usually there is a lack of agreements on a common set of coding schemes and a common style to build expressions, and therefore information from different systems cannot be processed in uniform way.

Individual items may be marked according to the SOAP approach (Subjective, Objective, Assessment, Plan); for most statements this information is redundant to a professional reader (it can be derived from the nature of the statement itself). Nevertheless, this explicit information can be used as a secondary key by computers.

Some constraints can perhaps be enforced; for example the presence of a result of a diagnostic activity implies that the life cycle of that activity has a "status = performed".

4.2. Attitude oriented to health issues

The record system provides an organisation of entries, supporting memory and decision making. In fact, most record systems of GPs are organised by health issues, i.e. collections of nearly complete statements are assigned to health issues. They correspond to a "local EPR" in fig. 1, and a *list of health issues* is a natural function that collects all the names of the health issues and their status. Relations among problems may remain implicit.

Historical data can be arranged in a chronological order under each appropriate health issue; or there is may be a heading related to the history before the assignment of care mandate (i.e. an history that provides a summary of major events and a family history in the period before the assumption of responsibility by the professional or service).

Note that for a GP the duties continue after the conclusion of a single episode of care (i.e. until the patient is in charge to him/her); therefore a GP will not have a "history related to the present episode of care" (see next paragraph). Moreover, a GP can consider many problems as simultaneously active during the same period for a particular patient, and the EPR may extend over many episodes of illness.

Usually activities are recognised (as well as some sub-category, as prescription of drugs, laboratory observation) and their life cycle is handled. This implies the handling of the relations between statements with different statuses (e.g. ordered vs. performed)

Combined with the previous typology, this organisation allows for three different views: chronological, by problem, by SOAP or by kind of statement (for example, a dynamic view about "all orders still pending").

4.3. *Attitude oriented to episodes of care*

An episode of care determines the idea of past, present and future within the record.

A professional in a hospital could record information in relation to the reason for admission and the chronological log of activities (journal) during a series of close stays (planned contacts included in a single episode of care). The use of section headings and subsection headings is common to most records in this typology. Relevant information about the past could be collected from patient or extracted from available documents; a synthesis of information in diagnostic reports received by the clinician may be arranged in the record. The record is closed with final discharge.

For an hospital, the idea of patient record is typically limited to one episode of care (which may include a follow-up in co-operation with primary care). In fact, there is no continuation of mandate after the episode of care (i.e. a set of planned contacts). Therefore there is a "before", a "during" and an "after" with respect to that episode. Clinical information "before" the episode of care goes either into the (unique) "history related to the present episode" or into a "(unrelated) past history".

4.4. *Workflow-oriented attitude*

The focus of the record system is to document interactions and changes of responsibilities. Each phase of the workflow (i.e. request, negotiation, performance, acceptance of output) features a variable degree of regularity that can be systematised in message standards. Diffusion of standards on messages raises the relevance of this attitude in current computer-based clinical systems. In this case the record system should at least mimic the paper-based patient file as collection of documents. In fact, a patient file collects not only the *local annotations* about impressions, decisions and status of performed and planned activities, but also a series of documents *generated by the interaction* with other professionals, for clinical and administrative purposes. The internal structure of diagnostic reports and attested summaries from previous documents is typically complex and may remain implicit.

4.5. *Process-oriented attitude*

This kind of record system integrates clinical and organisational processing, and facilitates quality monitoring. A sequence of activities (and sub-activities) is described in a processable format, in relation to a main problem (and sub-goals) [3, 4, 5]. An activity produces clinical and organisational data, to support the organisation of the work, as well as audit and quality assurance. In fact, this attitude allows to relate data (and costs) to clinical actions and their goals and to use "clinical profiles" of the patients to view and organise the data.

Record systems with a process-oriented attitude are relatively more difficult to implement, as they do not simply mimic paper-based organisations, but are an extension of the other cases. In fact they may be able to consider:

- the temporal evolution of activities;
- the relations among activities and sub-problems and sub-goals, as well as relations of data with "decisions in context";
- the organization of activities and nested sub-activities into the coherent framework of an episode of care;
- the communication for synchronization of activities by different professionals, also to regulate responsibilities.

Process-oriented record systems could be considered as extensions of an Act Manager (see the A-HCCs in [22]). Act Managers are typically oriented towards the management of the workflow about services of care provision (i.e. mainly to manage planning, scheduling, performing, reporting); the idea of service must be extended to include also activities of information handling, e.g.:

- prescribing, where physicians plan a drug therapy;
- collecting subjective information from the patient;
- producing decisions, impressions and plans from existing documents:
    - taking decisions from available data, including making a diagnosis;
    - expressing a second impression on data collected by other professionals;
- producing summaries from existing documents:
    - write a discharge letter;
    - extract relevant information about a given problem (perhaps on request by other physicians).

Moreover, with respect to an Act Manager, a process-oriented record systems must provide additional functionality for organising and presenting information.

5. Sharing clinical information from heterogeneous documentation sources

In §2.3, we defined the attested transactions and the electronic messages as basic documents. In the left zone of fig. 1, they are included in folders of growing complexity. Presence of documents with incompatible organisation within the same folder hampers optimal handling of clinical information and interoperability of applications.

In principle, advanced semantic processing [2, 14-19] could allow for rule-based transformations among different views, to reconstruct the virtual clinical statements in the basic documents. Nevertheless this kind of complete integration of clinical information is a huge task, perhaps unnecessary in most cases.

5.1. What — structures that may be shared (payload, header, envelope)

For most tasks, it is not necessary to share completely structured data. For example, a document or a significant part of it (e.g. a section) may be indexed or retrieved in effective ways just by processing its header.

In fact, the information to be shared may belong to three kinds of structures:

a) a <u>payload</u>, that could be managed for example as (i) a blob, until an peculiar application is launched for either display or processing it, (ii) a narrative piece, suitable for text-based search, (iii) a page with appropriate XML mark-up, (iv) a structured composition of data elements according to a standard format.

b) a header, that describes some of the following items pertaining to a document or to a section as a whole: the author, his/her organization, the subject of care, the date of recording, the overall level of security, the kind of healthcare event and its date, the kind of document/section. A header — independently of the availability of its payload — allows
   1. to generate a common directory across different legacy systems;
   2. to manage security at the level of the whole document or section;
   3. to find the pertinent documents, through queries to directories *about* the documents (i.e. not directly performed on their payload);
   4. to guide the presentation of the payload of a document as a blob to a reader;
   5. to guide machine interpretation of the payload.

c) an envelope, that provides information pertaining to a particular instance of a document or section, e.g. a pointer to its location (either the original one or to a suitable mirror), or message features such as date of transmission, sender, receiver, etc.

A notification is a particular kind of message, where the payload coincides with the header.

Within each information system, various strategies about sharing of clinical information (i.e. how much information should be made available to whom and why) are possible in principle, for example by using one or more of the following approaches:

1. a collection of documentation-based pointers to
   - access services to data storages of involved organizations, or
   - a record of an individual patient, or
   - a single document of a patient, or
   - a single section within a document
2. servers based on event notifications, with patient-related lists on
   - active / inactive health issues;
   - current / former care mandates;
   - ongoing / former activities;
3. servers based on synthetic information, containing for example HTML or XML pages about:
   - summary of each contact;
   - present state summaries, historic overviews;
   - care plans;
   - alerts;
   - motivated extracts.
4. a physically centralised record, e.g. accessible through a web-based secure interface;
5. an set of identical EPR (possibly by the same vendor and with the same object dictionary);
6. a federated record system, based on the mapping from the structured information elements contained in the heterogeneous feeder systems to a reference object dictionary.

5.2. Where — co-operation of local and remote applications

Different healthcare situations require specific levels of integration and interoperability.

Therefore another aspect to consider is the heterogeneity of applications and organisations involved. Co-operation may be requested at various degrees of performance:

1. Inner interoperability and local coherence on views within the same EPR

- how to rearrange the same data (i.e. data on the same patient) under different views, for different tasks;
- how to preserve coherence for people with the same clinical role (i.e. different doctors, different patients) and across different episodes of the same patient;

2. Outer interoperability across EPRs;

- on similar professional context (e.g. from a GP to another one);
- on different professional context (e.g. inpatients vs. outpatients, different medical specialties, allied professions);

3. Integration across multiple information sources;

- how to include a synthesis/the whole reports of examinations;
- how to select and include relevant data from previous encounters/episodes.

5.3. Why — goals for computer-based handling of clinical information

Each healthcare situation requires particular functions, and the mechanisms used to assure homogeneity of disparate statements within the same folder must be coherent with these needs. Getting clinical information from external sources is only an intermediate step in a complex chain of information handling. Depending on situations, users may have various goals about handling the clinical content of multiple documents (table 2).

Table 2. Computer-based handling of clinical information [8]

#	goal	computer-based handling of clinical information
1	layout-based presentation	display, print information (without healthcare-specific constructs)
2	healthcare-aware presentation	present information using healthcare-specific kinds of constructs
3	reorganization of information	browse with variable criteria, prepare multiple views, select, index; aggregate data from diverse patients (epidemiology, audit, QA)
4	trigger to reference knowledge	use pointers in look-up tables and knowledge bases (e.g. on drugs, on guidelines, on statistical tables for QA)
5	update content	write and amalgamate information into a different record system

5.4. How — needs for standards

Each goal implies a set of requirements on EHR systems, that corresponds to different kinds of standards. In general, standards are inevitable for envelopes and headers.

With respect to goal #1, no additional healthcare-specific standards on payload are needed. In fact, a set of generic transmission standards are nowadays available, e.g. ISO-OSI standards on Open Systems and the W3C standards about Web-based communication (including mark-up languages, as HTML and XML, and their derivatives).

They allow for transmission of multimedia documents and for their presentation to end-users with appropriate formatting, but they are not aware of healthcare constructs.

The easier way is to link a file or a part of a document with a precise application, able to interpret it correctly (and display it, and print it).

Receiving applications can find titles and list elements within a document and perhaps they can reproduce the textual content (and multimedia objects, not further considered here) for humans, according to original layout structure, but they are not able to intepret that structure nor the content for further processing.

Moreover, it is not possible to assure that the sender is providing the minimal amount of information, that could be adequate in the particular healthcare context for faithful interpretation of the data by the receiver.

Some awareness of healthcare semantics is instead required to handle heterogeneous clinical information according to goals from #2 to #5. Controlled phrases or annotations can be used to permit re-use of information at the requested level.

Most standards on healthcare messages are conceived to assure the usage of information according to goal #2. A set of messages was developed by standardisation bodies, for particular healthcare needs, e.g. laboratory orders and reports, specialist referrals [9, 7]. Each message is able to preserve the structure of a particular kind of clinical information. In this case semantic expertise is used during development of the standard (to decide the structure of segments and data fields) and by the sender application (to put content under the appropriate container). For presentation of information, no further semantic processing is required to the receiver. No interpretation is required to simply reproduce content under explicit section headings. If information about groupings of record components into record item complexes is preserved, the receiving application can present information according to the original organisation and propagate properties from complexes to components.

Awareness of semantics by receiving applications is required for the other goals. In goal #3 applications should be able to handle the relations among the section headings. In goal #4 they should map received section headings with the ones predefined in the knowledge source, then rearrange and transfer a standard content. In goal #5 applications must handle the content, to be sure that it is homogeneous with existing information.

The EHCR-"Domain Term list" standard [20, 21 part 2] provides a simplified set of basic descriptors to assure the correct interpretation of clinical statements, by proper annotations produced by look-up tables at the moment of generating the messages from an EPR. In this way messages may be able to satisfy goal #2 or to present a minimal level of interoperability suitable for goal #3.

5.5. When — operational context and task-oriented structures

If the operational context is well-defined, the environment is spontaneously simplified and integration is facilitated. Let us focus on primary tasks, *computer-based* usages of clinical information and the corresponding degree of awareness about handling needs.

Easiness of systematic structuring of basic documents (attested transactions and messages) depends on tasks:

- Primary task is *communication*. Data can either fit into a simple organization as in structured *standard messages* (e.g. orders, prescriptions, and claims), or they consist of complex unstructured narrative (referral/discharge letters, reports). The situation is well-defined before sending the individual electronic message, possibly with an international agreement on the set of useful data and their relations. Mandatory data elements in a standard assure the presence of the items needed by the receiver to accomplish safely and effectively its typical task.
- Primary task is *organizational effectiveness* (e.g. scheduling of internal activities, reminders). Transactions are well defined, and coded data can be used (and reused) to trigger information stored in *tables* (or knowledge bases). Data needed locally by a single application can be generalized to fulfil widely implemented functions, e.g.

consultation of drug data bases. Data elements and their contents must be standardized to allow plug-and-play installation of databases and tables (not for actual communication).

- Primary task is *local documentation*, even if users may be aware of potential *further usages* (e.g. when they record a plan). Transactions have a relative freedom, although some constraint is given by expected reuses. Some minimal structure is needed, in order to achieve advanced handling of data. Additional usages are envisaged for "predetermined" tasks (e.g. most activity-related clinical information is either exchanged among different users, as in shared care, or processed by the same user using various applications over time). Independent applications may require to access stored clinical information, or at least the subset needed for patient's care by different healthcare organizations or by different local applications during the same series of contacts for the same illness. This situation demands for *independence of data from applications*.
- Primary task is *local documentation*, but additional usages are not predetermined (e.g. collect data for patient history, during possible further contacts). Transactions cannot be forced towards a precise structure.

In summary, primary uses of information in a particular environment, and planned additional uses, further determine the organisation of data within either the transaction or the message, for a particular typology of EPR systems, and also the kind of coding schemes to be adopted, influencing the performance of the corresponding EHRs.

6. Conclusion

The unavoidable presence of different incompatible implementation strategies for EPR systems — to satisfy users' requirements in different environments — hampers reuse and interoperability of clinical information into EHR systems.

Semantic processing could in principle be able to perform adequate transformations among different typologies of record systems, for planned reuse of clinical information, but at huge costs. An EPR can be seen as a set of structured documents, made of interrelated statements. Principles for their organisation depend on primary tasks and uses that characterise a particular professional environment and on the modalities of healthcare provision. Understanding these principles enables us to progress in reconstruction of the organisation of information within the EPR and of nearly context-independent statements. This is the substrate for semantic conversion of clinical information from one organisation to another, i.e. to achieve faithful handling of semantics and interoperability among disparate systems according to tasks.

Sharing clinical information can be achieved at different levels, i.e. full semantic interoperability is expensive and perhaps unnecessary in most cases. The level that is suitable for a given environment has to be carefully decided by considering a number of criteria, related to tasks, presence of well-defined situations and easiness to structure the documents from involved EPR systems in a uniform way, closeness of expressions to "complete" clinical statements.

Acknowledgements.

Work partially financed by the EU Projects C-CARE and WIDENET.

References

[1] Tomelo (an European Project) see documentation at http://www.ehm.kun.nl/tomelo/#Workshops

[2] GALEN and GALEN-IN-USE. documentation (1992-98), available from AL Rector, Medical Informatics Group, Dept. Computer Science, Univ. Manchester, Manchester M13 9 PL, UK e-mail galen@cs.ac.man.uk ; see also http://www.cs.man.ac.uk/mig/galen

[3] Grifoni P et al, "Modelling the management of protocols as the kernel of a health-care information system", Proc. of 8th World Congress on Medical Informatics, MEDINFO '95, 1995.

[4] Rossi-Mori A et al "A model for structured description of healthcare activities and related data" in Gordon C, Christensen JP (eds) Health telematics for clinical guidelines and protocols, IOS Press 1995

[5] Luzi D, Ricci FL, "Shared care: workflow management for medical treatment improvement", Proc. of Health Telematics '95, 1995.

[6] HL7 Health Level 7 Documentation available at http://www.hl7.org

[7] Rossi Mori A, Consorti F. Exploiting the terminological approach from CEN/TC251 and GALEN to support semantic interoperability of healthcare record systems. Int J Med Inform 1998; 48:111-124

[8] Rossi Mori A (ed) Preliminary material for ENV13606-part 2 Communication of Electronic Health Care Record — Domain Term list (available on request by the Authors)

[9] CEN/TC251. Work plan of Technical Committee 251 "Health Informatics" of the European Committee for Standardization (CEN). Available from http://www.centc251.org

[10] Rector AL, Nowlan WA, Kay S. Foundations for an Electronic Medical Record. Methods Inf Med 1991;30:179-86

[11] Rector AL, Nowlan WA, Kay S, Goble CA, Howkins TJ. A framework for modelling the Electronic Medical Record. Methods Inf Med 1993; 32:109-19

[12] Andover Working Group. Accelerating the Movement Toward Standards-Based Interoperability in Healthcare. Available from http://www.dmo.hp.com/mpginf/whitepaper.html

[13] Sokolowski R (ed.). Integration services for clinical data exchange. White Paper draft, 1997. Available from http://www.omg.org/corbamed/cprcdr.htm

[14] Rossi Mori A, Consorti F, Galeazzi E. Standards to support development of terminological systems for healthcare telematics. Methods Inform Med 1998; 37: 551-563

[15] Rossi Mori A, Galeazzi E, Consorti F, Bidgood WD Conceptual schemata for terminology: a continuum from headings to values in patient records and messages. J Am Med Inform Assoc; Symp Suppl 1997:650-4

[16] ENV 1828. Medical informatics — Structure for classification and coding of surgical procedures. Brussels: CEN, 1995

[17] ENV 1614. Medical informatics — System of concepts for systematic names, classification, and coding for properties, including quantities, in laboratory medicine. Brussels: CEN, 1995

[18] ENV 12611. Medical informatics — Categorial structure of systems of concepts — Medical devices. Brussels: CEN, 1997

[19] Rossi Mori A, Consorti F. Integration of clinical information across patient records: a comparison of mechanisms used to enforce semantic coherence. IEEE Transactions on Information Technology in Biomedicine, 1998; vol.2, 4:243-253

[20] Rossi Mori A, Consorti F, Galeazzi E. A tagging system for section headings in a CEN standard on patient record. J Am Med Inform Assoc Symp Suppl 1998

[21] ENV13606. Health Informatics — Communication of Electronic Health Care Record, Brussels: CEN, 1999

[22] ENV 12967-1. Medical informatics — Healthcare information system architecture (HISA) — Part 1: Healthcare Middleware Layer. Brussels: CEN, 1998

Corresponding address:

Angelo Rossi Mori, angelo@itbm.rm.cnr.it
Istituto Tecnologie Biomediche, Consiglio Nazionale delle Ricerche, viale Marx 15, I-00137 Roma, Italy

Electronic Health Records and Communication
for Better Health Care
F. Mennerat (Ed.)
IOS Press, 2002

The Industrial Forum

Jacques E. ANDRÉ PhD
Consultant in Hospital Computing
5 traverse Clérambault
F - 13830 Roquefort-La Bédoule (France)
hoptimis@aol.com

The purpose of this Forum is to give the Industry the opportunity to express its opinion about the market and its financial, political and cultural problems. It should give the users and the developers a chance to dialogue and to exchange ideas, opinions, experiences and requirements.

The industry has recently faced significant environment changes:

⇨ The market has moved from an individual, departmental, mono-organisational computerisation to the implementation of integrated health networks; the objective being to secure the CONTINUITY of CARE with its potential qualitative and quantitative benefits. It means that the new health information systems have to be centred on and organised around the citizen and his health record. At the end of 2000, we made for PROREC-France a survey on "The Status of Medical Records in the French Public Hospitals". One of the most interesting results was to find out that 90 % of the 50 participating hospitals, representing 50,000 beds, were planning to implement a health network (see Appendix).

⇨ In order to allow the various partners of such networks (hospitals, clinics, GP's, specialists, nurses, pharmacists, nursing homes, etc.) to access and to share the citizen's record, to optimise the planning of activities, to understand each other and to benefit from the large amount of stored historical data, these new systems must include new sophisticated software modules such as:
- an ENTERPRISE ACCESS DIRECTORY (EAD) which, in the absence of a national identification number (like in France), allows the consolidation of the various identities given by different systems to the same person;
- a COMMON VOCABULARY ENGINE, to solve semantic problems;
- a patient wide SCHEDULING System;
- an INTEGRATION ENGINE, to facilitate the interface and the communication between the various systems linked to the network.

The industry is thus facing complex and costly developments when public authorities did not give any kind of guidelines concerning the creation, the management or the financing of such networks. If their qualitative advantages may seem obvious, a global evaluation of their benefits in terms of economy and productivity has never been made, as far as we know.

With very few exceptions, the same situation exist for Hospital Information Systems.

As, in order not only to expand but also very often to survive, software houses have to become international ,and as a hospital is a hospital, a health network is a health network and a medical record is a medical record wherever you are, the European Commission should sponsor some Return-on-Investment studies. This would help the vendors to justify their offers and the buyers to obtain a budget or a credit.

So far, in the Information Systems domain, the most significant international offers came from North-American companies. Few of them have been successful in Europe but not for the reasons given by their opponents who persistently claim that the main problem lies in the cultural differences between Europe and USA.

As we said already: a hospital is a hospital, etc.

These opponents exist at national level and at European level and their motivation is almost always the same: protectionism.

In France the situation is even more complex as public authorities are not only favourable to local solutions but continue to allow public-funded developments to compete against the private industry. In order to fight against such a behaviour, the industry has created some years ago the SNIIS, a national syndicate, which has recurrently threatened the Ministry of Health with legal proceedings at European level..

But the best example of protectionism as well as distrust against the private industry in general was given by CEN when the TC 251 was created in 1991 and declared: "The international standardisation work may not take into account the requirements, the interests, the cultures and the legislation of Europe. An European public support is needed in order to stimulate the competitiveness of the European industry. Europe is in favour of a systematic approach opposed to the industry-lead US approach".

No doubt that this negative attitude has been the major cause of the TC251 lack of concrete results.

In 1997, the Commission wrote : "The standardisation process must correspond to the market requirements. Some published standards show a lack of specificity. Other working methods should be applied"...

In spite of this realistic declaration and of a conference "for industrial suppliers of ICT solutions and healthcare organisations" organised by CEN and DG XIII on December 1998, the industry is still not involved and the recent attempts to build a fruitful co-operation with HL 7 have failed.

As chairman of the ICT Standards Board, Massimo Rusconi (OLIVETTI RICERCA) has perfectly summarised the problem : "The standardisation process must never interfere with commercial imperative to develop competitive products and release them into the market. ICT is a fast expanding sector that represents the new frontier of the global economy. Standardisation must complement the ICT industry's innovations and time-to-market, not hinder them".

To conclude, we may say that Medical Informatics Industry in Europe is underdeveloped, fragmentary, precarious and hyper-cautious.

The main reasons are:

- ⇨ the survival of protectionism at national and at European levels;
- ⇨ the lack of vision and of expertise of the decision-makers;
- ⇨ the lack of means, specially in hospitals, in terms of budget and people;
- ⇨ the individualism and the traditionalism of the medical profession;
- ⇨ the scientific, academic and theoretic attitude of the standardisation bodies and of the national and international Medical Informatics Associations;
- ⇨ the traditional "Reinvent-the-wheel" European intellectual approach.

We would like to stress the merit of Prorec-France which did not hesitate to give the industry a whole session in this high-level, high quality Conference.

In his welcome speech, the President of PROREC-France, Dr. F. Mennerat, said : "The broad objective assigned to PROREC is to identify, and subsequently try and help solve the issues opposing or slowing down the process of widely implementing high quality EHRs in Europe", we do hope that our contribution will help in the understanding of these issues.

APPENDIX

A survey by PROREC-France on the status of the Medical Records in French public hospitals

Jacques E. ANDRÉ PhD
Consultant in Hospital Computing
5 traverse Clérambault
F - 13830 Roquefort-La Bédoule (France)
hoptimis@aol.com

The Objectives

In order to have a better knowledge of the hospital environment and therefore to better direct its actions, the PROREC-FRANCE association decided last year to make a survey on the status of medical records in French public hospitals and on a certain number of associated projects like hospital-GP's networks.

The form

The survey was made with a short, simple and easy-to-fill in questionnaire sent by mail either to the CIO, either to the CEO, either to the CMO, following the size and/or the organisation of the hospital. The questionnaire was sent to 150 short-term public hospitals.

The results

The percentage of answers was pleasantly high: 33 %, representing 50,000 beds.
The questions and the answers were the following:

Question 1:

Do you have	centralised archives?	72 %
	departmental archives?	14 %
	both?	14 %

Question 2:

Are you using a Permanent Patient Identifier (PPID)?	Yes:	96 %
	No:	4 %
Is a national PPID necessary?	Yes:	82 %
	No:	6 %
	No answer:	12 %

Question 3:

Do you have a computerised Medical Records System

installed?	- common:	40 %
	- by department:	8 %
	- both:	8 %
being installed?	- common:	22 %
	- by department:	2 %
	- both:	2 %
planned?	- common:	20 %
	- by department:	6 %
	- both:	2 %

Question 4:

Is your Medical Record System aimed at containing **ALL** information pertaining to the patient or part of it?

All:	58 %
Part:	22 %
No answer:	20 %

Question 5:

Do you have a Health Network (Hospital to GPs link)

operational?		4 %
being implemented?		2 %
planned?		86 %
forecasted?		4 %
	No answer:	4 %

With what kind of communication?

Results server:	yes:	70 %
	no:	8 %
Access to the hospital medical records:	yes:	62 %
	no:	14 %
Exchange of records:	yes:	64 %
	no:	6 %

Question 6

Are you aware of the existing and/or coming standards?

yes:	44 %
no:	54 %
no answer:	2 %

What are, following your understanding, the objectives of these norms?

The presentation and the understanding of information:	32 %
The exchange of information:	68 %

Some conclusions:

1. The fifty hospitals that participated were obviously actively involved in the implementation or the planning of computerised medical records; therefore the large number of comments and remarks which we received in addition to the formal answers.
2. A large majority of hospitals are requesting a national patient identification number. It means that they have reached a certain level of complexity which requires integration, coherence and traceability.
3. The COMMON medical record has overtaken the DEPARTMENTAL medical record which implies several professional, ethical and cultural changes.
4. The answers to the questions 6 and 7 show that hospitals are willing to play a leading role in the implementation of health networks.

Electronic Health Records and Communication
for Better Health Care
F. Mennerat (Ed.)
IOS Press, 2002

A message model designed by EDISANTÉ WG 11

Pascal Charbonnel, François Rougerie
EDISANTÉ Association

Abstract. WG 11 is one of the Working Groups of the EDISANTÉ Association. First, his mission was to define message models with two parts :

- The envelope of the message, including a header, the characteristics of the transmitter, of the receiver, and of the patient concerned
- The contents of the message, including medical data which could be exchanged between different middleware.

This second part was halted by the « Réseau Santé Social », public network for all the healthcare professionals, who want to have a structured content for his « medical message format »
The prupose of EDISANTÉ is essentially to promote the use of EDI in health care. In a second time, this association decide to include work about envelope in a larger domain concerning all exchanges in medical domains.
so the GT 11 centred his action on content.

1. Framework

The starting point of the work has been an existing model —"MEDDOS"— developed by a software vendor to make his proprietary internal messages EDI-compatible.

It has been thought more efficient to start with existing material, and adapt them in order to have them:

- in the one hand compatible with EHRcom (ENV 13606),
- in the other hand accepted by the industrial parties.

Currently, Version 0.7 is completed. It is acknowledged that this version still have parts missing: for example, relationships between data items are not implemented yet.

2. What it is not about

- A patient or a healthcare professional identifier model, this issue being specifically addressed by another French organisation.
- A medical folder: it is only a message model in which it is possible to insert a medical record.
- A multiple patient message: even if it remains possible to further concatenate messages concerning several patients, for example in the view of epidemiological research.
- While this message model is fully compatible with EHRcom, it is not entirely an EHRcom message.
- It is a one way message. There is no processing of the data UID in the original system: if ever the information is transferred back within another message, it is then impossible to identify its previous origin.

3. What it is about

- A message model to transfer medical information between two health record systems.
- The health record system should be able to write, transfer and read the message. If it cannot read it, the message content should still remain readable using a standard browser.
- Health care data are collected over the course of a contact, during which it was first written in the original health record system.
- Optionally, it is possible to make use of an Original Component Complex, in order to signal the grouping of data written during the same contact that have identical semantics: for example all the clinical signs should be grouped into an OCC "clinical exam".
- Optionally, it is possible to make use of a Selected Component Complex, in order to signal the grouping of data not written during the same contact, while they have identical semantics: for example all the drugs prescribed should be grouped into a SCC "usual treatment".

4. Message architecture

```
Patient1

      Contact1
            composition1
                  item11
                        attributes
                  /item11
                  item21
                        attributes
                  /item21
                  item31
                        attributes
                  /item31
            /composition1
            composition2
                  item12
                        attribute
                  /item12
                  item22
                        attribute
                  /item22
                  item32
                        attribute
                  /item32
            /composition2
      /contact1

      Sélection 1
            Item 11
            Item 22
      / Sélection1

      Sélection 2
            Item 12
            Item 32
      /sélection 2

/patient1
```

5. Message elements

5.1 Patient

"Patient" corresponds here to "PatientMatching" in EHRcom

signid	CDATA	#REQUIRED
patid	CDATA	#REQUIRED
nom	CDATA	#REQUIRED
nom_usage	CDATA	#IMPLIED
prenom	CDATA	#IMPLIED
sexe	CDATA	#IMPLIED
datena	CDATA	#IMPLIED
datemo	CDATA	#IMPLIED

signid: identification of site, or of sending organisation
patid: identification of patient at site
nom: name at birth
nom_usage: usual name (for instance, married name)
sexe: 0 for a male, 1 for a female, and 2 if unknown
datena: date of birth, format: AAAAMMJJHHmm
datemo: date of death, format: AAAAMMJJHHmm

5.2 Contact

Each interaction between a Health Care Professional and the health record of the Subject of Care is made explicit by a segment "contact", followed by another segment identifying that Health Care Professional.

message_local_id	ID	#IMPLIED
timestamp	CDATA	#IMPLIED
type	CDATA	#REQUIRED
location	CDATA	#REQUIRED

timestamp: date and time, format: AAAAMMJJHHmmSS
type: type of contact
location: location of Health Care Professional at time of contact (see tables in annex 1 hereafter)

5.3 Health Care Professional

nom	CDATA	#REQUIRED
prénom	CDATA	# IMPLIED
spécialité	CDATA	#IMPLIED
adeli	CDATA	#REQUIRED

nom: name
prénom: first name
spécialité: medical speciality according to mentions on Health Professional Card (CPS), if Health Care Professional has one (see table in annex 1 hereafter)
adeli: professional ID number, if Health Care Professional has one

5.4 Item

LOCAL_MESSAGE_ID		
SEMANTIC_CLASS		
LABEL		
COMMENT	Free-text	
DATE PROCEDURE BEGAN OR WAS COMMENCED ON		
DATE PROCEDURE ENDED OR COMPLETED ON		
VALUE_TYPE		
VALUE		
TABLE_TYPE		
TABLE_CODE		
Unit		
SUBJECT OF INFORMATION	DS00	Patient
LIFE CYCLE	DY00	Concluded
NEGATION WARNING	DN00	Affirmative
CERTAINTY WARNING	DC00	Certain
RELIABILITY OF ANNOTATION	DE01	Validated by the Record Component author
KNOWING MODE	DK01	Observation or action by author
SYSTEM	DB15	Genital
FOCUS	DF15	Cancer screening

	Semantic Class
CO	DOCUMENT and MAIL
SY	SYMPTOM and SIGN
PA	Diseases or syndrome
AC	Act and procedure
ME	drug
XR	Measure and results examen
XBD	Examen asking
AM	Allergy
RI	Risk and exposure to risk
ET	Patient's condition
NCA	Not elsewhere classified *("non classé ailleurs")*

6. Original Component Complexes and Selected Component Complexes

Even though these two elements remain optional, it should be useful to find a consensus about how to name them.

Examples of OCCs are:
- "clinical examination"
- "prescription of medicinal products"
- "lab-test"

Examples of SCCs are:
- "usual treatment"
- "patient's statement"
- "planned preventive procedure"

7. Next steps

Next steps of this project will consist in:
- listing proposed thesaurus depending different data types
- testing exchanges between several middleware

- presenting a finalised work to AFNOR, in order to have it adopted as a French *de jure* standard
- including links between dates

8. Examples of items

8.1 The patient has received an intradermoreaction.

SUBJECT OF INFORMATION	DS00	Patient
LIFE CYCLE	DY00	Concluded
NEGATION WARNING	DN00	Affirmative
CERTAINTY WARNING	DC00	Certain
RELIABILITY OF ANNOTATION	DE01	Validated by the Record Component author
KNOWING MODE	DK01	Observation or action by author
SYSTEM	DB02	Blood, blood forming organs, lymphatics, spleen
FOCUS	DF09	- - observation of property by investigation
LABEL	IDR1	Intradermoreaction 10 UI
COMMENT	Free-text	
DATE PROCEDURE BEGAN OR WAS COMMENCED ON	19991010	Date of injection
DATE PROCEDURE ENDED OR COMPLETED ON		
VALUE_TYPE		
TABLE_TYPE	CISP2	
TABLE_CODE	A 70	Tuberculosis
SEMANTIC_CLASS	AC	Act or procedure
VALUE		Not applicable

8.2 A parent of the patient presented a cancer of colon.

SUBJECT OF INFORMATION	DS01	patient's parent	
LIFE CYCLE	DY00	Concluded	
NEGATION WARNING	DN00	Affirmative	The elementary entry being annotated does not contain negative expressions (Whenever negative, excludes the risk)
CERTAINTY WARNING	DC00	Certain	
RELIABILITY OF ANNOTATION	DE01	Validated by the Record Component author	
KNOWING MODE	DK04	Reported by patient	
SYSTEM	DB03	Digestive	
FOCUS	DF02	patho-physiological condition or state	actual or potential state, including disease, symptom, function (including pregnancy)
LABEL	Past familial history of cancer of colon		
COMMENT	Free-text		
DATE PROCEDURE BEGAN OR WAS COMMENCED ON			
DATE PROCEDURE ENDED OR COMPLETED ON		Not applicable	
VALUE_TYPE		Not applicable	
TABLE_TYPE	ICD-10	ICD-10	
TABLE_CODE	C18.9	Malignant neoplasm of colon, unspecified	
SEMANTIC_CLASS	PA	Condition	
VALUE		Not applicable	

8.3 Patient immunised against tetanus (first injection) on 13/10/2000

SUBJECT OF INFORMATION	DS00	Patient
LIFE CYCLE	DY00	Concluded
NEGATION WARNING	DN00	Affirmative
CERTAINTY WARNING	DC00	Certain
RELIABILITY OF ANNOTATION	DE01	Validated by the Record Component author
KNOWING MODE	DK01	Observation or action by author
SYSTEM	DB02	Blood, blood forming organs, lymphatics, spleen
FOCUS	DF16	- - - - immunisation activity
LABEL	VAT	Tetanus vaccine
COMMENT	Free-text	
DATE PROCEDURE BEGAN OR WAS COMMENCED ON	20001013	Date Injection
DATE PROCEDURE ENDED OR COMPLETED ON		Not applicable
VALUE_TYPE	1	Rank of injection
TABLE_TYPE	ICD-10	
TABLE_CODE	Z23.5	Need for immunisation against tetanus alone
SEMANTIC_CLASS	AC	Immunisation act
VALUE		Not applicable

8.4 The patient asserts that he had not received his second booster injection of tetanus vaccine

SUBJECT OF INFORMATION	DS00	Patient
LIFE CYCLE	DY00	Concluded
NEGATION WARNING	DN00	Affirmative
CERTAINTY WARNING	DC00	Certain
RELIABILITY OF ANNOTATION	DE01	Validated by the Record Component author
KNOWING MODE	DK04	Reported by patient
SYSTEM	DB02	Blood, blood forming organs, lymphatics, spleen
FOCUS	DF16	- - - - immunisation activity
LABEL	VAT	Ttetanus vaccine
COMMENT	Free-text	
DATE PROCEDURE BEGAN OR WAS COMMENCED ON	20001013	Date of injection
DATE PROCEDURE ENDED OR COMPLETED ON		Not applicable
VALUE_TYPE	1	Rank of injection
TABLE_TYPE	ICD-10	
TABLE_CODE	Z23.5	Need for immunisation against tetanus alone
SEMANTIC_CLASS	AC	Immunisation act
VALUE		Not applicable

Annex 1: Tables

Contact

UID	Type of communication
A1	Communication in the presence of patient
A2	Communication out of the physical presence of patient, though synchronous
A3	Communication out of the physical presence of patient, though asynchronous
A4	No communication with patient

UID	Location of encounter
00	Not specified
01	Residence of patient
02	School
03	Location of occupation
04	Prison
05	Transportation mean
06	Open air location
29	Other non medical location
41	Ward
42	Bedroom
43	Bed
44	Ambulance carrier
61	Hospital
62	Outpatient clinic
63	Emergency department
64	Diagnostic<department
65	Clinical laboratory
66	Day care department
67	Nursing / convalescent home
68	Medical surgery
69	Rehabilitation centre
70	Location of holiday
99	Other health care organisation

UID	Type of contact
A1-68	Consultation (at the health care professional's practice location)
A1-01	Home visit (at the patient's residence)
A1-29	Other location, in the presence of patient
A2-29	Non physical contact with patient
A3-68	Message transfer
A4-68	Health record management

Annex 2 : Administrative content

What follows is a proposal based on "NEF" *de facto* standard, which is totally compliant with the data mandated for the use of SESAM VITALE cards.

Section INSURED

IPA	Permanent identification of insured
SS	National registration number
CLE	Key of National registration number
REGIME	Code régime
CAISSE	Code caisse
CENTRE	Code centre
NOM	Name of insured
PRENOM	First name of insured
DATE	Date of birth of insured

Sub-section ADDRESS

N_RUE	No and name of street
CODEPOSTAL	Postal Code
VILLE	City
Pays	Country

Section BENEFICIARY

IPP	Permanent ID of beneficiary (IPP)
IPA	Permanent ID of insured (IPA)
DATE	Date of birth
RANG	Rank of birth
QUALITE	Relationship with insured
CODE	Code profession beneficiary
PROFESSION	Profession of beneficiary (free-text)
ENTETE	Title of beneficiary

Sub-section ADDRESS

N_RUE	No and name of street
CODEPOSTAL	Postal Code
VILLE	City
Pays	Country

Sub-section Exemption from co-payment ("exonération du ticket modérateur")

Type EXO	Type of Exemption from co-payment
DATEDEBUT	Starting date
DATEFIN	End date
ALD	Long lasting condition (diagnostic of condition)

Closing Remarks to the EuroRec '01 Working Conference on the Electronic Health Record

Aix-en-Provence, November 2001

Niels Rossing, Chief Informatics Officer,
Copenhagen Hospital Corporation, Denmark
e-mail: nr@hsd.hosp.dk

As a European, one takes great pride in having followed the development in IT for Health and the work around EHCR since the mid 80'ies up till now. From the days when no more than a handful of visionary individuals caught the receptive minds of another handful of people within the European Commission to and together they made the sound foundation for IT in Health Care. They were so successful that they made an R&TD program because they convinced Member States that this was already a rich field for development and would become a demand driven necessity at some point in time. Exactly when nobody knew in those days. Congratulations to those few far-sighted persons. And congratulations to us jumped the band-wagon. Over the last couple of days we have witnessed a full-fledged realisation of visions and dreams turned realities to the benefit of European citizens. Certainly things are not perfect and they never will be.

Purposes were all clear from the very start:

- Bridge the gap between what is medically possible and what is affordable to society, in other words contribute to efficiency and productivity.
- Increase efficacy by access to evidence based medicine and documentation of quality.
- Improve service to citizens by continuity of care and de-institutionalise care by breaking down boundaries between sectors i.e. right information in the hands of the right persons at the right moment.
- Empower the professionals by access to appropriate information, decision support, collaborative work, and work flow charts.
- Create a market for health IT in Europe.

The means were clear:

- Create a community or communities of developers, users and industry that act according to the needs of care providers.
- Use bleeding edge technologies as they develop.
- Standardise, go for open standards, later in the course of events: Go for open source.
- Make Member States think globally and act locally.
- Identify and break barriers: cultural and professional resistance, linguistic differences and balance out the legal and ethical issues.

The political issues were subtle but real and fortunately gradually changed over time:

- There was an element of "Beat the Americans and the Japanese" later on to the benefit of us all: "If you cannot beat them, join them".
- Early on the mutual benefit of collaborating with non-EU Europe became clear as did collaboration with the rest of the World, as for example Canada, Australia, Latin America and Africa.

Many work programs and projects, concerted actions, clustering activities have been over the years, many names of EU offices, much red tape and much overhead for projects working in R&TD. I dare not bet what has been the stronger among driving forces:

- Enthusiastic contacts and bright ideas fostered by EU and sponsored researchers.
- Technology coming to us inevitably.
- The demand of the people.
- Centres of excellence and collaborating groups established.

The Electronic Record was always the focal point whatever the program because it is the ultimate apotheosis of all efforts and it absorbs all other developmental aspects.

In its lifetime in our minds as a vision or an ever-moving elusive reality it highlighted all the words we learned to love:

- Modelling
- Modularity
- Scalability
- Compliance
- Collaborative work
- Safety and confidentiality
- Business process engineering, etc. etc.

Challenges of implementation

Now fate caught up on us and all developmental work in programs and elsewhere has materialised in products.

Now, something like the EHCR is there we realise that

- We must before we start the system organise our minds and redefine our rational mode of work so that
- We can define and organise our requirements

Implementation in

- a mission critical environment operating around the clock 365 days a year
- with thousands of users who do not want to be left alone on
- isolated information islands but who
- need messages from systems in other places that are different
- with thousands of users at 2.00 a.m. with little training

are real challenges that take leadership, commitment and very clear minds.

It is 20 % technology and 80% organisational and educational processes.

EuroRec and the Conference

I sincerely wish to congratulate EuroRec for having fulfilled so many of the objectives, contributed to the realisation of the EHCR via the PRORECs. Above all this activity like some others - let me mention EHTEL – unite European vendors, developers and users. Only where communities of this kind exist do all benefit maximally. I am fully aware, though, that to vendors health care IT was not a gold mine and they are the heroes.

At this very conference the key issues have been addressed in a totally appropriate and inspiring manner. We can all go back not only with memories of a charming place, meetings with great people but also with specific information ready to use on the topics of the workshops.

Finally I wish to congratulate the European Commission for supporting this kind of activity. It testifies to its understanding of appropriate encouragement. It may also encourage the commission that sometimes, European taxpayers do get their money's worth and now the EU Commission may be the beacon for yet another decade of visionary people with dreams that may come out as well as that of the 80's.

Outcome of EuroRec '01, lessons drawn and Farewell!

Dr. François MENNERAT, MD PhD
Chairman of ProRec-France
mailto:presidence@prorec-france.org

Time has now come to summarise the numerous impressions gathered here and there over the past two days.

Over these two busy days, we have addressed the most important aspects of Electronic Health Records.

Cultural, ethical, economic, political, and technical issues have been successively studied.

A lot of significant, though sometimes generic, statements have been made. Insofar, however, few definitive conclusion have been reached. Let us bet that numerous ideas and proposals will still be actively exchanged during yet many years: there is much left to be said for the next EuroRec conferences!

Several statements, and emerging matters will be used as concluding remarks. Some lead to broad guidelines and several pieces of advice that should form the background for the future work.

1. In spite of their strong interdependence, it is not an easy task to reconcile users and providers

ProRec aims at bringing together users and providers of EHRs, and help them share their respective concerns. This conference has been a significant occasion to display a wide variety of opinions about the ways to follow to reach the ultimate goal of a widespread use of top quality EHRs. But this goal does not always prove a quiet promenade.

On the one hand, when users become interested in using all the potentialities of computers and telecommunication, they dream of infringing the limits of some proprietary solutions proposed by their providers.

On the other hand, the providers rightly contend that as long as the market has not grown up and developed more than today, they have very few degrees of freedom. They obviously keep suspicious of any initiatives —public or private— that are not driven by the sincere concern of a fair reward of their efforts to offer practical solutions that actually work. They often disregard specifications which they have not authored, and which they suspect at first of being too theoretical and unrealistic.

Meanwhile, many potential users adopt a passive spectator attitude, and remain perplex. They think it clever to content themselves in watching this inequitable struggle, and eventually cheer the winners. Inevitably this wait-and-see policy will have to come to an end.

2. Both the users' needs and the technical environment appear yet unstable

We have been willing to make it explicit here that the issues, and hence the solutions, are not technical only. Yet technology has proved, and still does, that it often brings the missing bits that prevented the development of satisfying solutions to take place.

However, the environment is ever changing. Previously identified problems evolve on their own, but the accelerating evolution of the solutions proposed also help to better identify and understand new issues unknown so far. And at the same time, the community of users keeps continuously learning on its own activity, and this pushes further and further the fulfilment of ever changing and increasing needs.

This being said, the greatest attention should always be paid to the uttermost importance of 1) the User, 2) the User, and 3) the User. The main implication of this is: do NOT attempt to computerise medicine, but instead strive to "medicalise" computers.

3. De facto, or de jure standards?

Many do not consider this statement to justify any longing suspicion over the willingness to facilitate the organisation of a more consistent context, by the development of several limited *de jure* standards. These actors have some good reasons to fear that no comprehensively satisfying solutions can be awaited from the market, given its current state. Standardisation should not be presented as some kind of the intrusion of undue and unfair planned economy in the forgotten paradise of free enterprise. But indeed it should rely of the skill of the industrial developers, not only on the valuable knowledge of researchers.

Against this background, designers and developers of EHR systems are advised to start with simple functions based upon users' requirements and priorities, but to keep the logical model in mind right from the beginning so that later progress can be made using the same basic infrastructure.

The right standards should be used, but standards should be instated with moderation, in order to avoid unnecessary rigidity, and do not sterilise innovation.

4. The revision of the European EHR pre-standard

EuroRec '01 has been the occasion to launch the revision of this pre-standard into a full reasonably stable standard. Under the aegis of CEN / TC251, a group has been convened in the hospital of Aix-en-Provence on Sunday, and the first basis for the revision has been laid. The next step is a Task Force that will be established in the coming months.

The principal matters that have emerged over this working conference are:

4.1 The European concept of Electronic Health Record

There is a much more obvious respect for the European concept of EHR, a deliberately created entity with its own characteristics and rules.

CEN / ENV 13606 ("EHRcom") is a unique European pre-standard for EHR communication. It is the most advanced work world-wide with regard to this concern, and so far the only standard, even if experimental yet.

4.2 *Health Level 7*

The European standardisation work and HL7 are not in competition. Though not addressing the same situation or entity as the EHR, HL7 has certainly an important part to play, among other initiatives. HL7 has generated some useful ideas that the European standardisation work can use for advantage. The Memorandum of Understanding between CEN / TC251 and the HL7 organisation already acknowledges this.

4.3 *The next phase of the CEN work should now follow a "dual model" approach: Reference Model, and Archetypes*

Recent insights into the 2-model views of the EHR have gained rapid acceptance here, and this will seriously influence the next phase of the CEN work.

1. A <u>Reference Model</u> can be agreed upon by pursuing convergence between the various approaches.
   However, and even if it appears somehow contradictory, this should be achieved without departing significantly from the existing specifications embedded in the pre-standard, in order to build upon the experience of the implementers of the pre-standard.
2. <u>Archetypes</u>, for which a generic model needs to be confirmed, related to the Reference Model. The future standard might offer (informative) default instances of some archetypes for commonly occurring clinical objects that might need to appear in EHRs, and also provide for the safe exchange of such data.

4.4 *Drawing the attention of the industry*

A simplification of the Reference Model, coupled with the introduction of the Archetype mechanism will make it <u>more</u> possible for implementers to be interested in EHRs standards.

4.5 *Dissemination of CEN standards*

Future CEN standards must undoubtedly be released in documentary forms that permit easy understanding of their purpose and content.

4.6 *Collect implementation experience*

Several instances of the implementation of EHRcom, at least in part, actually exist in several places throughout Europe. Some of these have been the subject of presentations, and demonstrations, at this conference.

Implementation experience must guide and inform the next stages of standardisation.

It is expected that all interested parties, in particular developers and implementers who have worked on the pre-standard, bring their experience, for the sake of all other solutions providers, and of health care professionals, patients, and citizens.

The ProRec network should actively pursue finding out about all such implementations, and a regular liaison should be established in order to inform CEN.

EFMI could also play a role here, as well as other organisations.

4.7 The Open source movement should not be neglected

Open source concepts are rapidly gaining acceptance. Software, specifications, requirements, implementation guidance are all included.

There are exciting opportunities for ProRec to be involved in promoting and progressing the EU Chapter of *Open*EHR. Ass announced hereafter, this has an immediate implication.

5. The EuroRec Institute

During the EuroRec '01 Working Conference, the WIDENET consortium has found the opportunity to hold two meetings.

Among others, two major decisions result from their works, that are worth an official announcement.

1. The EuroRec Institute (alias the European Institute for Health Records) is founded by the existing ProRec Centres.

2. Mandate is given to the EuroRec Institute to start talks immediately to take the role of the European Chapter of the *Open*EHR Foundation.

Have a nice and safe trip back!

EuroRec 2002,
the 5th European Working Conference on Electronic Health Records,
will take place in Berlin,
in December 2002.

Author Index

Cocina mejor día a día

Arroces y pasta

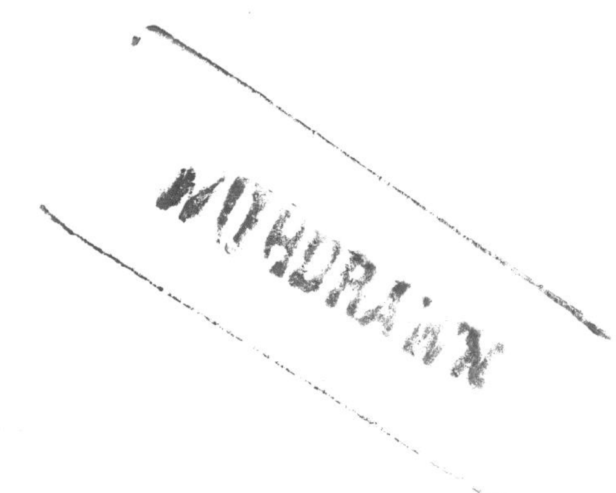

Cocina mejor día a día
Arroces y pasta

Diagonal 189, 08018 Barcelona
www.rbalibros.com / rba-libros@rba.es

Producción editorial: Bonalletra Alcompas, S.L.
Diseño y maquetación: Júlia Font i Cèl·lula
para Bonalletra Alcompas, S.L.
Fotografías: Becky Lawton (Imagen central
de la portada y todas las recetas);
Dreamstime (ingredientes y accesorios).
Textos y recetas: Iker Erauzkin
Ilustraciones: Mercè Iglesias

Ref.: RPRA023
ISBN: 978-84-929-8157-1
Depósito legal: B-13281-2011
Impreso por T.G.Soler

Cocina mejor día a día

Arroces y pasta

Las mejores recetas para triunfar en cualquier ocasión

RBA

Sumario

Atrévete a ir más allá

Desde tiempos remotos la pasta y el arroz han sido dos bases de cocina versátiles, que admiten múltiples acompañantes y que casan con prácticamente todos los ingredientes que les queramos añadir. No hay nada mejor que un puñado de pasta o de arroz para acabar con todos los restos huérfanos de una nevera. En salteado, como salsa o con cocciones de sofrito, admiten todos los acompañamientos. A la vez, pueden ser perfectos anfitriones de platos sofisticados, recetas originales y de sabor sorprendente. Como los grandes, se adaptan a lo que les queramos exigir.

Este recetario de cocina no es un manual al uso. Cada apartado se desarrolla en tres niveles, que van de lo sencillo a lo sofisticado. En el nivel 1 encontrarás recetas básicas y clásicas; son el punto de partida para formar una base culinaria. El segundo escalón exige un poco más de cuidado en la elaboración y la selección de ingredientes. Aquí aprenderás combinaciones ocurrentes y alguna presentación original. Entonces ya estarás preparado para llegar al nivel 3, el de los cocineros con solera, con imaginación y que cuidan el producto y el detalle. Las recetas no son más complicadas en este nivel, pero quizá sí más laboriosas y con unos resultados más espectaculares.

En definitiva, este es un libro apto para todos los cocineros. El novel aprenderá, de forma progresiva, que alcanzar la sofisticación no es tan complicado. El cocinero habitual podrá avanzar y descubrir nuevas ideas para preparar platos que tal vez ya domina, y el experto en cocina encontrará a lo largo de estas páginas sugerencias que quizá le resulten estimulantes o motivadoras.

Adelante pues, pasa la página y descubre cómo sacar el máximo partido a dos ingredientes que, por clásicos, a veces se quedan encallados en recetas aburridas o simples. ■

☛ Todas las recetas son para 4 personas.

P

asta

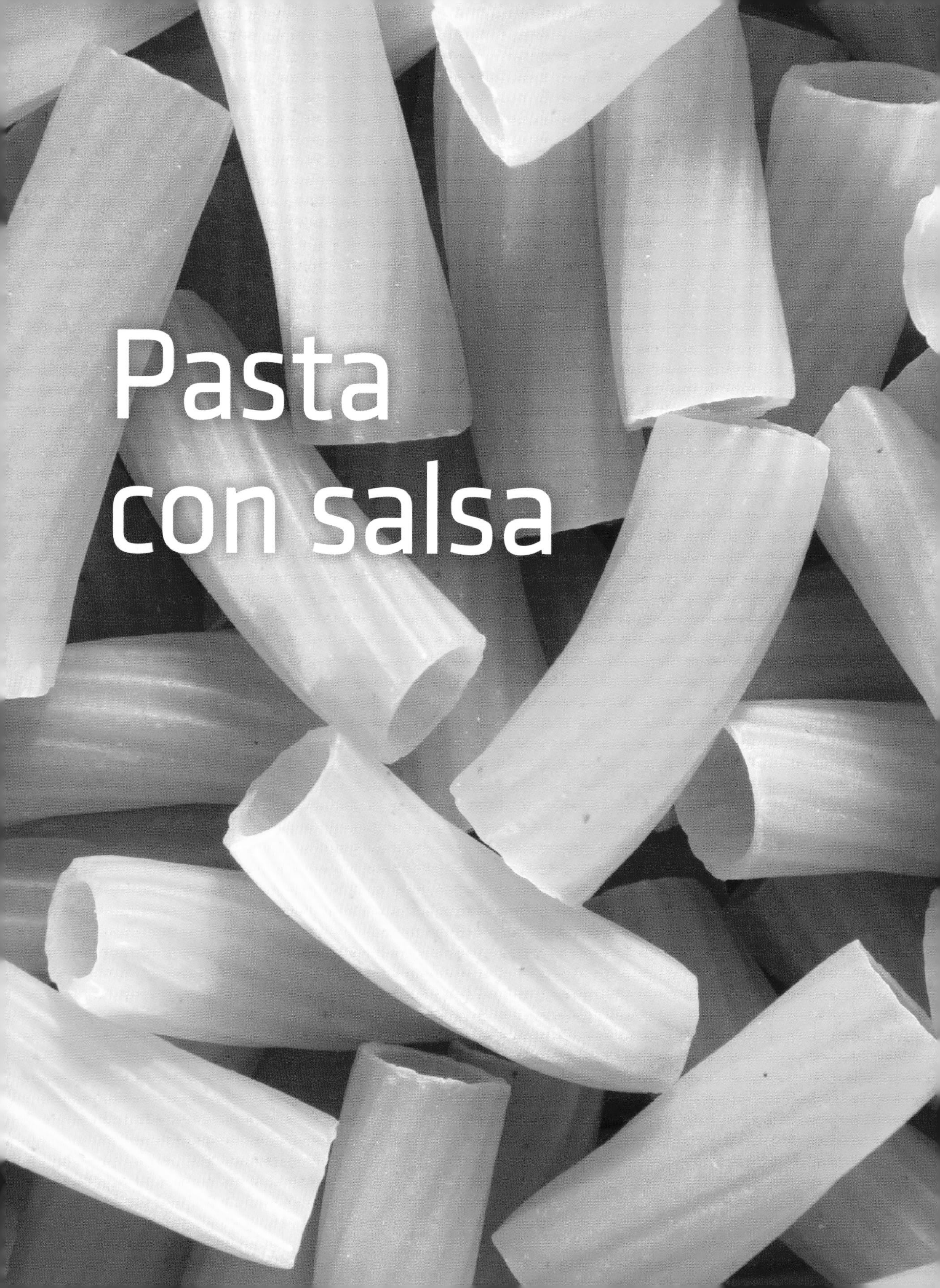

Pasta con salsa

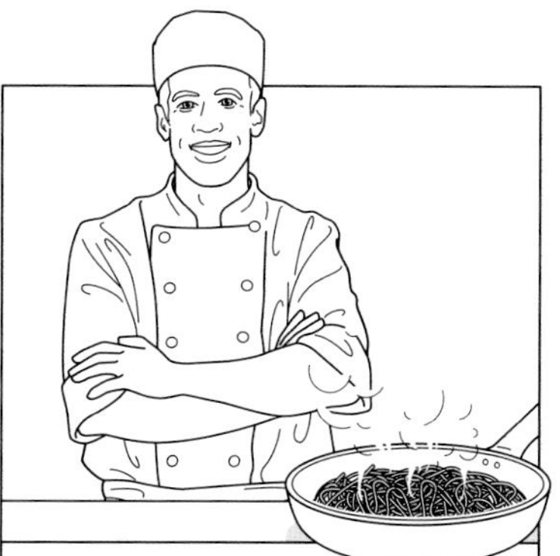
¡Hola! Os presentamos varias posibilidades para preparar deliciosos platos de pasta con salsa.

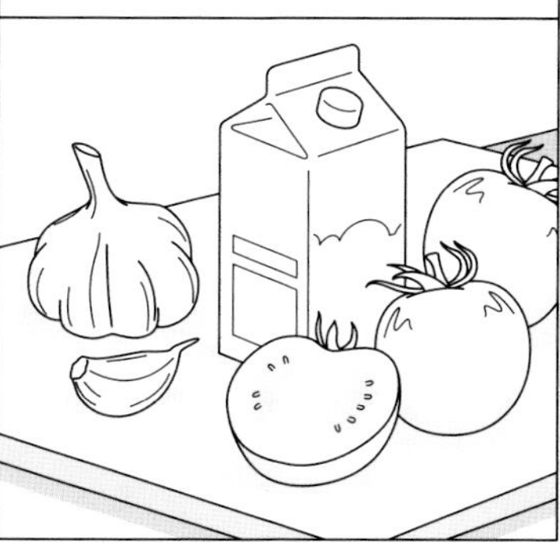
Primero, elaboraremos la pasta que elijamos a nuestro gusto.

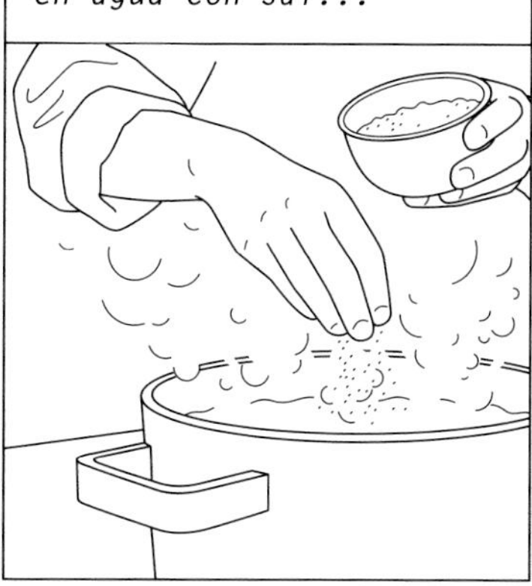
Podemos cocerla en agua con sal...

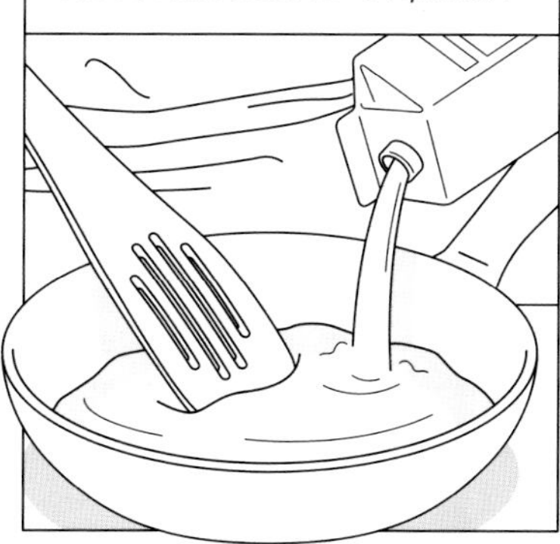
... o en la propia salsa; entonces esta deberá ser suficientemente líquida.

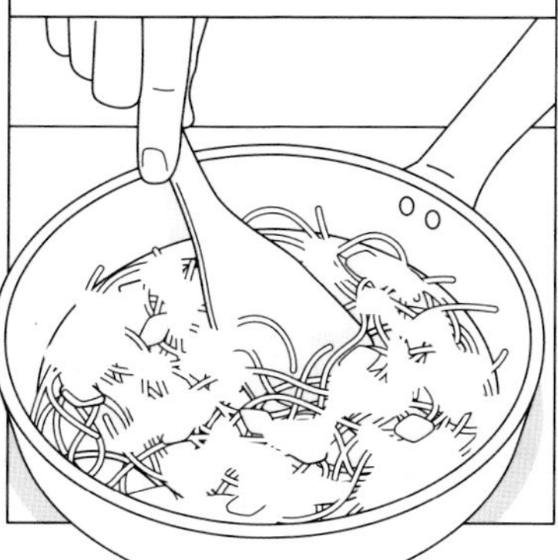
Verás cómo cocinar pasta larga con salsas de crema de leche...

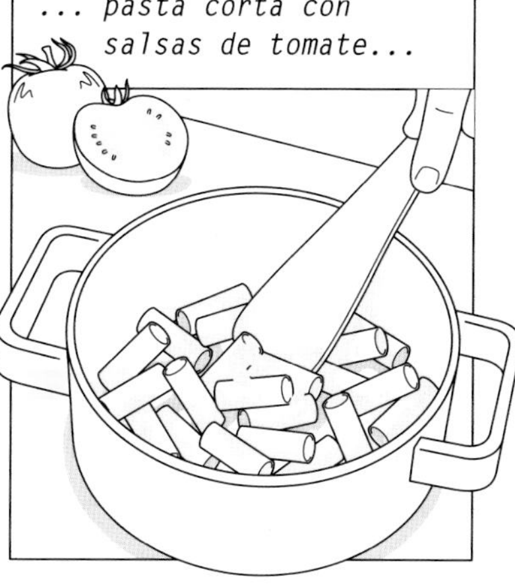
... pasta corta con salsas de tomate...

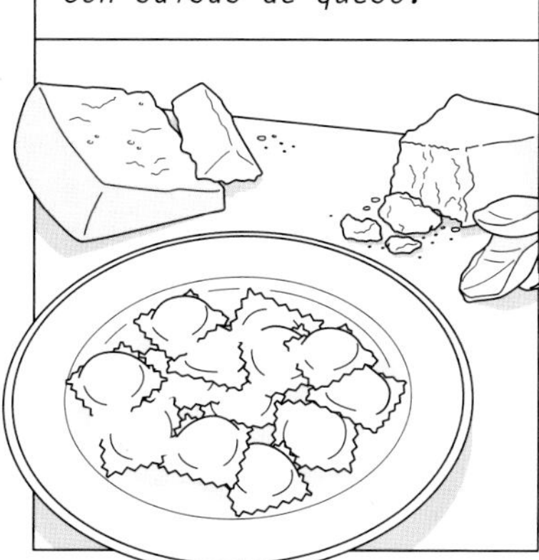
...y pasta rellena con salsas de queso.

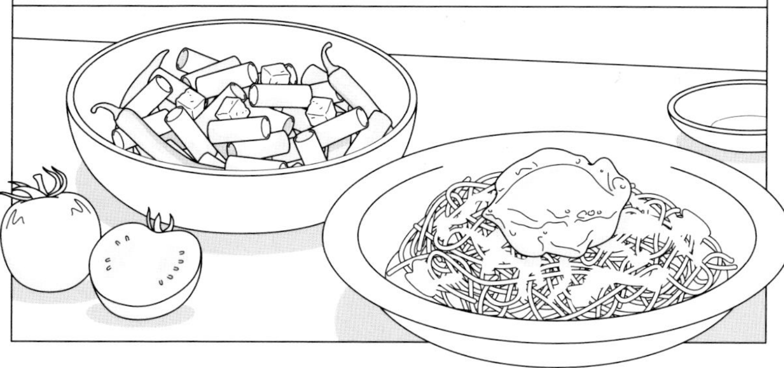
Las salsas pueden ser tan variadas como nos sugiera nuestra imaginación. Ligeras, cremosas, con carne, verduras... Una auténtica tentación.

Pasta con crema de leche

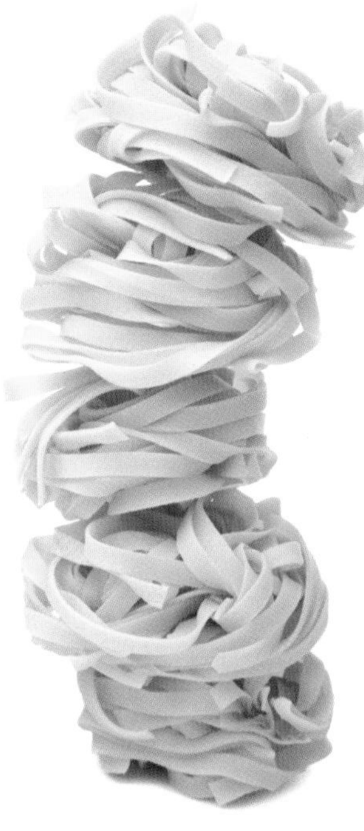

El ingrediente

La pasta, al menos en su origen, es la masa más sencilla que se puede preparar ya que solo consta de harina de trigo y agua. Se mezclan bien los ingredientes hasta formar una masa que pueda estirarse y cortarse, otorgándole la forma deseada. Al menos originalmente esa fue la fórmula de la pasta que, poco a poco, fue incorporando huevo, aceite de oliva, sal y otros ingredientes que aportan color y sabor a la masa. En este apartado se puede utilizar todo tipo de pasta larga: espaguetis, tallarines, *pappardelli, fettuccini, linguini*...

La técnica

Las salsas a base de crema de leche suelen ser muy sencillas de elaborar y por lo general no precisan de largos tiempos de cocción. No aptas para los alérgicos a la lactosa, la nata o la crema de leche son un buen medio para fundir otros sabores, como quesos, currys o especias de lo más variado.

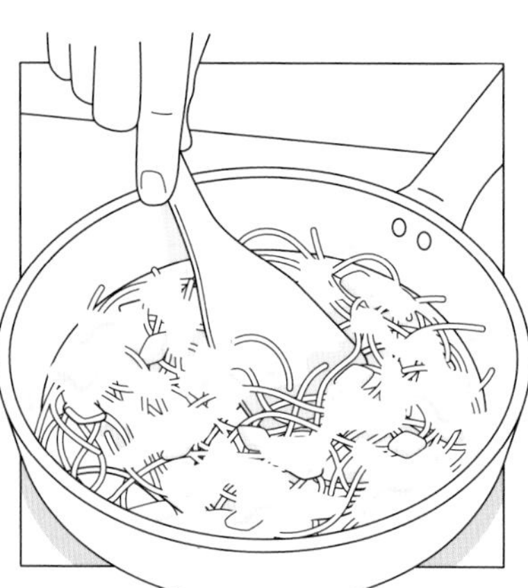

Plato a plato

Nivel **1** **Espaguetis a la carbonara.** Empieza con un clásico de la cocina italiana que se prepara rápidamente y sin demasiadas complicaciones.

Nivel **2** **Espaguetis con carbonara de trufa y huevo escalfado.** Añade un toque original a la carbonara de siempre con el inconfundible aroma de la trufa y un huevo al punto.

Nivel **3** **Cigalas en abrigo de pasta larga con carbonara de azafrán.** La pasta a la carbonara es el envoltorio de un exquisito fruto de mar con aroma de azafrán.

Nivel 1 Espaguetis a la carbonara

- **400 g de espaguetis secos**
- **200 g de jamón cocido o bacón**
- **400 ml de nata líquida**
- **2 dientes de ajo**
- **1 cebolleta tierna**
- **1 nuez de mantequilla**
- **Aceite de oliva**
- **Sal y pimienta**

10 min
20 min
1 €/persona
No prepares esta receta a personas con intolerancia a la lactosa.

- En una cazuela con abundante agua con sal y un chorrito de aceite de oliva, cuece los espaguetis durante el tiempo indicado por el fabricante hasta que queden *al dente*.
- Mientras se cuece la pasta, rehoga en una sartén con la mantequilla, la cebolleta y el ajo picados muy finos. Una vez la verdura se ablande, agrega el jamón cocido o el bacón cortado en pequeños tacos. Rehoga todo durante un par de minutos. Retira el exceso de grasa desprendido por el bacón y agrega la nata líquida, deja cocer 4-5 minutos a fuego lento y añade una pizca de sal y una de pimienta, blanca o negra, al gusto.
- Retira la pasta del agua, escúrrela y enfríala en agua con hielo o bajo el grifo. Cortarás de este modo su cocción. Agrega la pasta a la salsa y mezcla bien.
- Sirve la pasta acompañada de queso parmesano recién rallado.

Trucos

La receta tradicional prescinde de la nata líquida, que es sustituida por yema de huevo y mantequilla. Para los alérgicos a la lactosa, puedes elaborar esta receta con caldo de verduras o pollo.

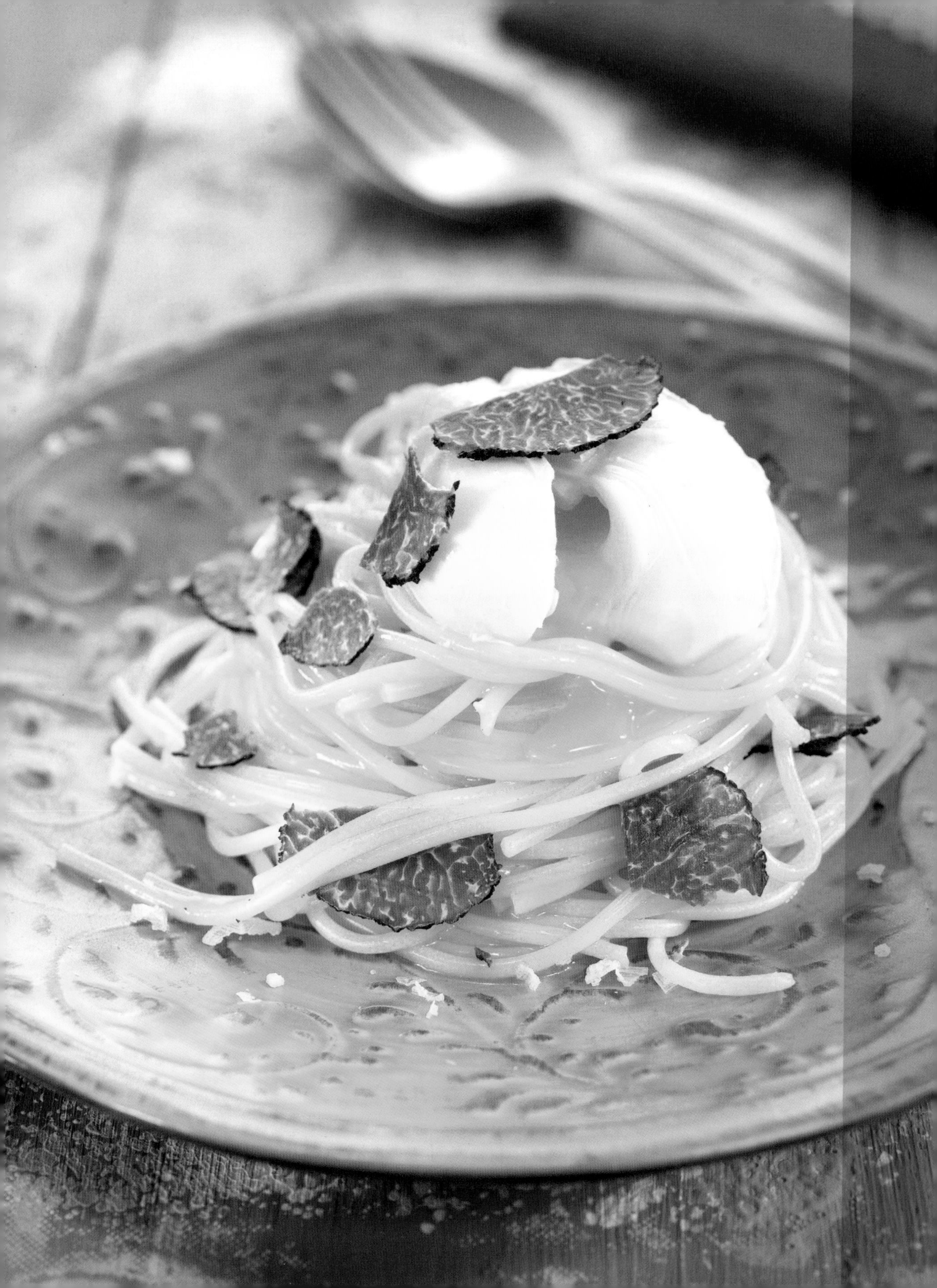

Nivel 2 Espaguetis con carbonara de trufa y huevo escalfado

- 400 g de espaguetis
- 100 g de mantequilla
- 4 huevos
- 1 trufa fresca de 10 g
- Sal
- Pimienta negra
- Aceite de oliva
- Vinagre

5 min
20 min
4 €/persona
Sin contraindicaciones, a no ser que alguno de tus invitados sea alérgico al huevo.

- En una cazuela con abundante agua con sal hirviendo y un chorrito de aceite de oliva, cuece los espaguetis durante el tiempo que indique el fabricante hasta que queden *al dente*.
- Mientras pon a hervir un cazo de agua con sal y un chorrito de vinagre. Rompe la cáscara de cada huevo, disponlos en un plato y después incorpóralos en el cazo. Cuece los huevos durante 3-4 minutos, escalfándolos. Después retíralos del agua y resérvalos.
- Retira la pasta del agua, escúrrela y enfríala en agua con hielo o bajo el grifo. Así cortarás su cocción. Resérvala.
- Ahora elabora la salsa. Derrite la mantequilla y una vez esta se ablande, ralla la mitad de la trufa sobre ella, agrega la pasta y mezcla bien. Salpimienta. Reparte la pasta entre los platos, coloca un huevo en cada uno. Ralla el resto de la trufa sobre los huevos.

Trucos

Remueve el agua cuando vayas a introducir los huevos para que la yema quede bien centrada.

Si no tienes trufa fresca puedes aromatizar la pasta con un chorrito de aceite de trufa.

Nivel **3** Cigalas en abrigo de pasta larga con carbonara de azafrán

- 100 g de espaguetis
- 30 g de queso parmesano
- 200 ml de nata líquida
- 8 cigalas grandes
- 1 pizca de azafrán
- Mantequilla
- Sal
- Pimienta
- Aceite de oliva

25 min
20 min
6 €/persona
Las personas con intolerancia a la lactosa deben evitar esta receta.

- En una cazuela con abundante agua con sal y un chorrito de aceite de oliva, cuece los espaguetis durante el tiempo indicado por el fabricante hasta que queden *al dente*.
- Mientras se cuece la pasta, pela las cigalas y conserva los cuerpos de las mismas. Una vez cocida, saca la pasta del agua y enrolla las cigalas con los espaguetis aún calientes. Reserva en una bandeja de horno durante 4-5 minutos.
- Después ralla el queso sobre la pasta y hornéala a 190 °C durante 4 minutos hasta que la cigala quede cocida. Retira la pasta del horno y reserva.
- Para elaborar la salsa, derrite una nuez de mantequilla a fuego lento en una sartén y sofríe el azafrán. Transcurridos unos segundos, sin que el azafrán se queme, agrega la nata líquida y deja cocer durante 6-8 minutos. Salpimienta.
- Distribuye la pasta en los platos, salsea y sirve de inmediato.

Trucos

Cuando prepares la salsa puedes agregar las cabezas de las cigalas a la sartén para aromatizarla aún más.

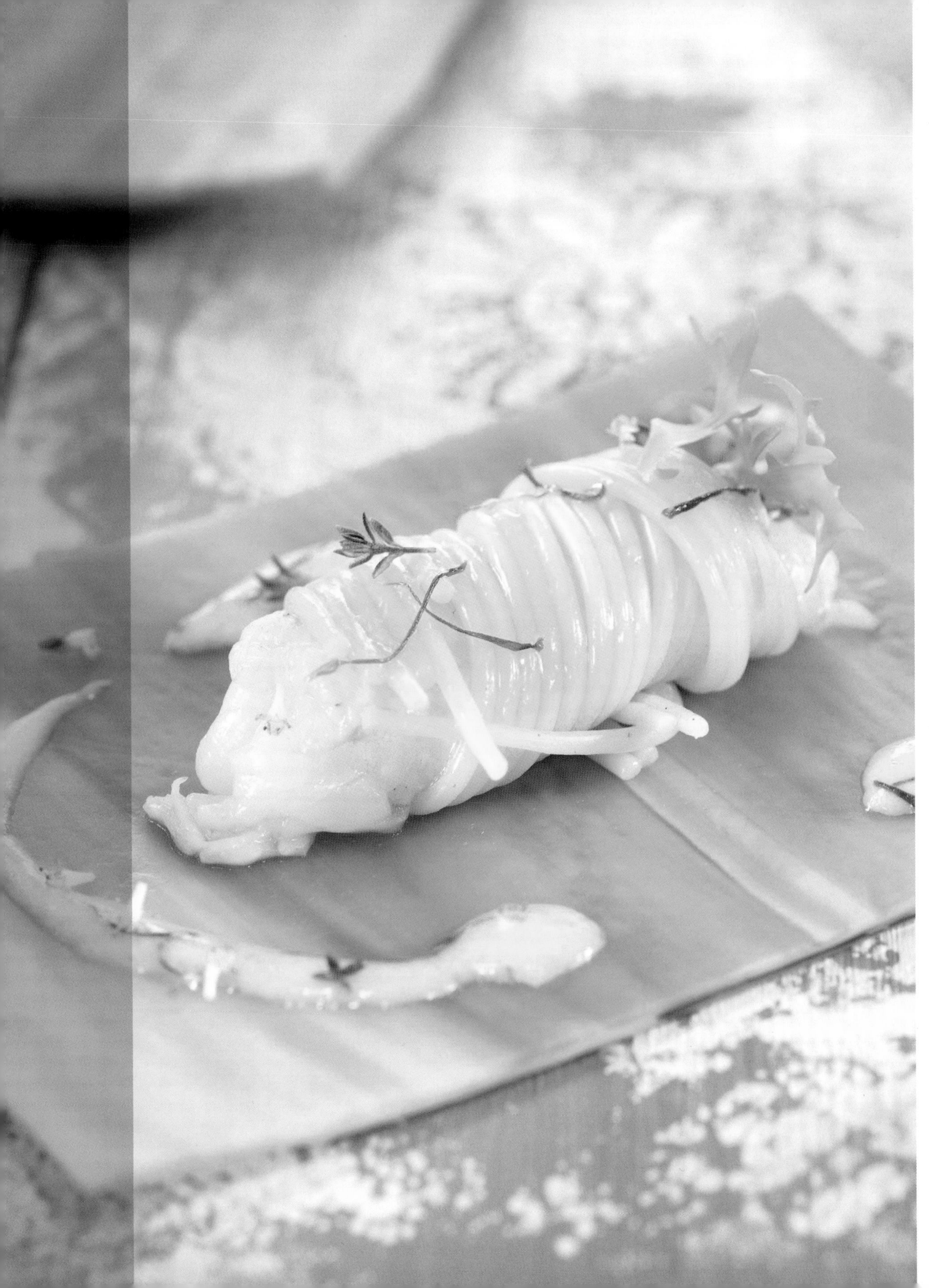

Pasta con tomate

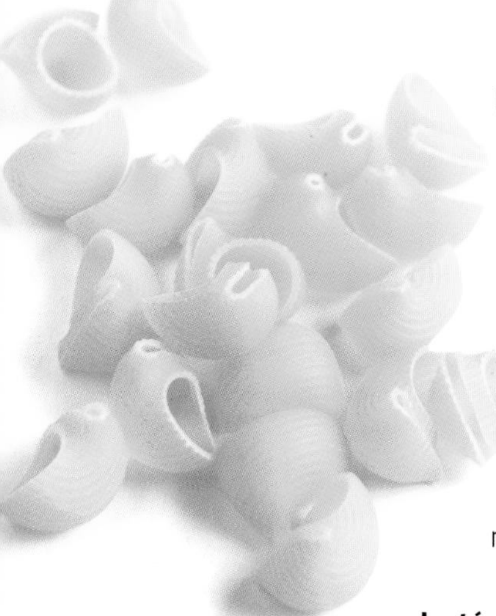

El ingrediente

La pasta aporta 340 kcal cada 100 g y es una de las principales fuentes de hidratos de carbono que existen. En el mercado se ofrece gran variedad de formas de pasta. En el caso de la corta, encontrarás desde los clásicos macarrones, las pajaritas, las plumas y los fideos, hasta otras ideales para sopas, como la maravilla, las letras o las estrellas.

La técnica

Necesitas tomates muy maduros, tipo pera o rama, carnosos y con abundante pulpa. Para preparar el sofrito, sofríe primero la cebolla, a fuego lento, hasta que esta caramelice. Luego incorpora el tomate, ya sea triturado o troceado. Compensa la acidez de ciertos tomates agregando una cucharadita de azúcar a la salsa.

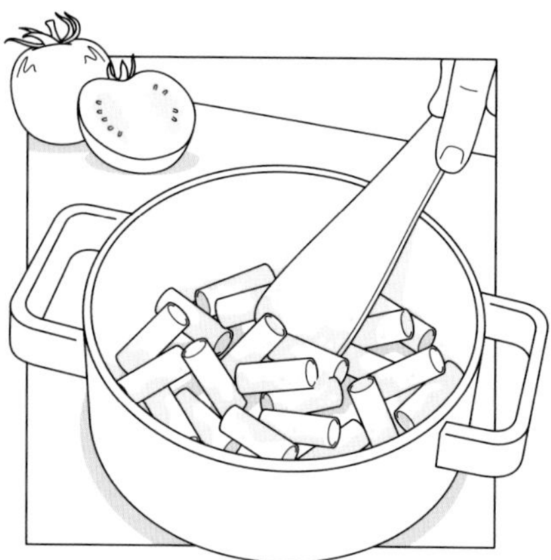

Plato a plato

Nivel **1** **Macarrones a la *puttanesca*.** El punto de partida son unos macarrones de sabor fuerte gracias a la presencia de las sardinas y las alcaparras.

Nivel **2** **Macarrones con tomate confitado, chiles, mozzarela y aceite de albahaca.** Sigue con una versión actualizada de la clásica *puttanesca*. El chile y la mozzarela ponen su toque único.

Nivel **3** **Macarrones rellenos de crema de olivas, miel, tomates en aceite y navaja al horno.** Acaba con la forma más sofisticada: unos macarrones rellenos acompañados de unas deliciosas navajas aromatizadas con miel.

Nivel **1** # Macarrones a la *puttanesca*

- 300 g de plumas
- 50 g de olivas de Kalamata
- 30 g de alcaparras
- 200 ml de salsa de tomate ya frita
- 12 sardinas en salazón
- 4 tomates secos
- 2 cebollas
- 1 pimiento verde
- 1 pimiento rojo
- 1 manojo de orégano
- Aceite de oliva
- Sal y pimienta

25 min
20 min
2 €/persona
Prescinde de las sardinas para adaptar esta receta a una dieta vegetariana.

■ En una cazuela o en una olla con abundante agua hirviendo con sal y un chorrito de aceite de oliva cuece la pasta durante el tiempo indicado por el fabricante. Transcurrido este tiempo escúrrela y enfríala en agua con hielo. Reserva. Mientras la pasta se cuece, desala las sardinas limpiando sus lomos bajo el grifo.
■ En una sartén sofríe la cebolla junto a los pimientos. Una vez la verdura se ablande, añade el tomate frito, deja cocer unos 5 minutos y agrega entonces las olivas, las alcaparras, las sardinas desaladas y troceadas, el orégano troceado, los tomates secos previamente hidratados y una pizca de sal y pimienta. Cuece durante 5 minutos, mezcla la salsa con la pasta y ya podrás servir el plato.

Trucos

Si preparas esta receta con pasta fresca, la puedes cocer en la misma salsa de tomate.

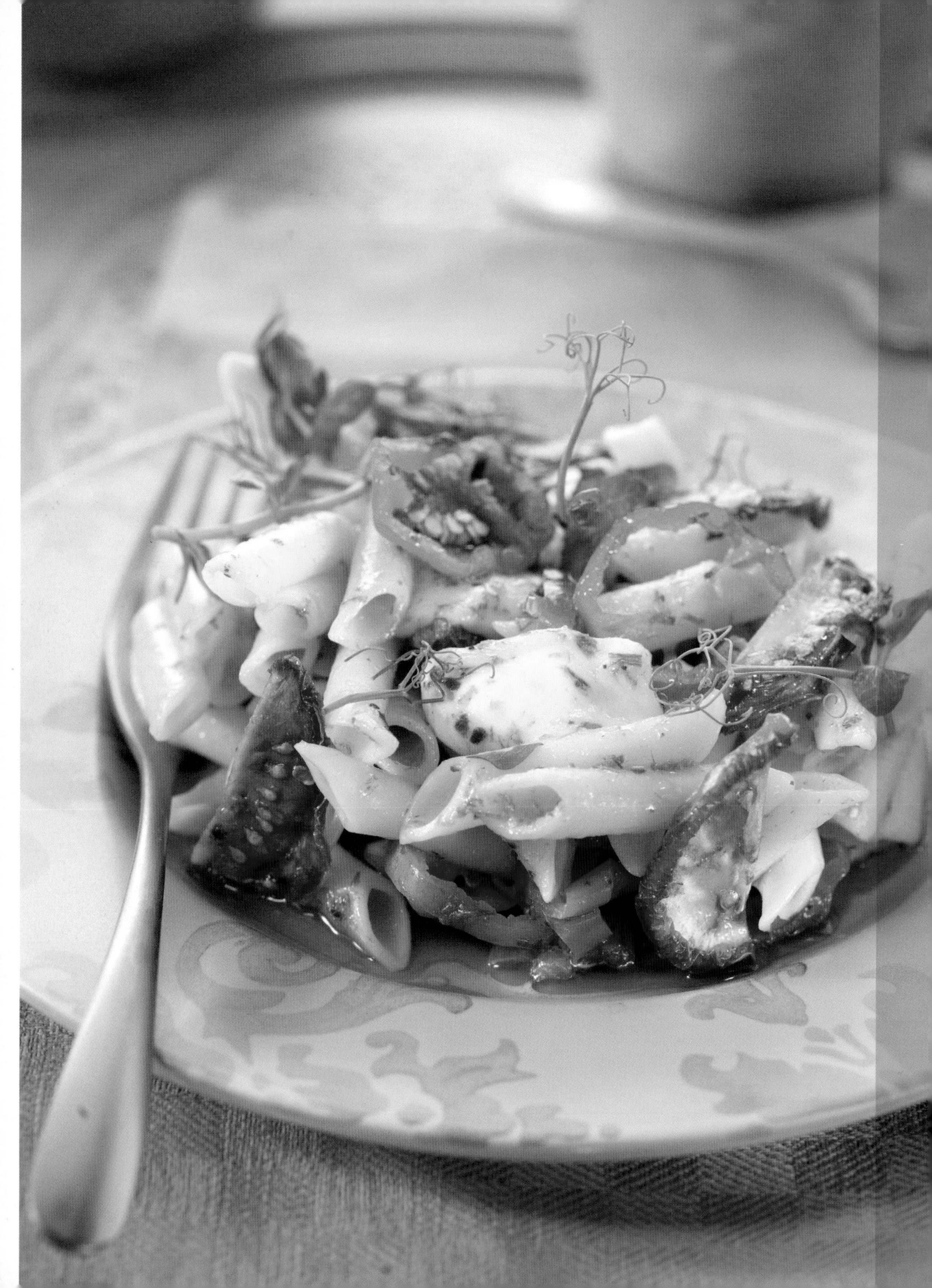

Nivel **2** Macarrones con tomate confitado, chiles, mozzarella y aceite de albahaca

- **400 g de macarrones**
- **200 ml de aceite de oliva**
- **4 tomates pera**
- **2 trozos de mozzarella de búfala**
- **2-4 chiles dulces**
- **1 cebolla tierna**
- **1 manojo de albahaca**
- **1/2 manojo de cebollino**
- **Sal y pimienta**

30 min
20 min
2 €/persona
Si alguien tiene intolerancia a la lactosa, no incluyas la mozzarella.

■ En una cazuela o en una olla con abundante agua hirviendo con sal y un chorrito de aceite de oliva cuece la pasta durante el tiempo indicado por el fabricante. Transcurrido este tiempo, escurre la pasta, enfríala en agua con hielo y resérvala.

■ Mientras se cuece la pasta, pela los tomates, elimina las semillas y resérvalos. Si tienes dificultades para pelar los tomates, puedes escaldarlos ligeramente en agua hirivendo durante 20 segundos. Luego deja que se enfríen y podrás retirar la piel con facilidad.

■ En una sartén con un chorrito de aceite de oliva caliente, saltea la cebolla cortada finamente, hasta que empiece a dorarse. Agrega entonces el tomate troceado a cuartos y los chiles cortados en rodajas. Saltéalo y agrega la pasta.

■ Tritura la albahaca con el aceite de oliva y el cebollino hasta obtener un aceite de color verde intenso, cuélalo y resérvalo.

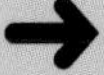

Nivel 2 Macarrones con tomate confitado, chiles, mozzarella y aceite de albahaca

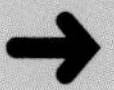

■ Corta la mozzarella en medallones. Puedes calentar la pasta al horno y fundir así al mismo tiempo el queso. Sírvelo acompañado del aceite de albahaca.

Trucos

☛ Si lo prefieres, puedes elaborar esta receta con tomate seco en aceite.

☛ También puedes servir este plato de pasta con un queso de tipo cherne, provolone o incluso una mozzarela ahumada. Prepara estos quesos a la plancha hasta que queden dorados y ligeramente fundidos, y córtalos en dados antes de servir.

Nivel 3 Macarrones rellenos de crema de olivas, miel, tomates en aceite y navaja al horno

- 200 g de macarrones
- 100 g de tomates en aceite
- 100 g de olivas de Kalamata sin hueso
- 16 navajas
- 1 cucharada de miel
- 1 manojo de ajos tiernos
- Aceite de oliva
- Sal y pimienta

30 min
20 min
2 €/persona
Sin contraindicaciones.

■ En una cazuela o en una olla con abundante agua hirviendo con sal y un chorrito de aceite de oliva cuece los macarrones durante el tiempo que indique el fabricante. Una vez cocida la pasta, escúrrela y enfríala en agua con hielo. Reserva.
■ En el vaso de la batidora tritura las olivas con la miel hasta obtener una pasta espesa. Rellena los macarrones con esta pasta con la ayuda de una manga pastelera de boca estrecha y reserva.
■ Limpia las navajas. Para ello, déjalas en remojo unos minutos. Cuando veas que se abren ligeramente, con la ayuda de una puntilla de cocina, recupera su carne y lávala bajo el grifo con agua fría.
■ En una sartén saltea los ajos tiernos con las navajas ya limpias y los tomates en aceite cortados en juliana. Cuando ya esté cocido, agrega los macarrones para calentarlos. Salpimienta y sirve de inmediato.

Trucos

Puedes agregar también anchoas a la pasta de olivas para enriquecer su sabor. Para darle un toque final al plato, puedes añadir unas hojitas de albahaca u orégano.

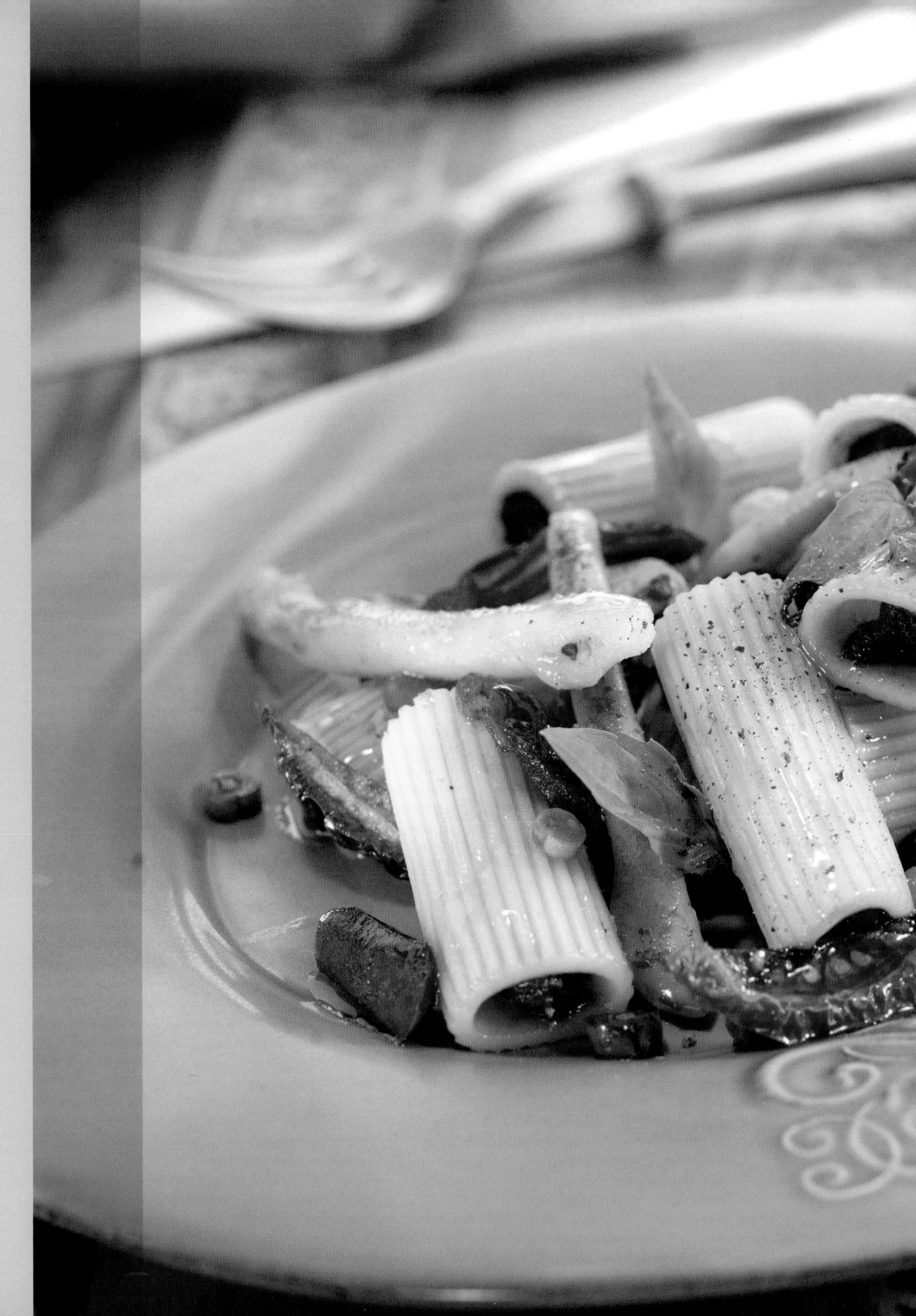

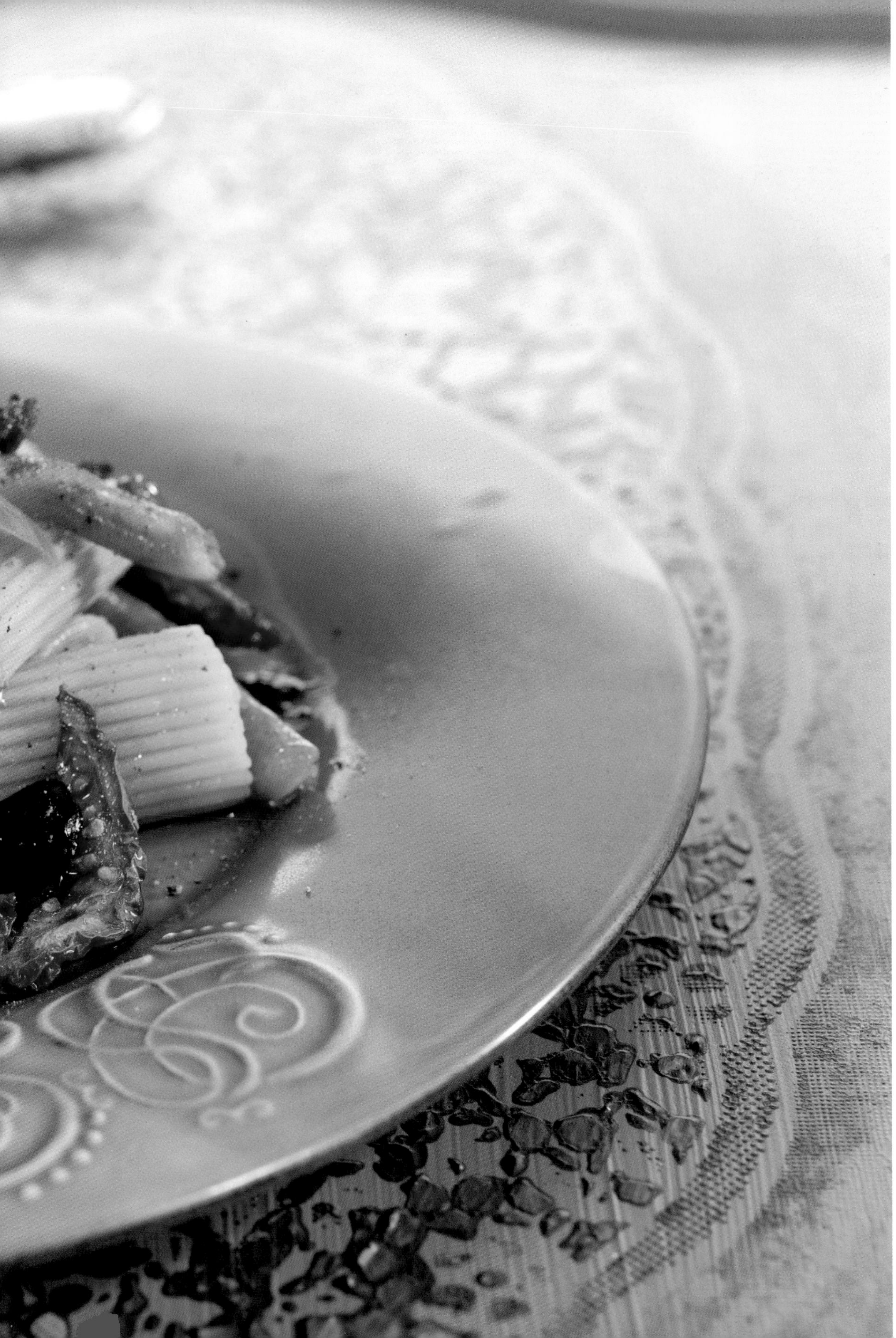

Pasta con salsa de queso

El ingrediente

Ya sea de carne, pescado, verdura, marisco, legumbres o incluso de frutas, la pasta rellena ofrece siempre excelentes y sorprendentes resultados. Puedes rellenar la pasta deseada con los ingredientes que quieras y acompañarla posteriormente con una salsa acorde con el relleno. Raviolis, *tortellini*, canelones o caracolas son algunos de los formatos más conocidos.

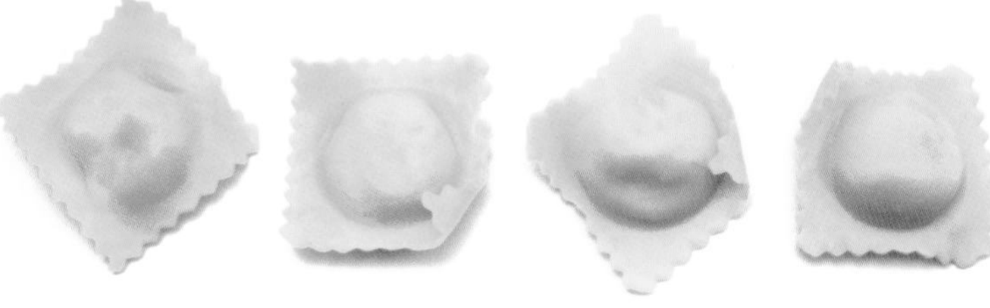

La técnica

Te propongo emplear el queso para acompañar platos de pasta por su excepcional cualidad para fundirse, ya sea integrándolo en salsas o directamente sobre la pasta. También se emplea como ingrediente de relleno de la pasta, para conseguir bocados de textura cremosa.

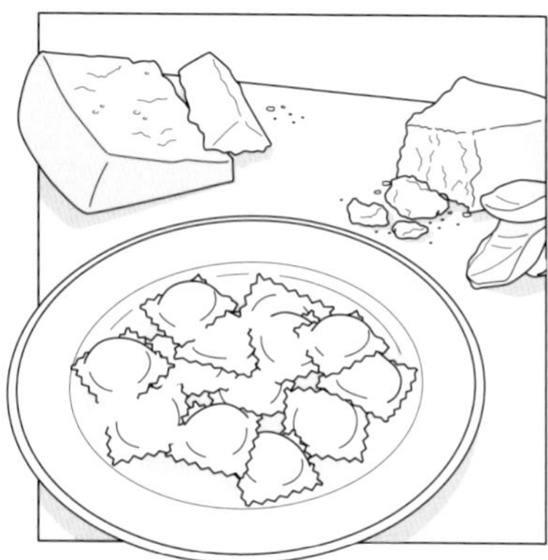

Plato a plato

Nivel **1** **Raviolis de nueces y gorgonzola.** Te proponemos elaborar en casa una pasta rellena tradicional con un dúo de queso y frutos secos que no falla jamás.

Nivel **2** ***Tortellini* de espinacas con crema de parmesano.** Una vez sepas hacer raviolis, atrévete a darles un toque de color con el verde de las espinacas. Pura energía envuelta en pasta de harina.

Nivel **3** **Raviolis de cigalas con sopa de coco, lima y citronela.** Acaba con una propuesta sofisticada: rellena la pasta con la princesa de los mariscos y báñala en una sorprendente sopa tropical.

Nivel **1**
Raviolis de nueces y gorgonzola

- 400 g de pasta para lasaña fresca
- 200 g de gorgonzola
- 100 g de nueces enteras peladas
- 1 manojo de cebollino
- 1 huevo
- Aceite de oliva
- Sal en escamas y pimienta

30 min
5 min
2 €/persona
Las personas con intolerancia a la lactosa, presente en el queso, deben evitar este plato.

■ Sobre una mesa de trabajo estira las láminas para lasaña fresca. Sobre la lámina y dejando espacio entre ellos, forma pequeños montoncitos de queso gorgonzola. Sobre el queso dispón media nuez pelada y una pizca de cebollino picado finamente.

■ Pinta con huevo batido alrededor del queso y cubre el relleno de queso con otra lámina de pasta fresca. Presiona para sellar la pasta, que debe pegarse con la ayuda del huevo. Después corta los raviolis con un molde corta-pasta. Reserva.

■ En un cazo con agua hirviendo, una pizca de sal y un chorrito de aceite de oliva, cuece la pasta durante 4-5 minutos hasta que quede tierna. Sácala del agua, escúrrela y sírvela directamente aliñada con un chorrito de aceite de oliva, una pizca de sal en escamas, una pizca de pimienta y cebollino picado.

Trucos

También puedes adquirir los raviolis ya preparados.

Puedes elaborar una salsa de gorgonzola fundiendo el queso en nata hervida o en caldo de verduras.

Acompaña el plato con nueces picadas y trocitos de queso.

Nivel **2**

Tortellini de espinacas con crema de parmesano

- 400 g de pasta fresca para lasaña
- 200 g de espinacas frescas
- 50 g de piñones
- 50 g de queso parmesano
- 30 g de pasas
- 400 ml de nata líquida
- 1 huevo
- Aceite de oliva
- Sal y pimienta

20 min
20 min
2 €/persona
Las personas con intolerancia a la lactosa deben evitar este plato.

- En una sartén con un chorrito de aceite de oliva saltea ligeramente las espinacas con las pasas y los piñones hasta que queden tiernas durante aproximadamente 4 minutos. Reserva.
- Sobre una mesa de trabajo estira las láminas de pasta fresca. Sobre la pasta y dejando espacio entre ellos, forma pequeños montoncitos de espinacas salteadas.
- Pinta la lámina alrededor de las espinacas con huevo batido y cubre con otra lámina de pasta fresca. Presiona para sellar la pasta, que debe pegarse con la ayuda del huevo, y forma los *tortellini*. Primero pliega la pasta formando un triángulo, enrolla la base de éste sobre sí misma y finalmente junta los extremos más distanciados, moldeando con delicadeza. Reserva.
- Cuece los *tortellini* durante 4-6 minutos en abundante agua con una pizca de sal y un chorrito de aceite de oliva.
- Mientras se cuece la pasta, en una sartén cocina la nata liquida durante 6 minutos, agrega el queso recién rallado y deja que se disuelva en la nata. Corrige el punto de sal y pimienta y retira del fuego. Sirve con los *tortellini*.

Trucos

Puedes adquirir los *tortellini* ya rellenos. Sigue las indicaciones del elaborador para cocerlos.

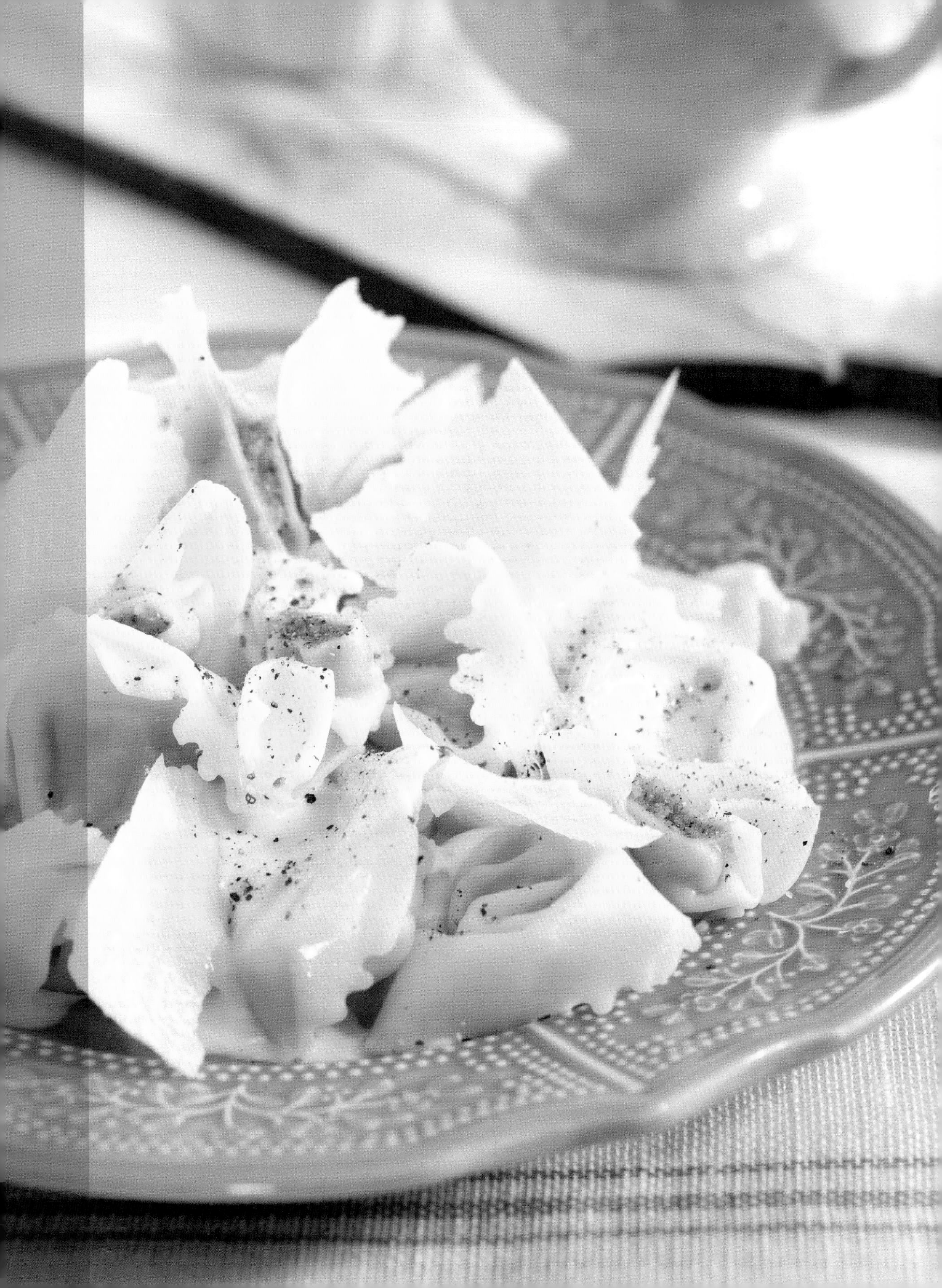

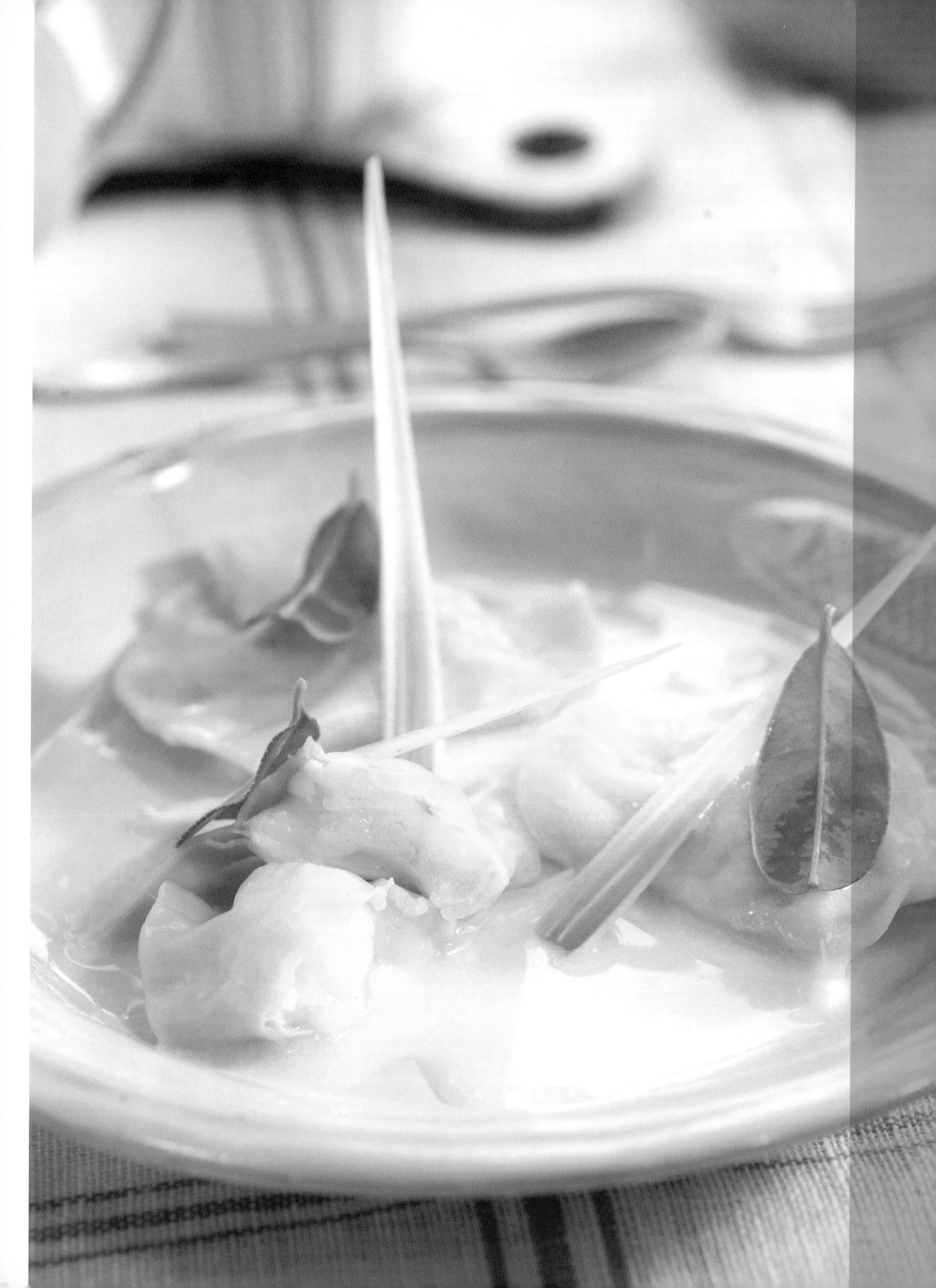

Nivel 3 Raviolis de cigalas con sopa de coco, lima y citronela

- 24 hojas de pasta *won-ton*
- 12 cigalas medianas
- 6 hojas de lima *kaffir*
- 200 ml de leche de coco
- 1 ramita de citronela
- 1 cebolla tierna
- 1 huevo
- 1/2 puerro
- Sal y pimienta
- Azúcar
- Aceite de oliva

20 min
20 min
5 €/persona
Sin contraindicaciones.

■ En una mesa de trabajo estira 12 hojas de pasta *won-ton*. Sobre las hojas, en el centro, dispón las cigalas peladas y una cucharadita de puerro y cebolla, previamente cortados finos y ligeramente salteados.

■ Pinta con el huevo batido la pasta, alrededor de las cigalas, y cúbrela con otra hoja de pasta *won-ton*. Presiona hasta sellar la pasta y corta los raviolis con la ayuda de un molde corta-pasta. Reserva.

■ Para elaborar la sopa de coco, cuece la leche de coco con las hojas de lima, la rama de citronela, una pizca de sal y una de azúcar. Cuece durante 5-6 minutos a fuego lento y deja enfriar.

■ En un cazo con agua hirviendo, una pizca de sal y un chorrito de aceite de oliva, cuece los raviolis durante 4 minutos. Una vez cocidos sírvelo acompañados de la sopa de coco. Es mejor servir esta salsa tibia, con los raviolis bien calientes.

Trucos

Si no tienes hoja de lima utiliza piel de lima. Si no encuentras citronela, puedes prescindir de ella.

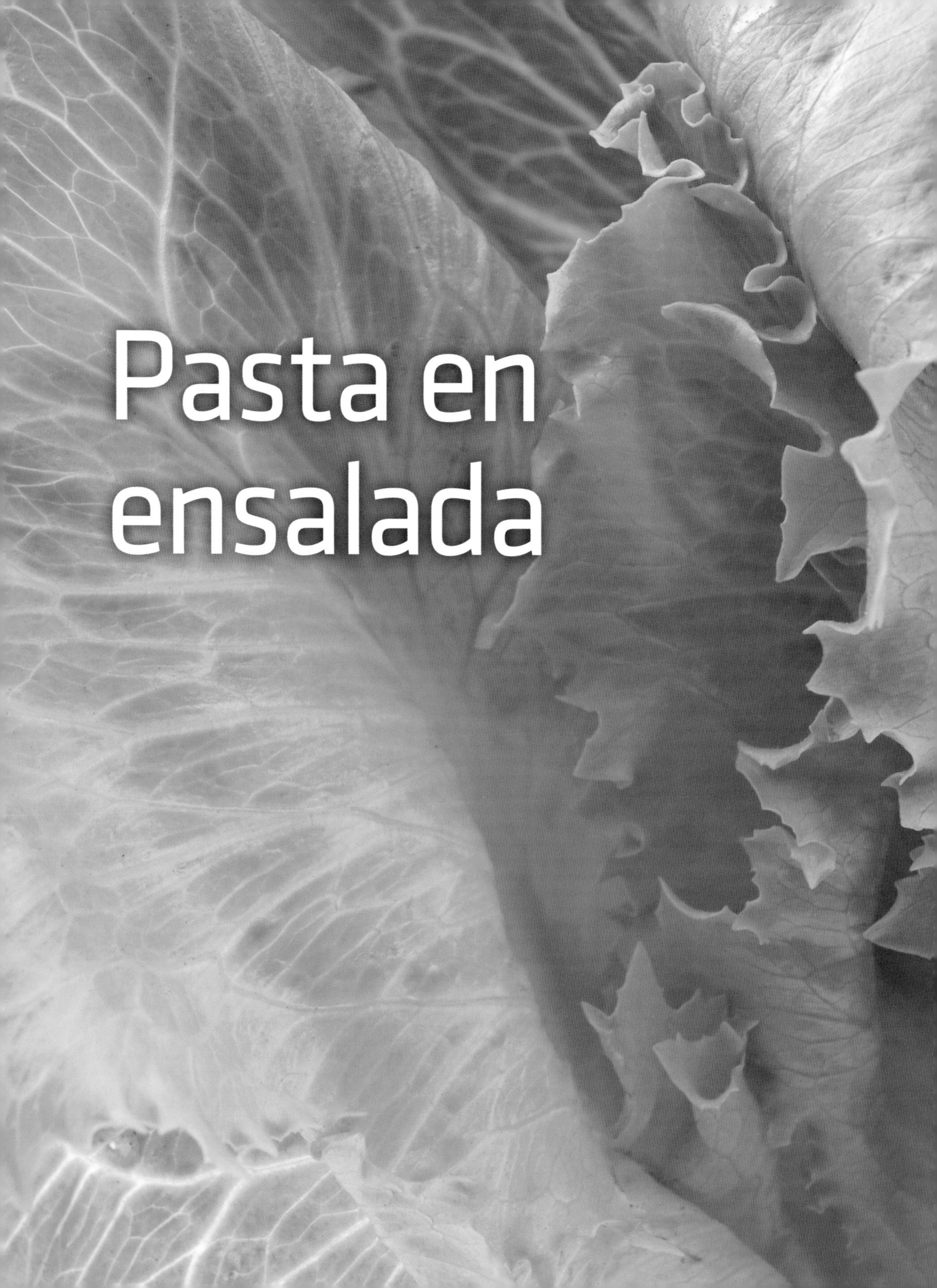

Pasta en ensalada

La pasta da un carácter personal a las ensaladas y además enriquece nuestra dieta.

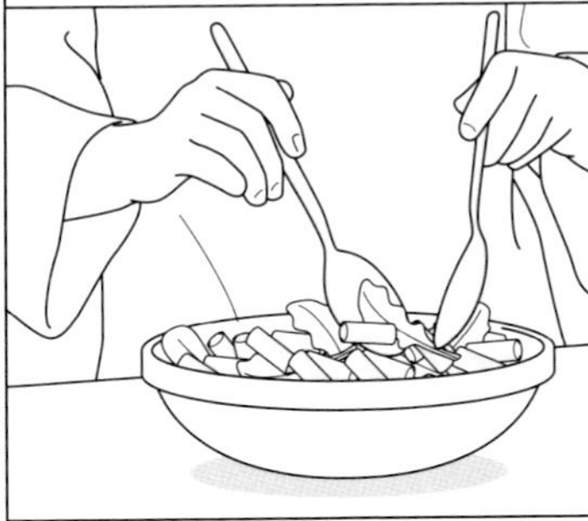

Después de cocerla es importante enfriarla en abundante agua con hielo. Así se frena su cocción, ya que aun fuera del agua conserva parte del calor de la cocción.

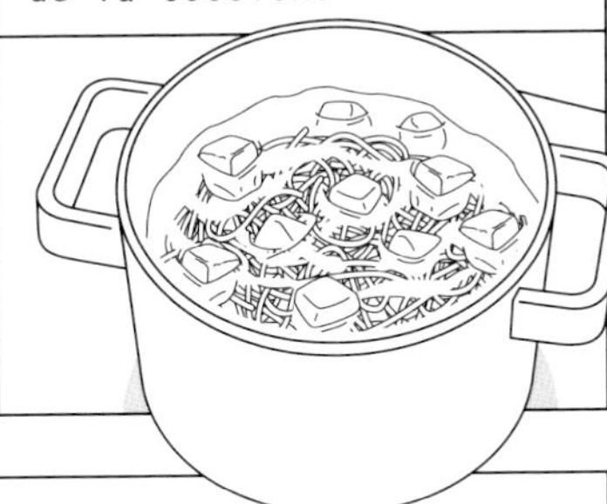

Aprenderás a elaborar pasta con vinagreta en ensaladas con pescados y carnes...

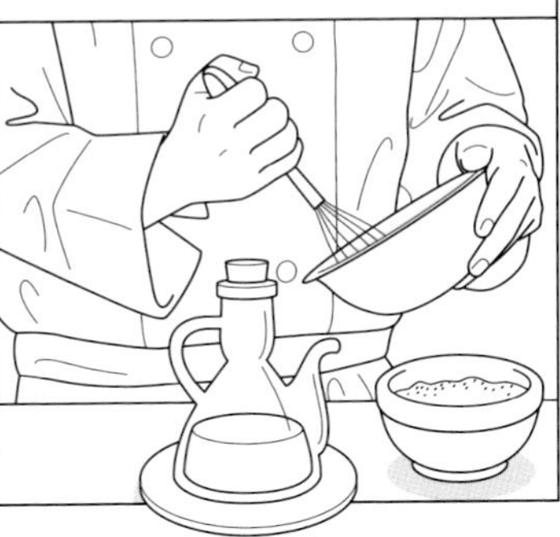

... pasta con mayonesa...

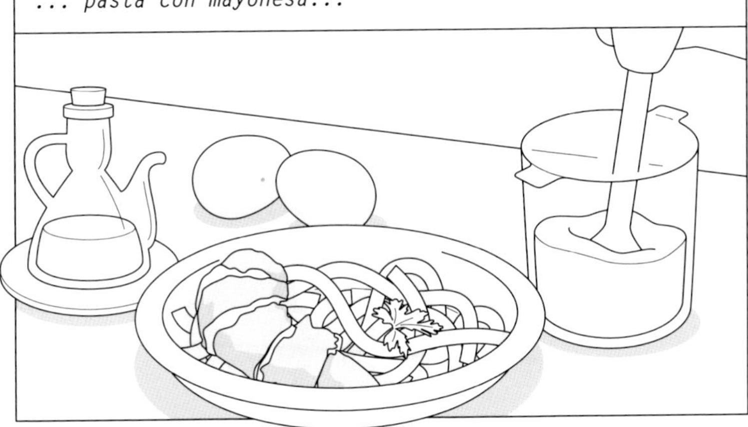

... o pasta con carácter mediterráneo.

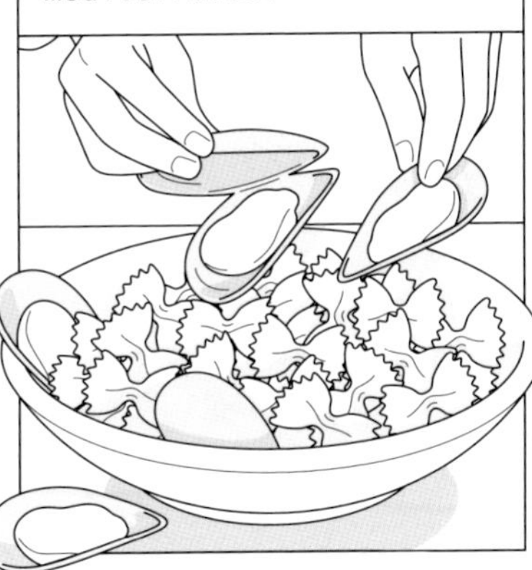

Los acompañamientos quedan a tu elección: verduritas hervidas, trozos de fruta, carnes y pescados...

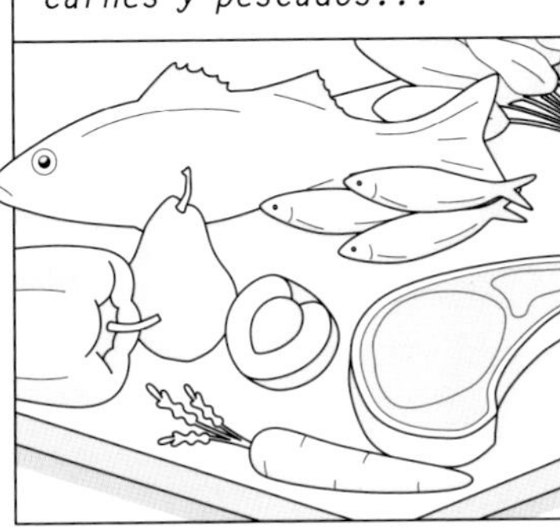

También puedes contar con infinidad de aderezos, que pueden ser de tu propia creación...

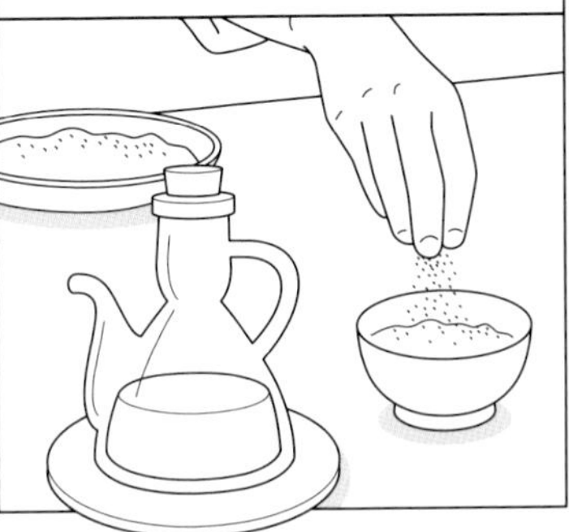

... o simplemente un buen chorro de aceite de oliva virgen.

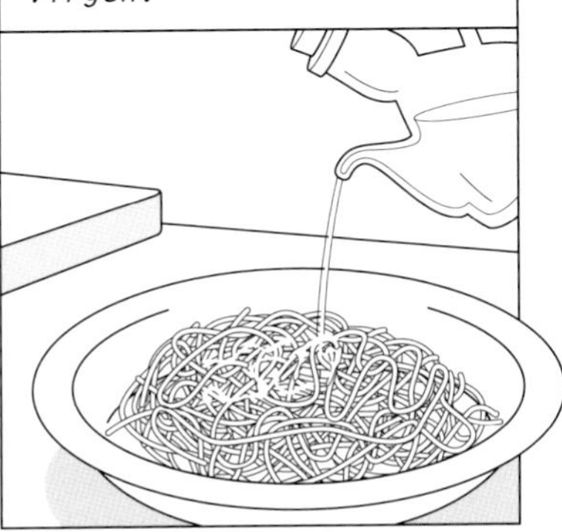

Pasta con mayonesa

El ingrediente

La mayonesa es una salsa idónea para aderezar ensaladas de pasta de todo tipo, pues puedes aromatizarla a tu gusto, ya sea con hierbas aromáticas o especias, o aligerarla para obtener una salsa lisa, homogénea y fluida.

Partiendo de una base de mayonesa puedes enriquecer su sabor agregando un diente de ajo a su elaboración y obtener así una mayonesa de ajo. También puedes elaborar una salsa rosa añadiendo un par de cucharadas de tomate frito y un chorrito de coñac y zumo de naranja; prueba también con unas gotas de tabasco. Además, si elaboras tu mayonesa con un aceite aromatizado, con trufa, setas, hierbas aromáticas, etc., obtendrás una mayonesa con el gusto del aceite empleado.

La técnica

Para elaborar una sencilla mayonesa, tritura en el vaso de una batidora un huevo entero con un chorrito constante de aceite de oliva, hasta obtener la densidad deseada. Rebaja entonces con un chorrito de leche o de zumo de limón. Tanto los ingredientes como los instrumentos deben estar a temperatura ambiente, de ese modo evitarás que la mayonesa se corte.

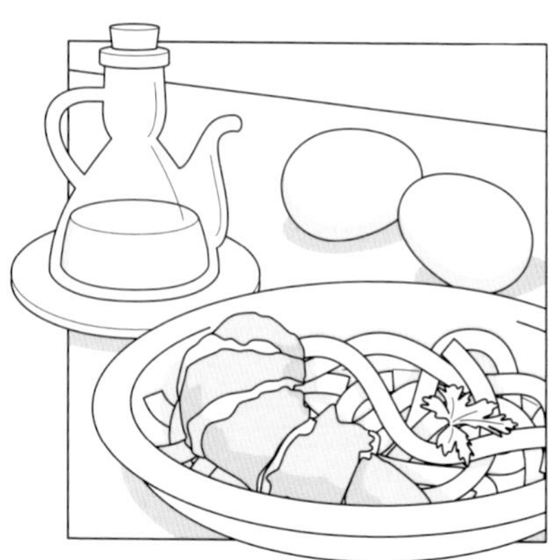

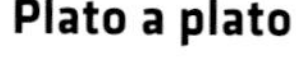

Plato a plato

Nivel **1 Ensalada piamontesa.** Haz la prueba con una sencilla ensalada de pasta con pimientos y ajo y aderezada con una clásica mayonesa.

Nivel **2 Ensalada de pasta corta con rúcula, tomate, orégano y alcachofa.** Añade un toque crujiente a la ensalada de pasta con la alcachofa frita y aderézalo con el toque aromático del orégano.

Nivel **3 Ensalada de cintas de pasta con bogavante y mayonesa de marisco.** Da un toque sofisticado a tu plato de pasta con el refinado bogavante. Una mayonesa especial con naranja y tabasco le dará el toque personal.

Nivel **1** # Ensalada piamontesa

- 150 g de pasta corta, tipo caracolas, lazos, etc.
- 1 pimiento rojo asado
- 1 pimiento verde de tipo italiano
- 1 diente de ajo
- 1 cebolleta tierna
- 3 huevos
- 50 g de olivas verdes sin hueso
- Aceite de oliva
- Sal y pimienta
- Un poco de leche o medio limón (opcional)

30 min
20 min
2 €/persona
Sin contraindicaciones.

■ Cuece la pasta en un cazo con abundante agua hirviendo con sal, siguiendo las indicaciones del fabricante. Una vez cocida, enfría la pasta bajo el chorro de agua fría. Resérvala.
■ En otro cazo con agua hirviendo con sal cuece 2 huevos durante 8 minutos. Retíralos del agua y enfríalos. Pélalos y resérvalos.
■ Para elaborar la mayonesa, tritura en el vaso de la batidora un huevo fresco con un chorrito constante de aceite de oliva hasta obtener la densidad deseada. Puedes aligerarla con un chorrito de leche o el zumo de medio limón.
■ Mezcla en una fuente la pasta con los huevos cocidos cortados en cuartos, las olivas, los pimientos, el ajo y la cebolleta, todo picado tan fino como te sea posible. Salpimienta y agrega 2 cucharadas de salsa mayonesa.

Trucos

Enriquece la ensalada a tu gusto agregando atún en aceite, anchoas o marisco. También puedes aromatizar la mayonesa con un chorrito de coñac.

Nivel 2 Ensalada de pasta corta con rúcula, tomate, orégano y alcachofa

- 150 g de pasta corta de tipo caracolas, lazos, etc.
- 100 g de rúcula
- 2 alcachofas
- 1 bandeja de tomates cherry
- 1 ramita de orégano
- 50 g de jamón ibérico (opcional)
- Aceite de oliva
- Vinagre de Jerez
- Sal y pimienta

30 min
20 min
2 €/persona
Sin contraindicaciones.

■ Cuece la pasta siguiendo las indicaciones del fabricante hasta que esté *al dente*. Enfríala bajo el chorro de agua fría y resérvala.
■ Limpia las alcachofas y córtalas en cuartos. Fríelas en aceite de oliva bien caliente hasta que queden crujientes, y déjalas sobre papel de cocina absorbente. Resérvalas.
■ Mezcla en un recipiente la pasta con los tomatitos cortados por la mitad, el jamón ibérico (opcional) y las hojas de rúcula. En el momento de servir añade las alcachofas crujientes y adereza.
■ Para aderezar la ensalada tritura en un mortero una pizca de sal con una de pimienta, la ramita de orégano, 3 cucharadas de aceite de oliva y una de vinagre de Jerez.

Trucos

Puedes sustituir el orégano por unas hojas de albahaca. También puedes cambiar el jamón ibérico por jamón de pato o salmón ahumado.

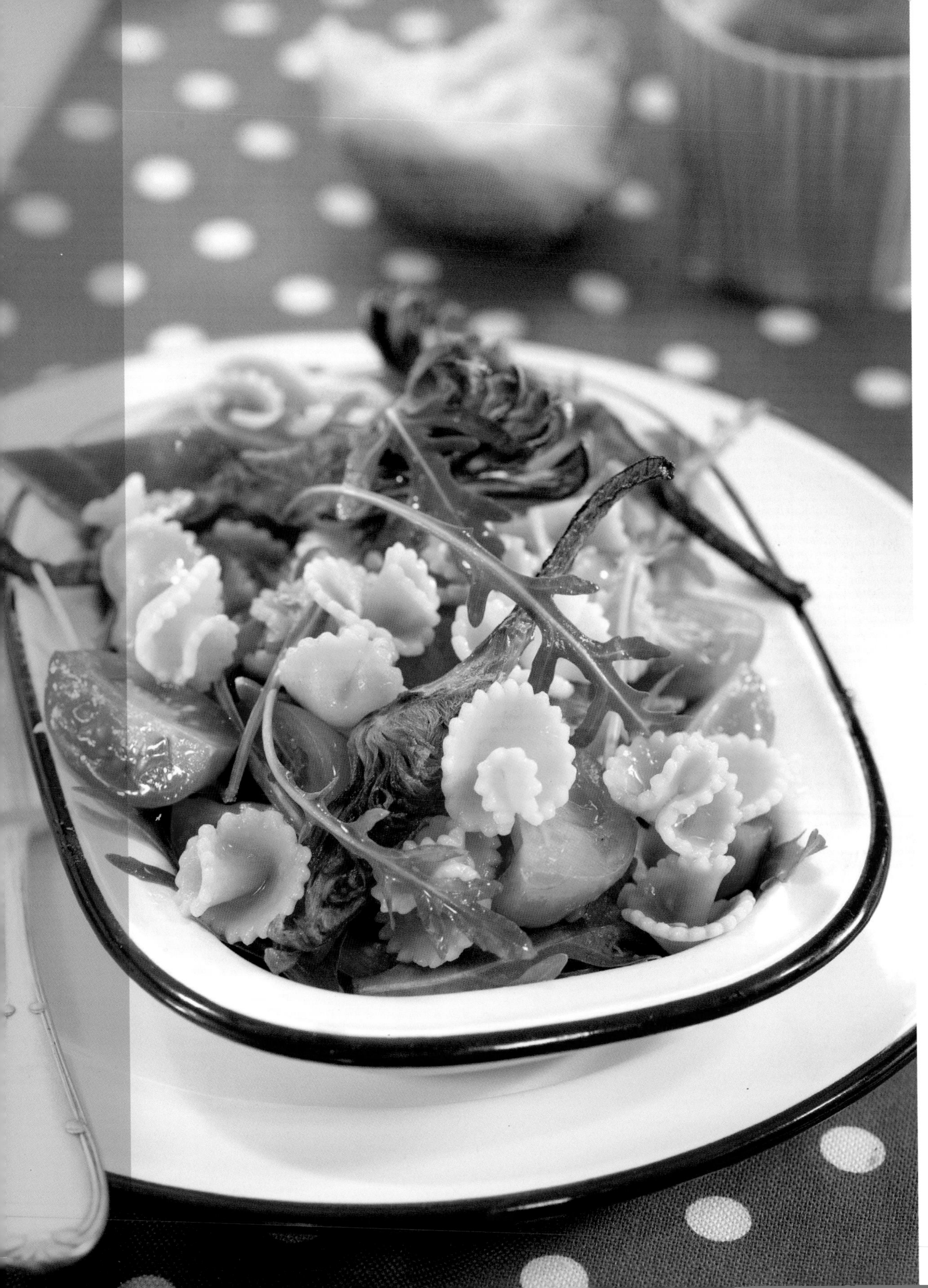

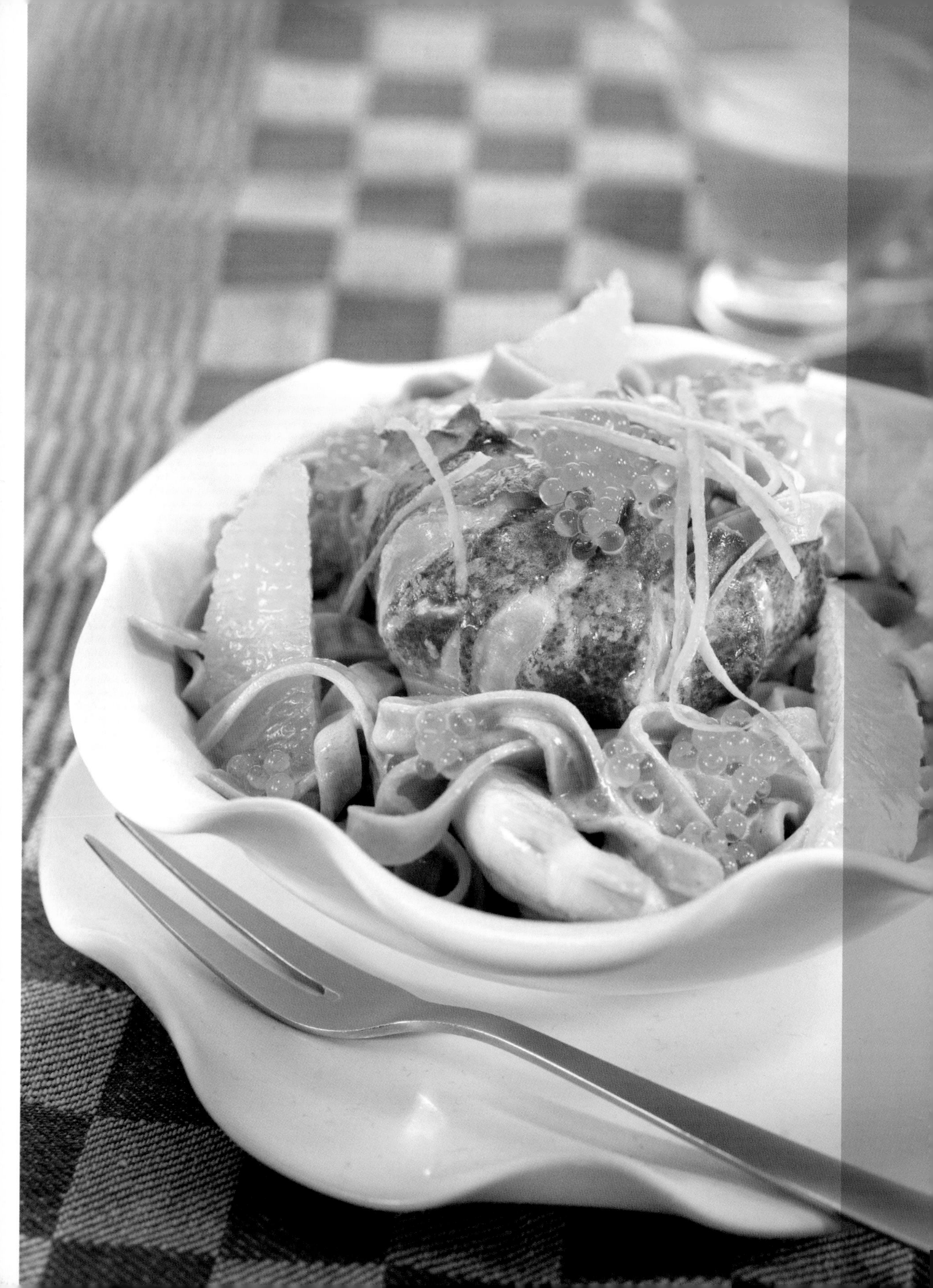

Nivel **3**

Ensalada de cintas de pasta con bogavante y mayonesa de marisco

- 150 g de pasta larga de tipo *tagliatelle* de espinacas
- 1 bogavante de 600 g
- 12 langostinos cocidos
- 2 naranjas
- 1 zanahoria
- 100 ml de salsa mayonesa
- 2 cucharadas de tomate frito
- Huevas de trucha
- Tabasco
- Sal y pimienta

45 min

20 min

4 €/persona

Receta no indicada para alérgicos al marisco.

- Cuece la pasta siguiendo las indicaciones del fabricante hasta que esté *al dente*. Una vez cocida, enfríala bajo el chorro de agua fría. Resérvala.
- Cuece el bogavante durante 10-12 minutos en una olla con abundante agua hirviendo con sal. Una vez cocido, enfríalo en abundante agua con hielo. Pela el bogavante y reserva el cuerpo y las pinzas.
- Mezcla en un recipiente la pasta con las huevas de trucha, la zanahoria rallada, los gajos de una naranja, los langostinos pelados y un poco de piel de naranja rallada. Reserva.
- Con la ayuda de unas varillas de cocina, mezcla en otro recipiente la mayonesa con el zumo de media naranja, unas gotitas de tabasco y el tomate frito. También puedes agregar el jugo de la cabeza del bogavante para enriquecer el sabor de la salsa mayonesa. Se trata, sencillamente, de elaborar una salsa rosa enriquecida con el sabor del marisco. Añade una cucharadita de coñac para potenciar el sabor.

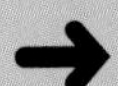

Nivel 3 Ensalada de cintas de pasta con bogavante y mayonesa de marisco

➜ ■ Distribuye el cuerpo del bogavante en dos platos y reparte las dos pinzas en otros dos platos. Acompaña con la ensalada de pasta y langostinos y adereza con la mayonesa de marisco.

Trucos

☛ Puedes prescindir del bogavante y agregar a esta ensalada el marisco que desees. Emplea gambas o langostinos o combina estos con mejillones abiertos al vapor, patas de cangrejo cocidas, cigalas, o combinando el marisco con carne, como trozos de pechuga de pollo salteados.

Pasta con vinagreta

El ingrediente
La vinagreta es, por definición, una salsa compuesta de aceite, cebolla y vinagre, que se consume fría con los pescados y con la carne. Sin embargo, en la cocina de hoy en día se trata de algo más, pues es una salsa que adaptamos a nuestro capricho y que destinamos también a ensaladas de todo tipo, pasta, aperitivos, etc.

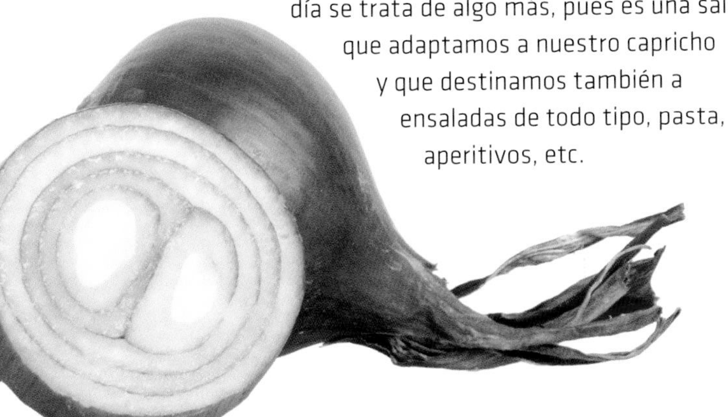

La técnica
Cuida de picar finamente los ingredientes de tu vinagreta para tener una sensación agradable a la hora de degustarla. Las vinagretas pueden servirse también tibias, como un escabeche, y albergar infinidad de posibilidades e ingredientes.

Plato a plato

Nivel **1** **Ensalada de pasta corta con salmón, nueces y eneldo.** Salmón y frutos secos combinan a la perfección en este plato de salida. El toque aromático del eneldo es un añadido al particular sabor de esta receta.

Nivel **2** **Ensalada de pasta con gambas y vinagreta de cítricos.** Atrévete en este segundo paso a aliñar la pasta con naranja y lima y dale un toque sofisticado con unas deliciosas gambas con huevas de trucha.

Nivel **3** **Ensalada tibia de pasta con *carpaccio* de pato caramelizado.** Pasta y carne casan bien, si además sustituimos la ternera por un *magret* de pato, daremos un tumbo a las notas gustativas del comensal.

Nivel 1 Ensalada de pasta corta con salmón, nueces y eneldo

- 150 g de pasta corta de tipo caracolas, lazos, etc.
- 150 g de salmón ahumado
- 75 g de nueces peladas
- 50 g de queso fresco
- 1 rama de eneldo fresco
- 150 ml de nata líquida
- Aceite de oliva
- Sal y pimienta blanca

25 min
15 min
3 €/persona
Esta receta no está indicada para personas con intolerancia a la lactosa.

- Cuece la pasta siguiendo las indicaciones del fabricante hasta que esté *al dente*. Una vez cocida, enfríala bajo el chorro de agua fría. Resérvala.
- En un recipiente mezcla la pasta bien fría con el salmón cortado en tiras y las nueces peladas. Salpimienta y reserva.
- Bate muy despacio la nata con el queso fresco y el eneldo picado finamente. Se trata de deshacer el queso en la nata y no montar la nata con el queso. Una vez este se haya disuelto, agrega un chorrito de aceite de oliva. Adereza la ensalada con esta preparación.

Trucos

Si lo prefieres, puedes calentar ligeramente esta ensalada en el microondas y degustarla como un entrante caliente.

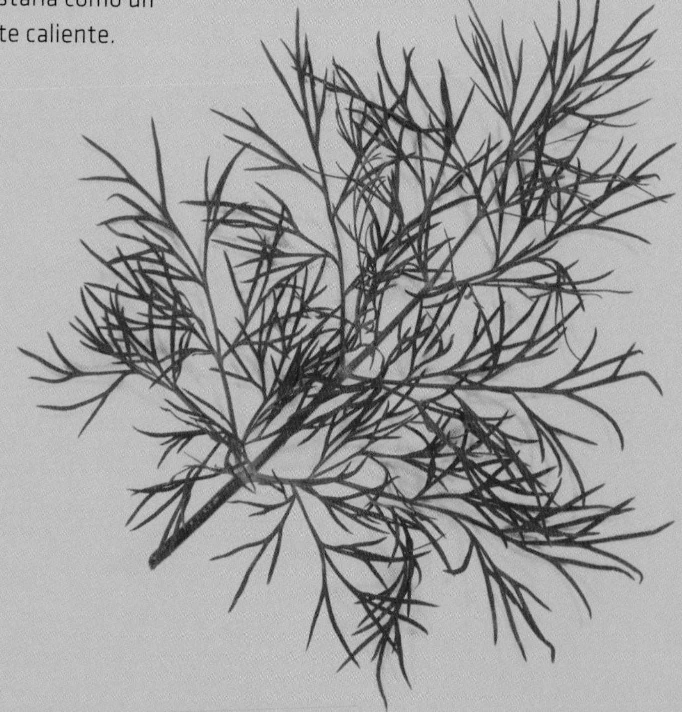

Nivel **2**

Ensalada de pasta con gambas y vinagreta de cítricos

- 150 g de pasta corta de tipo caracolas, lazos, etc.
- 16 gambas o langostinos cocidos
- 1 calabacín
- 1 cucharadita de jengibre fresco picado
- 1 manojo de espárragos trigueros
- 1 naranja
- 1 lima
- 1 cebolleta tierna
- 1 zanahoria
- Huevas de trucha o salmón
- Sal y pimienta rosa
- Aceite de oliva

25 min

15 min

3 €/persona

Esta receta no es apta para personas alérgicas al marisco.

■ Cuece la pasta siguiendo las indicaciones del fabricante hasta que esté *al dente*. Una vez cocida, enfríala bajo el chorro de agua fría. Resérvala.

■ Con la ayuda de un pelador de patatas haz finas tiras de espárragos y calabacín. Cuécelas en un cazo con agua hirviendo durante 2-3 minutos, sácalas y enfríalas en agua con hielo. Resérvalas.

■ Pela las gambas o los langostinos y agrégalos a un recipiente con los gajos de la naranja, unas tiras de piel de naranja y de lima, una cucharada de huevas de trucha o salmón, las tiras de calabacín y espárragos, la pasta cocida y la zanahoria rallada. Reserva.

■ En un recipiente mezcla la cebolleta picada finamente con el jengibre, 3 cucharadas de aceite de oliva, el zumo de media lima y el zumo de media naranja. Mézclalo todo bien, salpimienta y sirve acompañando la ensalada.

Trucos

Si lo prefieres puedes dejar reposar durante media hora las tiras crudas de espárragos y calabacín en agua con hielo, para que queden *crocantes*, y servirlas así como *crudités*, sin necesidad de cocerlas.

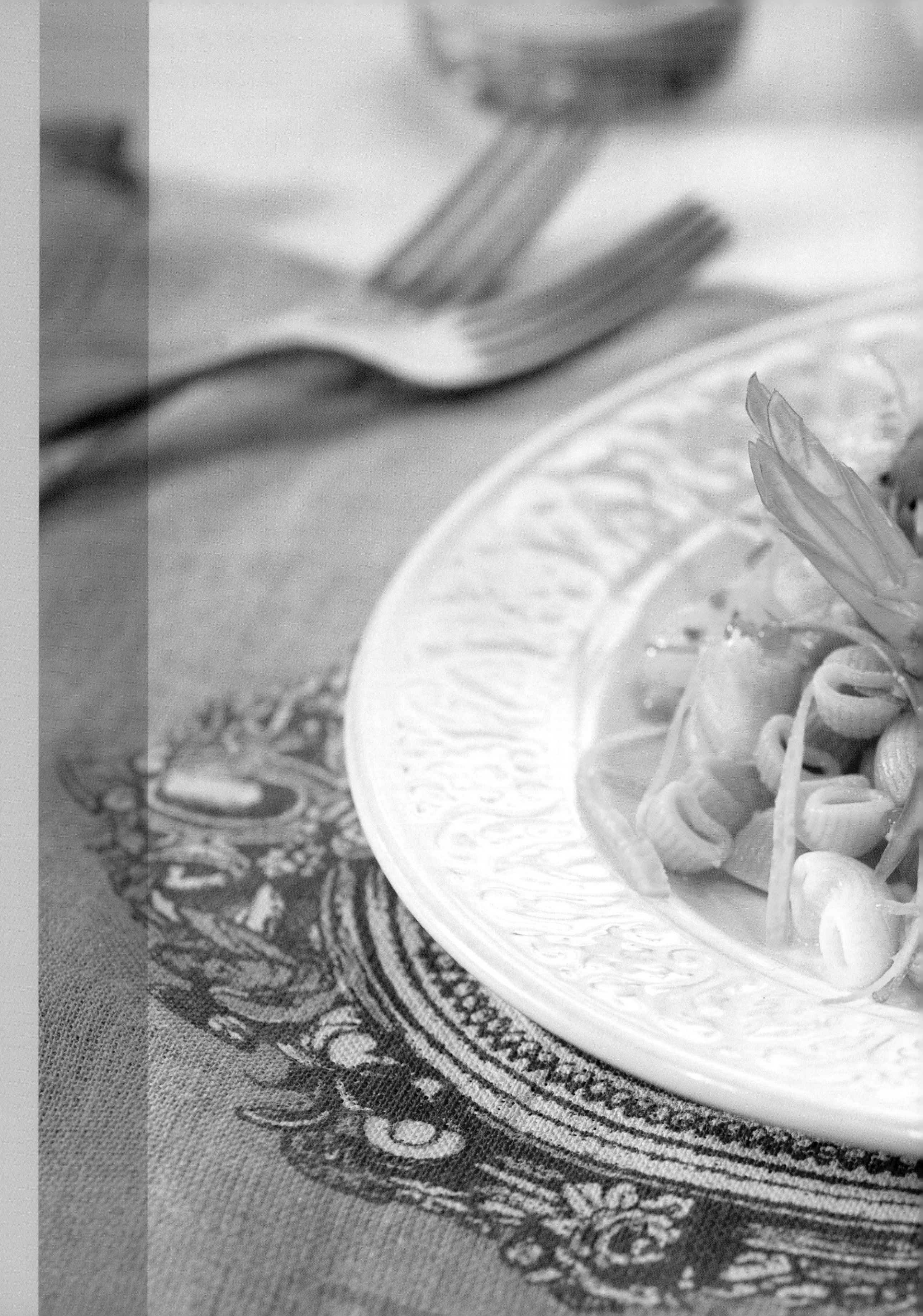

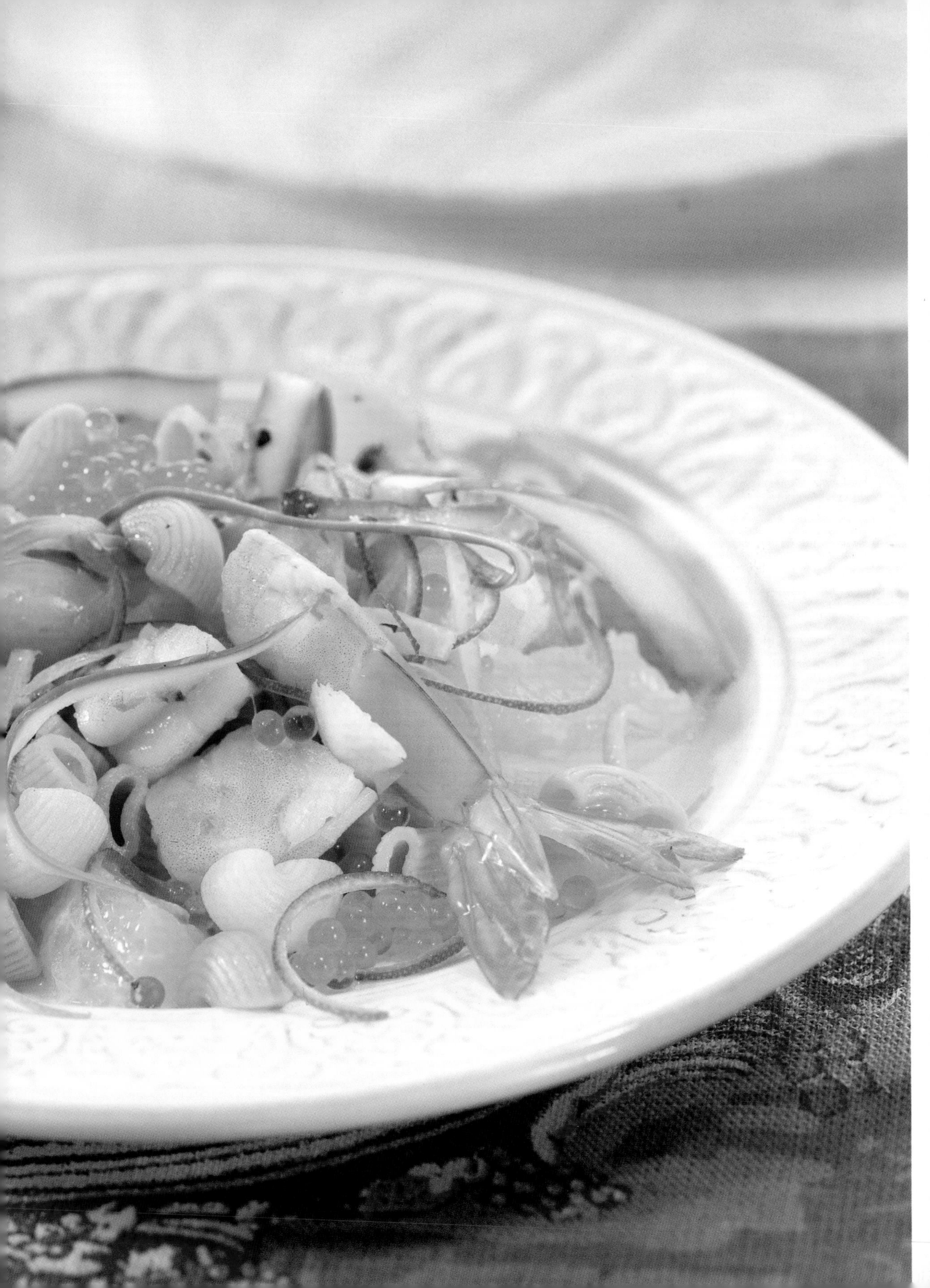

Nivel **3** Ensalada tibia de pasta con *carpaccio* de pato caramelizado

- 150 g de pasta corta de tipo caracolas, lazos, etc.
- 1 pechuga de pato (*magret*)
- 1 granada
- 1 mango
- 1 cucharada de mostaza en grano
- 1 cucharada de salsa de soja
- 2 cucharadas de miel
- Germinados
- Aceite de oliva

25 min
15 min
3 €/persona
Sin contraindicaciones.

■ Cuece la pasta siguiendo las indicaciones del fabricante hasta que esté *al dente*. Una vez cocida, enfríala bajo el chorro de agua fría. Resérvala.

■ En una sartén a fuego medio, sin aceite, fríe el *magret* de pato, primero por el lado de la piel durante 4-5 minutos, y luego dale la vuelta y déjalo cocer un par de minutos más. Transcurrido este tiempo, agrega la miel a la sartén y apaga el fuego, añade la salsa de soja y deja que el *magret* caramelice. Dale la vuelta repetidas veces para que el caramelo se adhiera bien mientras se enfría; esta acción puede llevarte varios minutos.

■ En un recipiente mezcla la pasta con los granos de granada, los germinados, el mango cortado en cuadraditos y la mostaza en grano y sírvela en 4 platos.

■ Una vez el *magret* se haya enfriado, córtalo en finas láminas y disponlas sobre la ensalada. Calienta ligeramente la salsa restante en la sartén, añade un chorrito de aceite de oliva y sirve acompañando la ensalada.

Trucos

Puedes añadir una cucharada de jengibre fresco picado a la sartén para aromatizar aún más el *magret*.

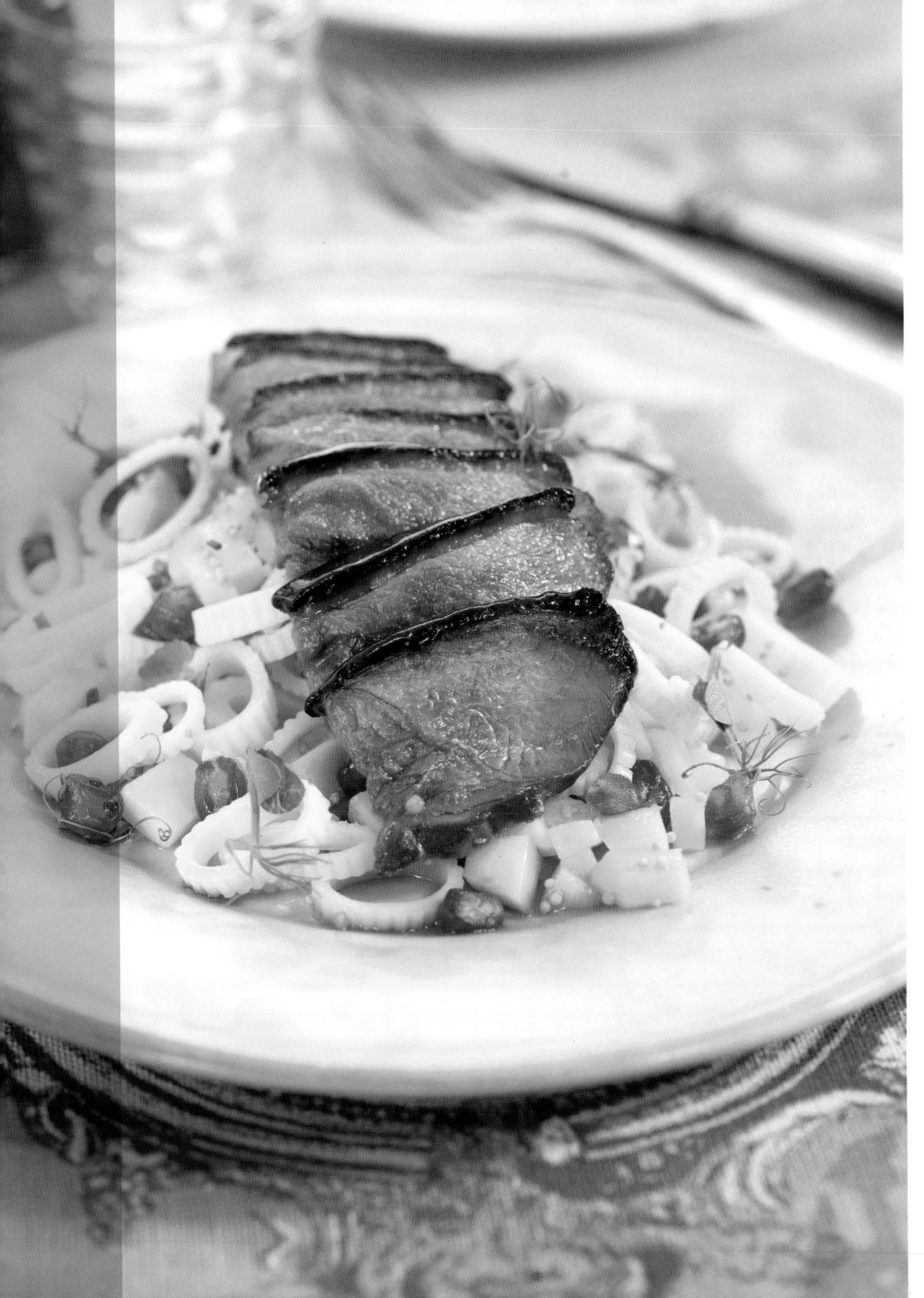

Pasta con carácter mediterráneo

El ingrediente
La dieta mediterránea es sin duda una de las más recomendables para seguir una alimentación equilibrada. Rica en productos del mar y de la tierra, bebe del Mediterráneo, que baña costas tan ricas en culturas como en cocinas distintas. Desde la tradición árabe, hasta la turca, pasando, cómo no, por la española, la griega o la italiana. Ofrece, en definitiva, una gran variedad de ingredientes con infinitas posibilidades.

La técnica
La cocina mediterránea está llena de sabores exóticos, conferidos por las numerosas hierbas y especias que se emplean en ella, platos salados con contrastes dulces, especias más o menos picantes...

Podrás conservar las hierbas propias de la temporada encurtidas en aceite de oliva, para su posterior consumo. También puedes adquirir aceites ya aromatizados para conferir a tus platos el delicioso sabor de las hierbas aromáticas. Algunas hierbas como el eneldo, el romero o el tomillo se pueden también secar y conservar así para añadir a tus guisos, ensaladas o vinagretas.

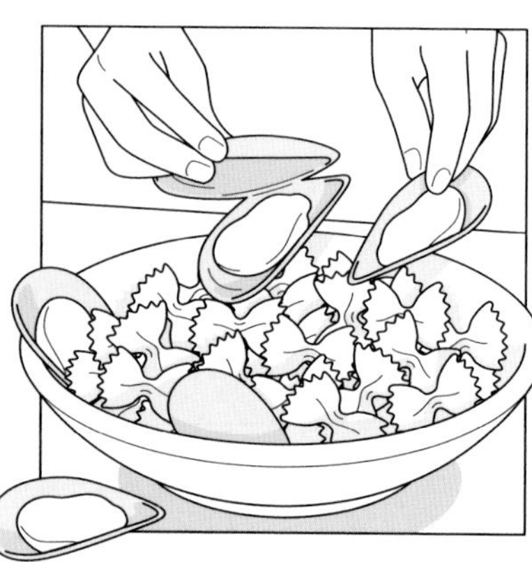

Plato a plato

Nivel **1** **Ensalada de pasta al estilo griego.** Viaja con los sabores de la costa griega de la mano del queso feta y la salsa Tzatziki, elaborada, cómo no, con yogur griego cremoso.

Nivel **2** **Ensalada de pasta como un *taboulé*.** Descubre los sabores de Oriente con un plato tradicional a base de pasta perla, servido frío y coronado con pasas y piñones.

Nivel **3** **Ensalada de pasta con escabeche de mejillones.** Remata la jugada con un plato con sabor a mar. Los mejillones y el calamar hacen las veces de carne para acompañar la pasta.

Nivel 1 Ensalada de pasta al estilo griego

- 150 g de pasta corta de tipo caracolas, lazos, etc.
- 100 g de olivas de Kalamata
- 150 g de queso feta
- 100 ml de salsa Tzatziki
- 1 bandeja de tomates cherry
- Aceite de oliva
- Sal y pimienta

2 5min
15 min
2 €/persona
Esta receta no está indicada para personas con intolerancia a la lactosa.

■ Cuece la pasta siguiendo las indicaciones del fabricante hasta que esté *al dente*. Una vez cocida, enfríala bajo el chorro de agua fría. Resérvala.

■ Mezcla en un recipiente la pasta bien fría con las olivas deshuesadas y picadas, el queso feta cortado en dados, los tomates partidos por la mitad y un chorrito de aceite de oliva. Mezcla bien, salpimienta y sirve acompañado de la salsa Tzatziki.

Trucos

Si no encuentras la salsa Tzatziki puedes elaborarla tú mismo mezclando un yogur cremoso (tipo griego) con un diente de ajo picado, una ramita de menta picada y un trocito de pepino troceado.

Nivel **2**

Ensalada de pasta como un *taboulé*

- 150 g de pasta perla
- 50 g de piñones
- 50 g de uvas pasas
- 50 g de olivas verdes deshuesadas
- 2 cucharadas de germinados de rábano
- 1 rama de menta
- 1 cebolleta
- 1 pimiento verde
- 1/2 pimiento rojo
- Aceite de oliva
- Sal y pimienta

25 min
10 min
2 €/persona
Sin contraindicaciones.

■ Cuece la pasta siguiendo las indicaciones del fabricante hasta que esté *al dente*. Una vez cocida, enfríala bajo el chorro de agua fría. Resérvala.

■ Pica la cebolleta y los pimientos tan finamente como te sea posible y resérvalos.

■ En un recipiente mezcla la pasta bien fría con las olivas picadas, los pimientos, la cebolleta, las pasas, los piñones, los germinados de rábano y unas hojitas de menta. Mezcla bien, salpimienta y aderézalo con un chorrito de aceite de oliva. Ya lo puedes servir.

Trucos

Hidrata las pasas en agua para que estén tiernas antes de ponerlas en la ensalada.

Si quieres, puedes espolvorear una cucharadita de azúcar lustre y canela sobre la ensalada antes de servirla para ofrecer un sabor más exótico si cabe.

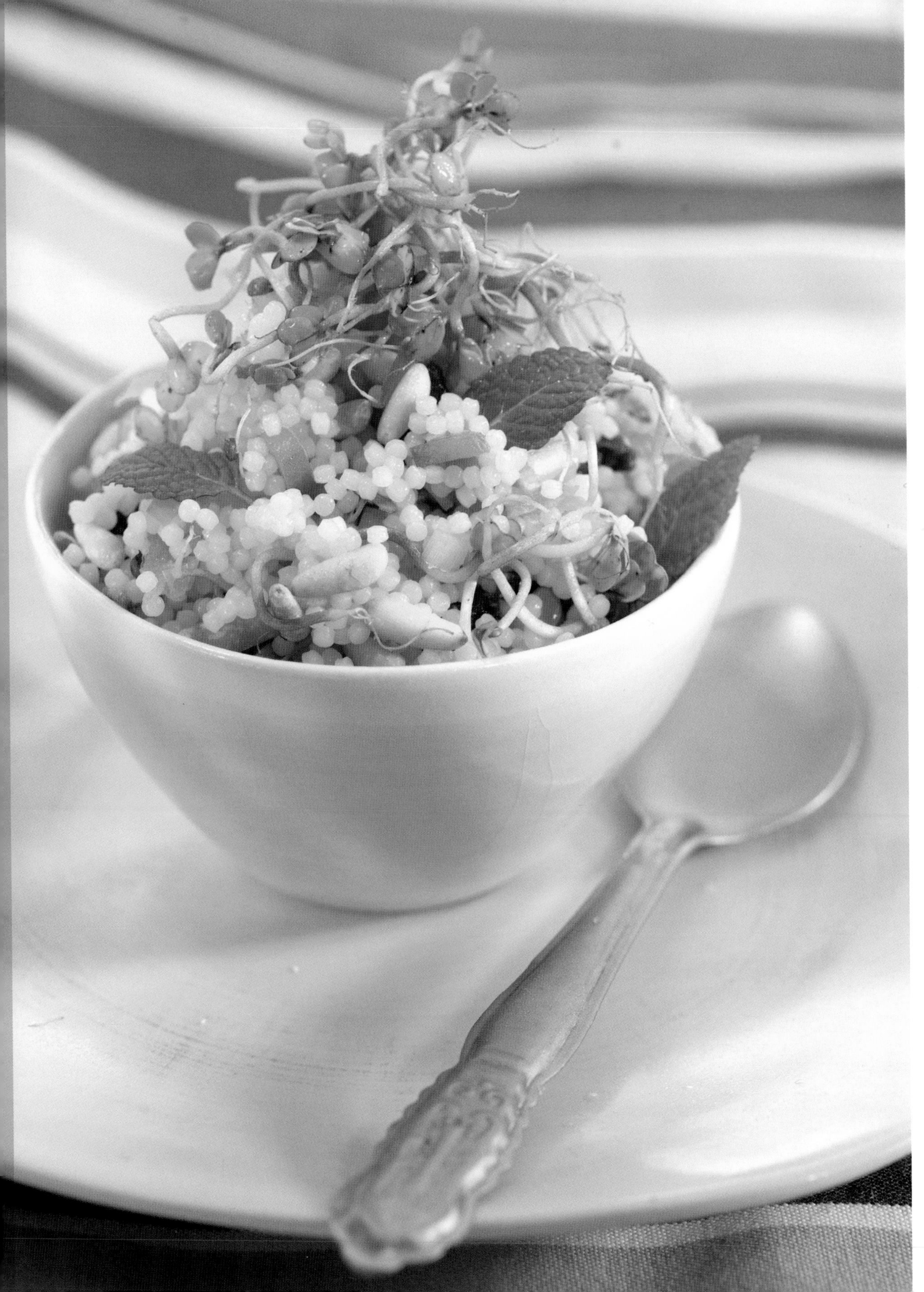

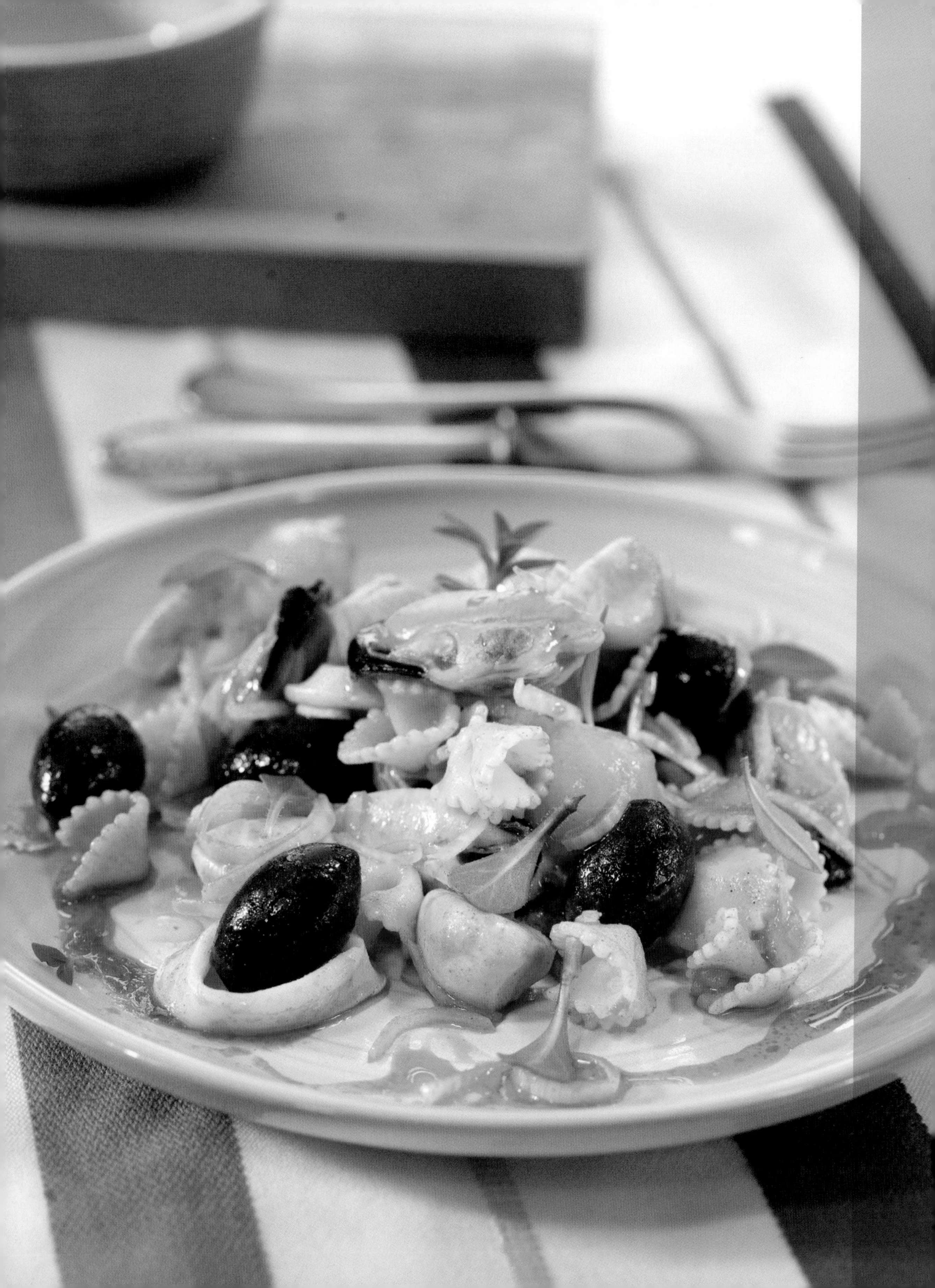

Nivel **3**
Ensalada de pasta con escabeche de mejillones

- 150 g de pasta corta de tipo lazos
- 500 g de mejillones
- 100 g de olivas de Kalamata o de Aragón
- 2 calamares de playa limpios
- 1 cebolla tierna
- 1 diente de ajo
- 1/2 puerro
- 200 ml de aceite de oliva
- 50 ml de vinagre de Jerez
- 1 cucharadita de pimentón dulce
- 1 ramita de orégano
- Sal y pimienta en grano

30 min
20 min
3 €/persona
Sin contraindicaciones.

■ Cuece la pasta siguiendo las indicaciones del fabricante hasta que esté *al dente*. Una vez cocida, enfríala bajo el chorro de agua fría. Resérvala.

■ Dispón un cazo al fuego con agua, sal y unas bolitas de pimienta. Hierve los mejillones hasta que se abran. Escúrrelos y deja que se enfríen.

■ Corta el puerro a medallones finos, la cebolla en juliana y lamina el ajo. Confita los tres ingredientes en un cazo a fuego lento. Una vez la verdura empiece a ablandarse, agrega los calamares bien limpios, cortados en anillas, y la carne de los mejillones. Pasados unos minutos, apaga el fuego y agrega el vinagre y el pimentón. Deja enfriar.

■ Mezcla la pasta con el escabeche de mejillones y las olivas y sírvelo con unas hojitas de orégano.

Trucos

Puedes modificar el sabor de tu escabeche empleando un pimentón dulce, picante o incluso ahumado.

Es importante que los calamares sean de playa y frescos para que queden tiernos con una cocción breve, como la del escabeche. También puedes agregar a tu escabeche gambas, almejas, navajas o el marisco que te guste.

Pasta al horno

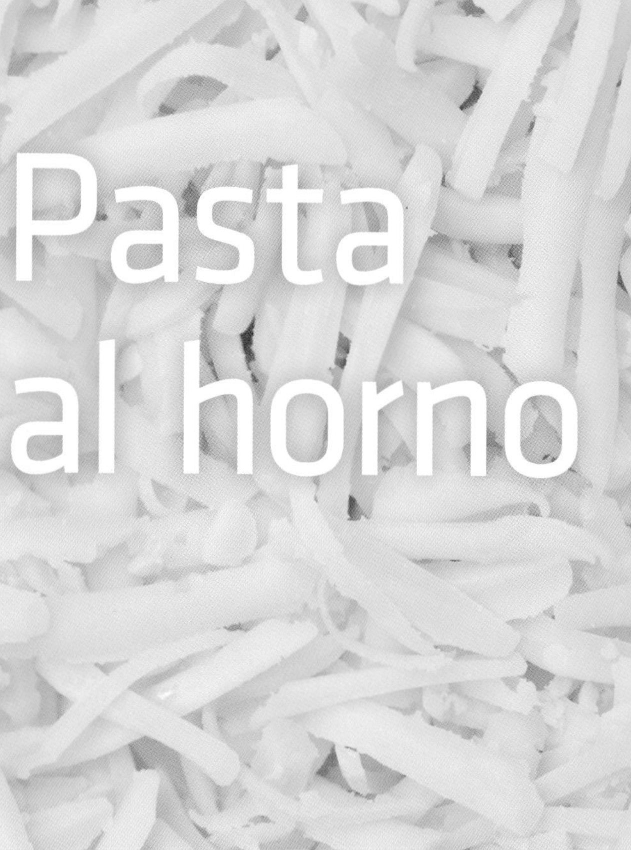

Podemos preparar casi cualquier tipo de pasta en el horno, no solo canelones o lasaña.

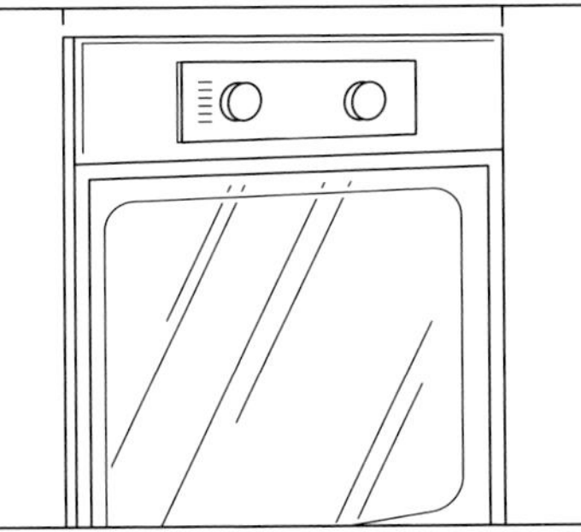

Sobre todo la que vaya acompañada de salsa de queso o bechamel.

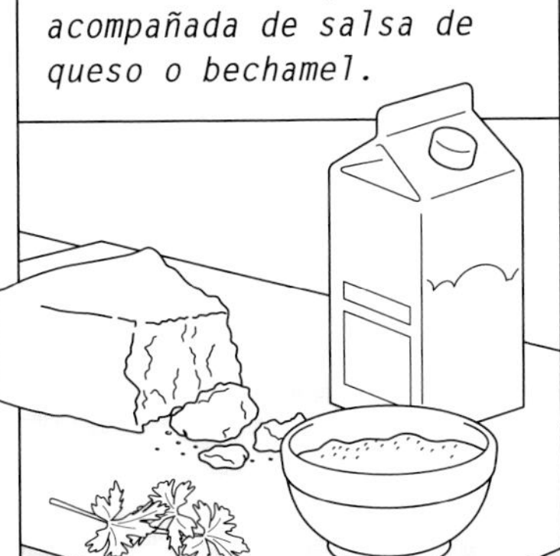

Alguna, como los fideos finos para fideuá, podemos cocerla directamente en el horno.

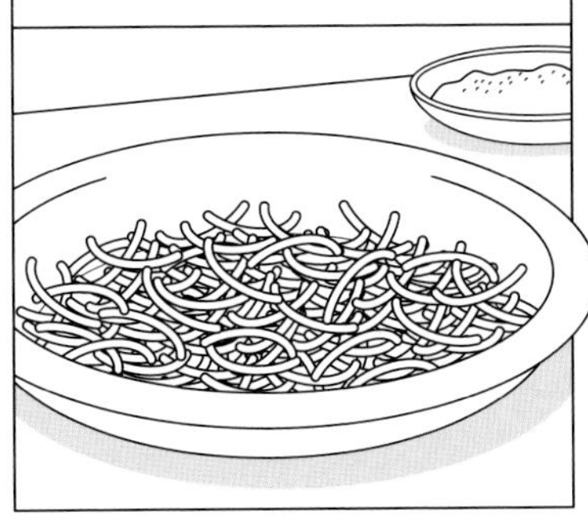

Podemos también gratinar simplemente, hasta que la salsa esté crujiente y dorada.

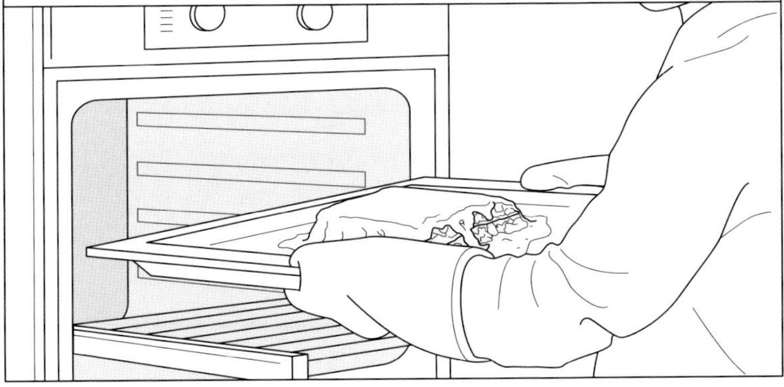

Te mostraré desde cómo preparar canelones con carne o verduras...

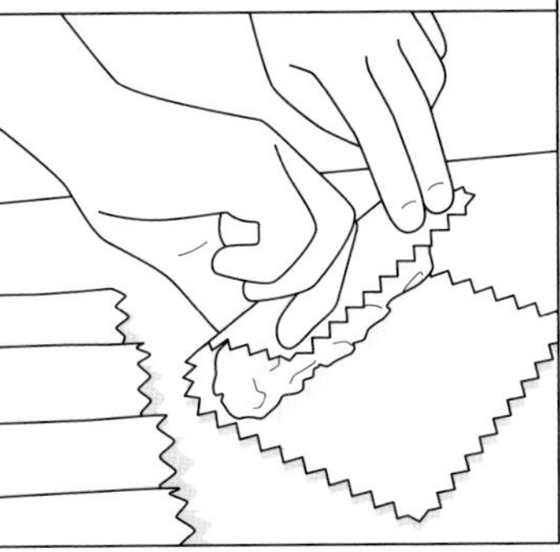

... hasta hacer unos canelones “de gala”, con setas, trufas y foie.

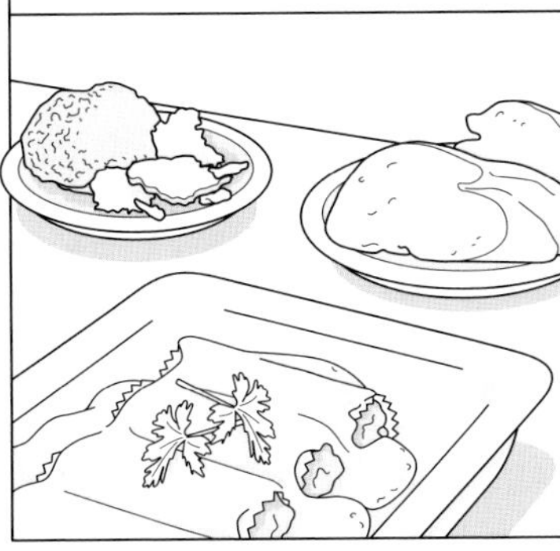

Te convertirás en el maestro de las lasañas...

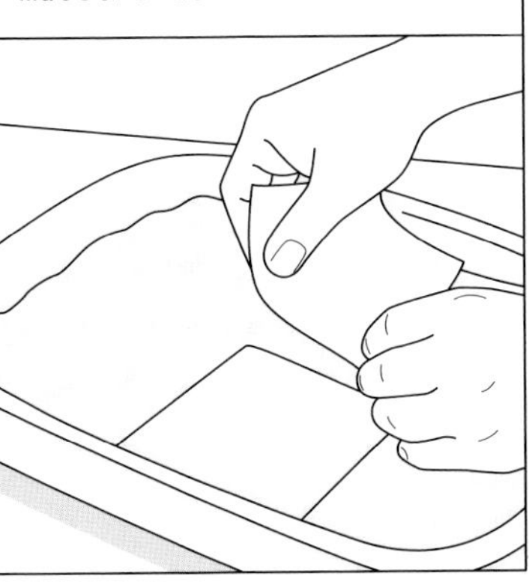

... y prepararás estupendos sofritos para tu pasta al horno.

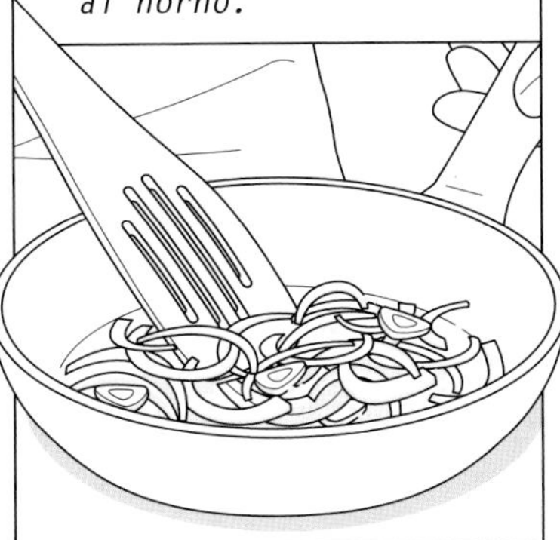

Canelones

El ingrediente

En principio, para elaborar canelones podemos emplear la misma masa que para la elaboración de las lasañas. Se trata de pasta fresca cortada en cuadrados, que en este caso enrollaremos para formar el canelón. Aun así, existen masas de pasta más modernas o exóticas con las que podemos elaborar nuestras preparaciones (masas ultrafinas como la pasta *won-ton*), masas de pasta a base de harina de arroz, o incluso alguna con la peculiaridad de ofrecernos una textura crujiente tras el horneado, como pueden ser la pasta filo o la pasta *brick*.

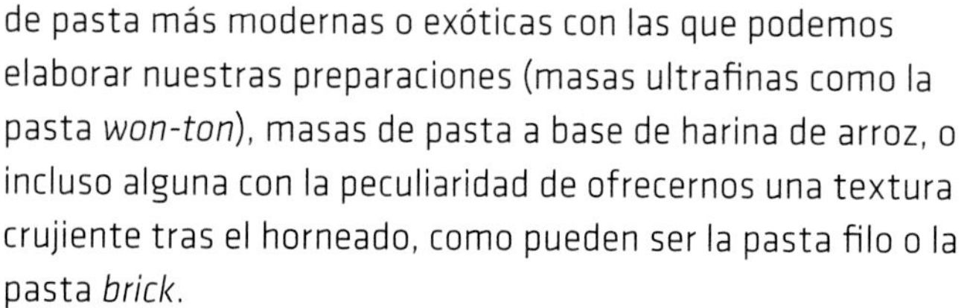

La técnica

Para poder rellenar canelones en serie, dispón un trapo de cocina bien limpio sobre una mesa de trabajo, pon los canelones sobre el trapo, superpuestos, uno encima de otro, formando algo parecido a una escalera, dejando la mitad libre donde dispondrás el relleno. Ya solo queda enrollar los canelones, cocerlos y servirlos en la bandeja de horno.

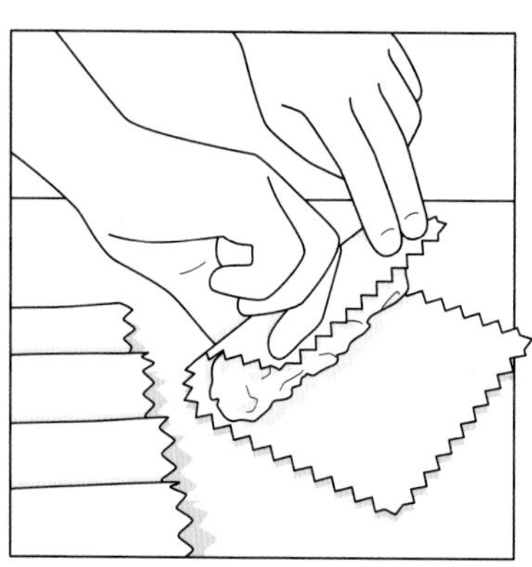

Plato a plato

Nivel **1** **Canelones a la boloñesa.** Empieza rompiendo un mito: preparar canelones no es laborioso ni difícil. Sigue los pasos de la receta y obtendrás unos jugosos canelones rellenos de carne.

Nivel **2** **Canelones de jamón, espinacas y alcachofas.** Dale la vuelta a un clásico de los canelones para vegetarianos combinando las clásicas espinacas con deliciosas alcachofas. Para los carnívoros puedes añadir unas tiras de jamón.

Nivel **3** **Canelones de setas y trufa con crema de *foie*.** Llegados a este punto, atrévete con la versión más sofisticada de los clásicos canelones. Albergan en su interior lo más delicioso del bosque en combinación con una exquisitez como el *foie*.

Nivel **1** # Canelones a la boloñesa

- 16 hojas de pasta para canelones
- 500 g de carne de ternera picada
- 75 g de mantequilla
- 125 g de harina + 1 cucharadita
- 1 cebolla
- 1 pimiento verde
- 2 dientes de ajo
- 200 ml de salsa de tomate frito
- 400 ml de leche
- Queso rallado
- Sal y pimienta

45 min

25 min

2 €/persona

Esta receta no está indicada para personas con intolerancia a la lactosa.

■ Cuece la pasta siguiendo las indicaciones del fabricante hasta que esté *al dente*. Una vez cocida, enfríala bajo el chorro de agua fría. Resérvala.

■ En un cazo a fuego lento rehoga la cebolla, el ajo y el pimiento picados finamente. Una vez la verdura se ablande, añade la carne picada y deja que se cueza, salpimienta y agrega una cucharadita de harina y medio vaso de leche. Déjalo cocer durante 3-4 minutos y retira del fuego. Deja enfriar y reserva.

■ Estira las láminas de pasta sobre una mesa de trabajo y dispón una cucharada de la carne preparada sobre cada una. Enrolla la pasta para formar los canelones.

■ Elabora la bechamel. Para hacerla derrite la mantequilla en un cazo a fuego lento, añade la harina y mezcla bien. Vierte entonces el resto de la leche poco a poco, integrándola a la harina con la ayuda de unas varillas de cocina, sin dejar de remover y a fuego muy lento, hasta obtener una salsa lisa y homogénea, sin grumos. Deja cocer 3-4 minutos y salpimienta.

■ Cubre una bandeja de horno con salsa de tomate y dispón los canelones encima. Cubre con bechamel, espolvorea con queso rallado y cuece en el horno a 180 °C durante 10-12 minutos, hasta que los canelones se gratinen bien.

Trucos

Puedes enriquecer la farsa o relleno de carne agregando hierbas aromáticas, setas, frutos secos, verduras o el ingrediente que desees.

Nivel **2**

Canelones de jamón, espinacas y alcachofas

- 16 hojas de pasta para canelones
- 250 g de espinacas frescas
- 100 g de jamón ibérico
- 50 g de piñones
- 75 g de mantequilla
- 125 g de harina + 1 cucharadita
- 6 alcachofas
- 1 cebolla
- 400 ml de leche
- Queso rallado
- Aceite de oliva
- Sal y pimienta

25 min
25 min
2 €/persona
Esta receta no está indicada para personas con intolerancia a la lactosa.

- Cuece la pasta siguiendo las indicaciones del fabricante hasta que esté *al dente*. Una vez cocida, enfríala bajo el chorro de agua fría. Resérvala.
- Limpia las alcachofas y córtalas a dados. Reserva. Rehoga en un cazo a fuego lento la cebolla picada muy fina. Una vez empiece a ablandarse, agrega las alcachofas y deja sofreír todo durante 10-12 minutos, hasta que las alcachofas queden tiernas. Añade entonces los piñones, el jamón cortado en tiras y las espinacas frescas. Mezcla todo bien y déjalo cocer hasta que las espinacas se ablanden. Salpimienta y reserva.
- Estira las láminas de pasta sobre una mesa de trabajo y dispón una cucharada del relleno sobre cada una. Enrolla la pasta para formar los canelones.
- Elabora la bechamel. Para hacerla derrite la mantequilla en un cazo a fuego lento, añade la harina y mezcla bien. Vierte entonces la leche poco a poco, integrándola a la harina con la ayuda de unas varillas de cocina, sin dejar de remover y a fuego muy lento, hasta obtener una salsa lisa y homogénea, sin grumos. Deja cocer 3-4 minutos y salpimienta.
- Rocía una bandeja de horno con un chorrito de aceite de oliva y dispón los canelones. Cúbrelos con la bechamel y espolvorea con queso rallado. Cuece en el horno a 180 °C durante 10-12 minutos, hasta que los canelones se gratinen bien.

Trucos

Añade una cucharadita de miel a las espinacas para enriquecer su sabor. También puedes incorporar uvas pasas o acompañar estos canelones con la tradicional salsa *romesco*.

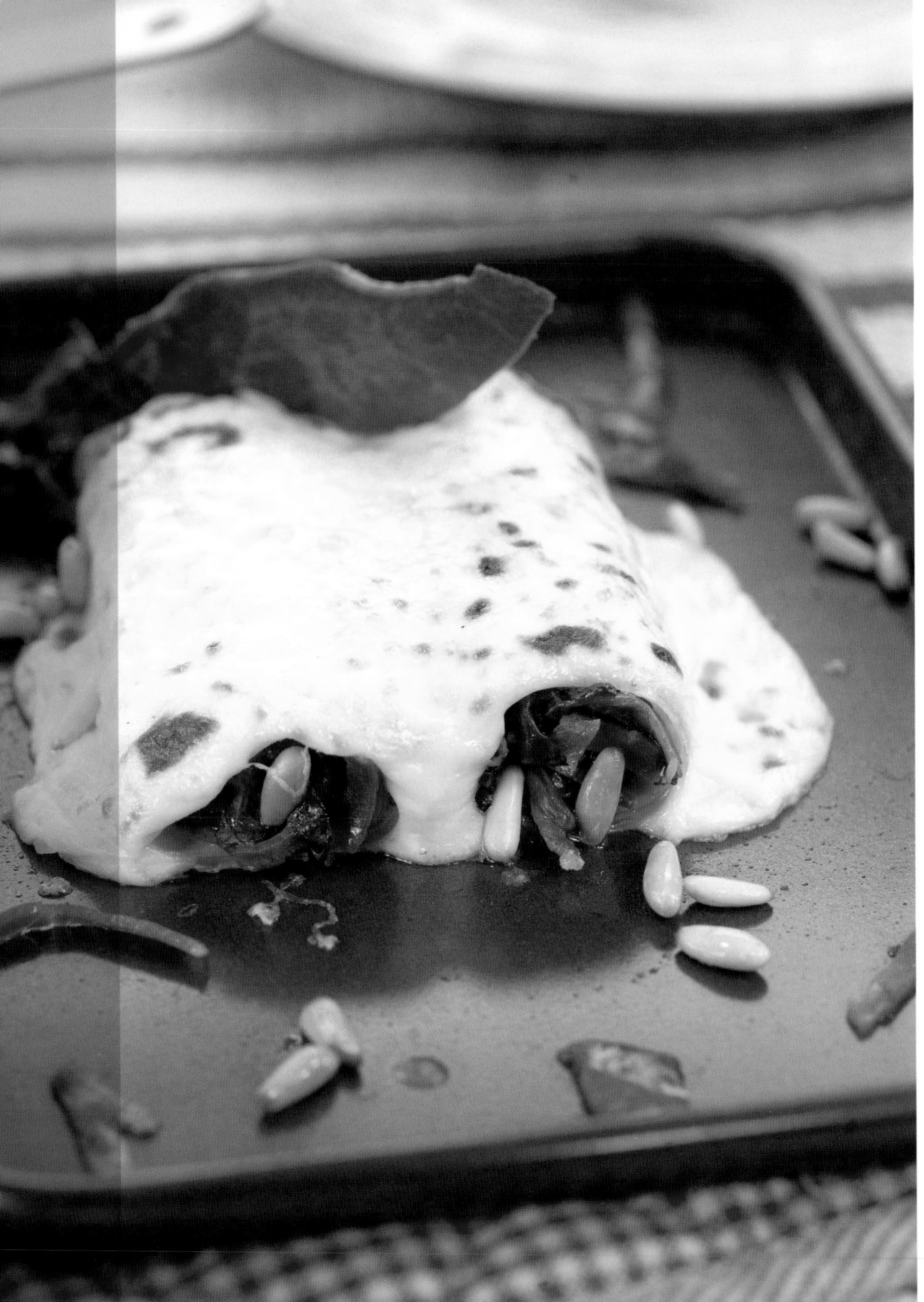

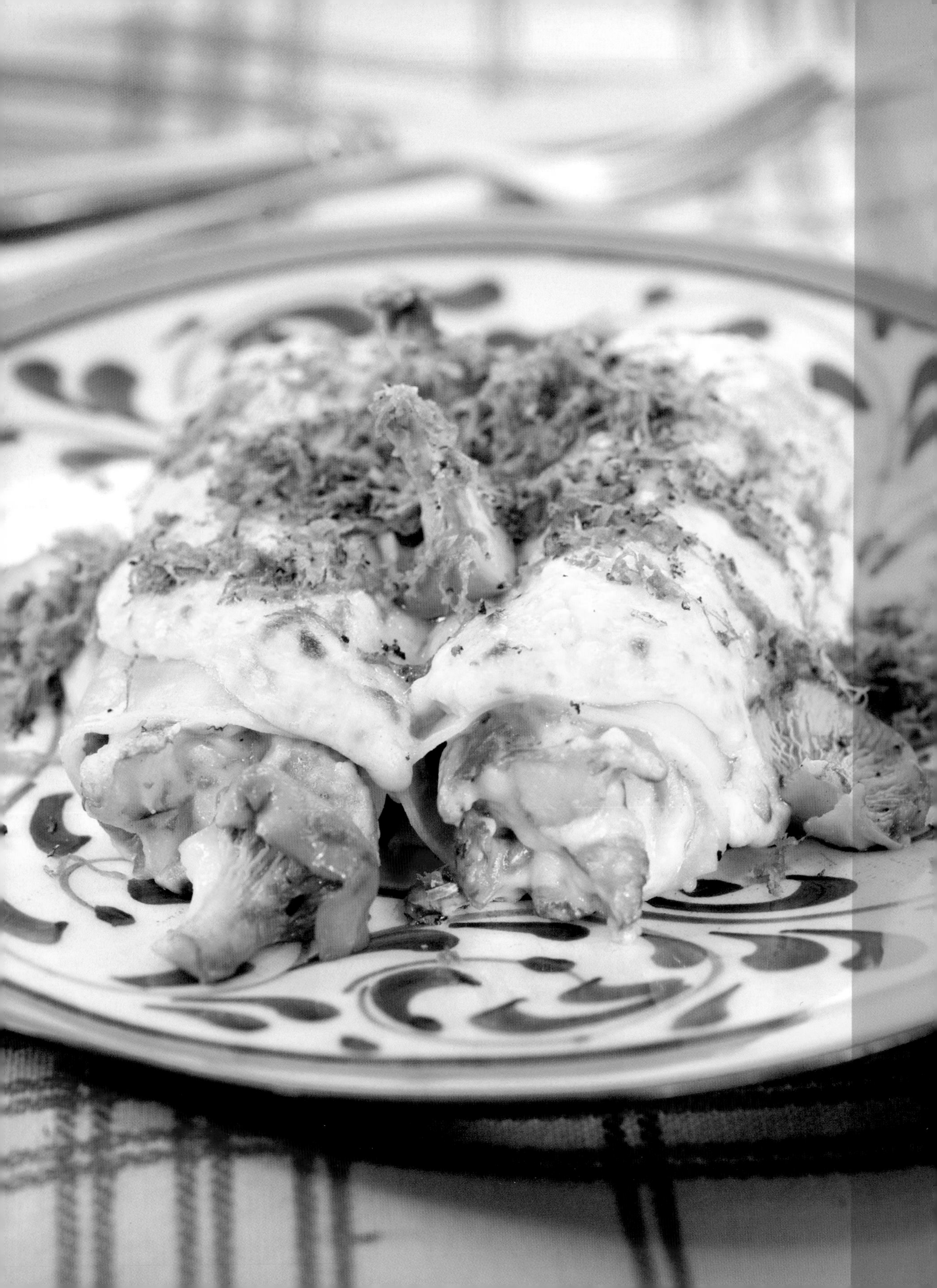

Nivel **3**

Canelones de setas y trufa con crema de *foie*

- 16 hojas de pasta para canelones
- 1 trufa de temporada (10-12 g)
- 400 g de setas de temporada
- 100 g de jamón ibérico
- 200 g de *foie* fresco
- 75 g de mantequilla
- 125 g de harina + 1 cucharada
- 1 cebolla tierna
- 1 puerro
- 2 dientes de ajo
- 400 ml de leche
- Queso rallado
- Aceite de oliva
- Sal y pimienta

30 min
25 min
6 €/persona
Esta receta no está indicada para personas con intolerancia a la lactosa.

- Cuece la pasta siguiendo las indicaciones del fabricante hasta que esté *al dente*. Una vez cocida, enfríala bajo el chorro de agua fría. Resérvala.
- En un cazo a fuego lento rehoga la cebolla, el puerro y el ajo picados muy finitos. Cuando empiece a dorarse agrega las setas limpias y troceadas y deja que se doren.
- Una vez la verdura y las setas estén doradas, incorpora el jamón cortado en tiras y mezcla bien. Agrega una buena cucharada de harina, mezcla con el resto de los ingredientes y añade un buen vaso de leche hasta formar una bechamel espesa de setas y jamón. Deja enfriar.
- Estira las láminas de pasta y dispón una cucharada del relleno sobre cada una. Enrolla la pasta para formar los canelones.
- Elabora la crema de *foie*. Para hacerla, derrite la mantequilla en un cazo a fuego lento. Añade la harina y mezcla bien. Vierte a continuación el resto de la leche poco a poco, agregándola a la harina con la ayuda de unas varillas de cocina, sin dejar de remover y a fuego muy lento, hasta obtener una salsa lisa y homogénea, sin grumos. Deja cocer la bechamel 3-4 minutos, agrega entonces el *foie* cortado a daditos y mezcla bien. Salpimienta.
- Rocía una bandeja de horno con un chorrito de aceite de oliva o aceite de trufas o setas y dispón los canelones. Cúbrelos con la crema de *foie*, y espolvorea queso rallado encima. Cuece en el horno a 180 °C durante 10-12 minutos.

Trucos

Una alternativa a la bechamel de *foie* consiste en triturarlo agregando poco a poco 200 ml de leche hirviendo hasta obtener una crema y cubrir con ella los canelones. No es necesario gratinar.

Lasaña

El ingrediente

Como ya hemos indicado, la pasta empleada para la elaboración de lasañas no dista mucho de la que utilizamos en la elaboración de los canelones. Sin embargo, al contrario que en estos, encontramos pasta para lasañas que no precisa de cocción previa y que puede hornearse directamente. Esta pasta precocida se hidrata con el calor desprendido por el resto de los ingredientes en el horno y resulta muy práctica para elaborar este tipo de propuestas. Existe también pasta fresca para lasaña que podemos adquirir precocida y congelada y que, tras su descongelación, resulta igualmente práctica.

La técnica

Elaborar pasta fresca no tiene por qué ser complejo. Partimos de 100 g de harina especial para pasta, que suele ser harina "00", a la cual agregaremos un huevo y una pizca de sal. Amasaremos bien hasta obtener una masa lisa y homogénea, con textura de plastilina, y la estiraremos sobre una mesa de trabajo enharinada. Ya solo falta cortarla y moldearla.

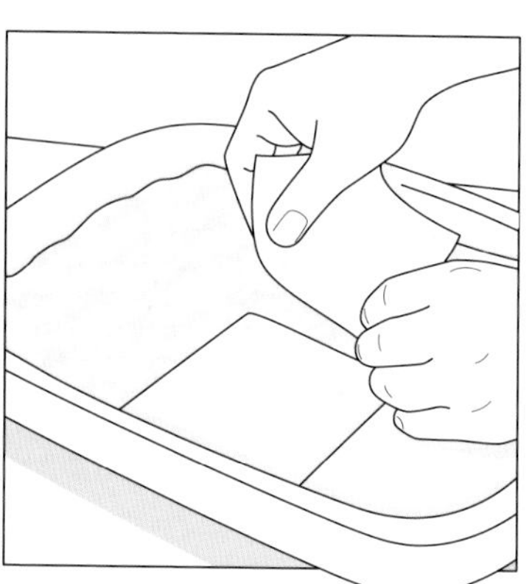

Plato a plato

Nivel **1** **Lasaña de verduras.** Empieza con una lasaña clásica en la que la pasta se intercala con deliciosos pisos de verduras cocidas. Descubrirás que es más fácil de lo que te imaginas.

Nivel **2** **Lasaña de salmón ahumado y queso tierno.** Prueba a hacer una lasaña sustituyendo la clásica pasta italiana por pasta *won-ton* y dale un toque original con el sabor del salmón ahumado.

Nivel **3** **Lasaña ligera de gambas y espárragos con salsa holandesa.** Gradúate en la escuela de la lasaña con una versión especial, con ingredientes sorprendentes y una salsa ligeramente distinta a la clásica bechamel.

Nivel **1** # Lasaña de verduras

- 2 paquetes de pasta para lasaña precocida
- 2 cebolletas
- 2 dientes de ajo
- 2 zanahorias
- 1 puerro
- 1 pimiento verde
- 400 g de champiñones
- 75 g de mantequilla
- 125 g de harina
- 250 ml de salsa de tomate frito casero
- 400 ml de leche
- Queso rallado
- Aceite de oliva
- Sal y pimienta

30 min

25 min

2 €/persona

Esta receta no está indicada para personas con intolerancia a la lactosa.

■ Lamina los ajos y corta las cebolletas, el pimiento y el puerro en juliana. Rehógalos todos juntos en un cazo o una sartén con un chorrito de aceite de oliva. Deja que la verdura se ablande y agrega entonces los champiñones laminados. Cuece durante 5 minutos más, hasta que todos los ingredientes queden tiernos.

■ Vierte el tomate frito en una bandeja de horno y dispón encima una primera capa de pasta fresca. Reparte encima una buena cucharadita de verduras y cubre con otra capa de pasta. Repite esta operación un par de veces hasta formar la lasaña.

■ Derrite la mantequilla en un cazo a fuego lento, añade la harina y mezcla bien. Vierte entonces la leche poco a poco, integrándola a la harina con la ayuda de unas varillas de cocina, sin dejar de remover y a fuego muy lento, hasta obtener una salsa lisa y homogénea, sin grumos. Deja cocer 3-4 minutos y salpimienta. Cubre la lasaña con la bechamel y queso rallado y cuécela al horno a 180 °C durante 18-20 minutos, hasta que la pasta quede cocida y la lasaña gratinada.

Trucos

Puedes variar las verduras de la lasaña a tu gusto, o emplear setas de temporada en lugar de champiñones.

Si lo deseas, puedes intercalar finas lonchas de jamón ibérico en tu lasaña para enriquecer y potenciar su sabor.

Nivel **2**

Lasaña de salmón ahumado y queso tierno

- 2 paquetes de pasta *won-ton*
- 500 g de queso fresco
- 100 g de nueces peladas
- 250 g de espinacas frescas
- 400 g de salmón ahumado
- 2 cebollas tiernas
- 1 bolsa de germinados (100 g)
- 1 puñado de *mezclum*
- 1 manojo de cebollino
- 1 manojo de eneldo fresco
- Mantequilla
- Aceite de oliva
- Sal y pimienta blanca

30 min
15 min
3 €/persona
Esta receta no está indicada para personas con intolerancia a la lactosa.

■ Corta las cebollas en juliana y rehógalas en un cazo o una sartén con un chorrito de aceite de oliva. Cuando se ablande agrega las nueces y las espinacas y saltea hasta que estas estén cocidas. Reserva.

■ Cuece las hojas de pasta *won-ton* en un cazo con agua hirviendo y sal durante 2-3 minutos. Pasado este tiempo saca las hojas del agua caliente y enfríalas en un recipiente con abundante agua y hielo.

■ Unta un molde de horno con una nuez de mantequilla y dispón una base de hojas de pasta *won-ton* hasta formar un rectángulo. Encima pon una fina capa de queso fresco y espolvorea una cucharadita de eneldo. Cubre con otra capa de pasta y dispón esta vez una capa de espinacas y de salmón ahumado. Repite esta operación un par de veces más.

■ Finaliza la lasaña dándole un ligero toque de horno a 180 °C durante 10 minutos. La puedes servir acompañada de un chorrito de aceite de cebollino, un puñado de germinados y *mezclum*. Salpimienta antes de servir.

■ Para elaborar el aceite de cebollino tritura 200 ml de aceite de oliva con un manojo de cebollino hasta obtener un aceite de un color verde intenso y un sabor ligeramente picante.

Trucos

Si no encuentras pasta de tipo *won-ton*, emplea pasta clásica y procede cociendo la pasta o empleándola siguiendo las instrucciones del fabricante.

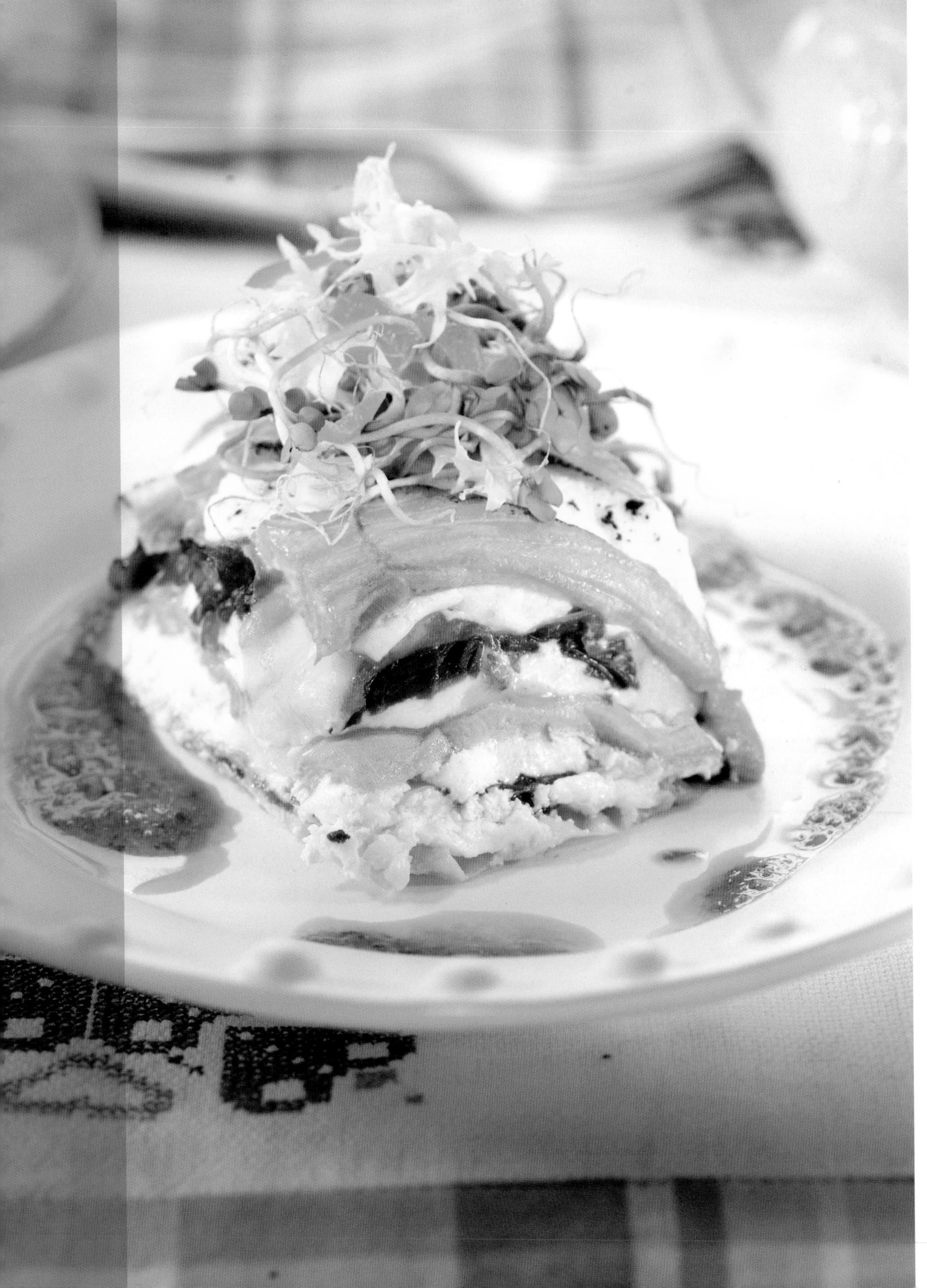

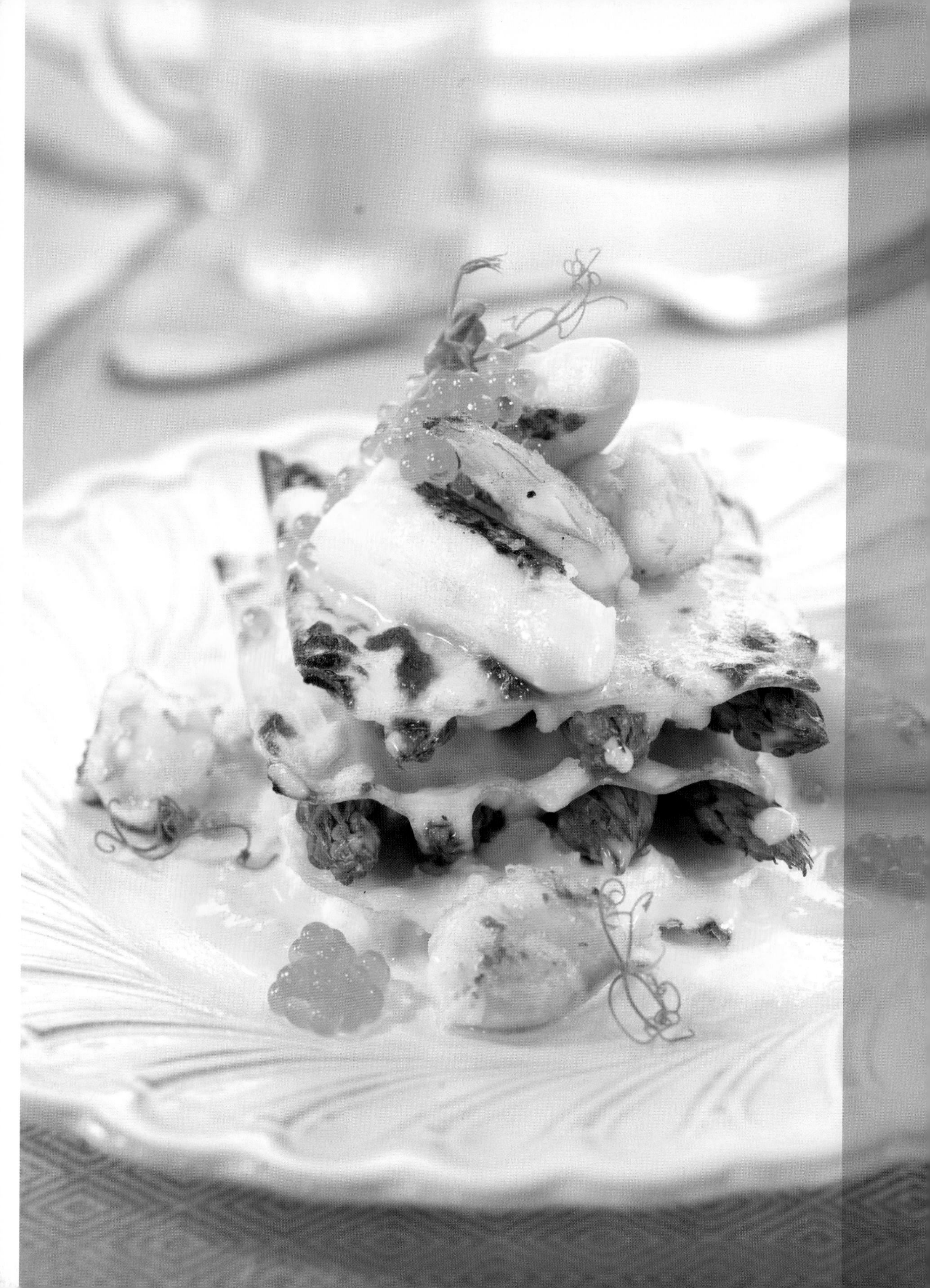

Nivel **3**
Lasaña ligera de gambas y espárragos con salsa holandesa

- 1 paquete de pasta de lasaña precocida
- 1 manojo de puntas de espárragos trigueros
- 12 puntas de espárragos blancos
- 16 gambas o langostinos
- 1 bote de huevas de trucha
- 200 g mantequilla + 1 nuez, para untar
- 4 yemas de huevo
- 2 cucharaditas de zumo de limón
- Sal y pimienta negra

20 min
10 min
4 €/persona
Sin contraindicaciones.

■ Para hacer la salsa holandesa derrite 200 g de mantequilla en un cazo a fuego muy lento. Déjala reposar unos minutos y elimina el suero que aparece en la parte inferior. Con la ayuda de unas varillas de cocina, emulsiona las yemas de huevo al baño María. Agrega la mantequilla de forma paulatina y sin dejar de batir la mezcla cuidadosamente. Debes obtener una emulsión, una crema con textura espumosa. Una vez montada la salsa, mezcla con el zumo de limón, una pizca de sal y otra de pimienta negra recién molida. Reserva. Si la salsa se cortase, vuelve a empezar el proceso de nuevo con instrumentos de cocina limpios y añadiendo la parte cortada a otra yema de huevo poco a poco, hasta que vuelva a ligar.

■ Cuece los espárragos trigueros durante 2 minutos en un cazo con agua hirviendo. Transcurrido este tiempo, saca los espárragos del agua y déjalos enfriar. Reserva.

■ Dispón una lámina de pasta precocida en una bandeja de horno previamente untada con mantequilla. Distribuye sobre la pasta 4 puntas de espárrago triguero, cubre con otra hoja de pasta y repite la operación. En la parte superior de la lasaña dispón las puntas de espárragos blancos y las gambas peladas.

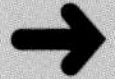

Nivel 3 Lasaña ligera de gambas y espárragos con salsa holandesa

➜ Cubre con la salsa holandesa y hornea a 190 °C durante 8-10 minutos, hasta que la salsa quede bien gratinada. Sirve acompañado de huevas de trucha y un chorrito de aceite de oliva.

Trucos

☛ Si tienes dificultades a la hora de elaborar la salsa holandesa, puedes servir esta lasaña con una bechamel ligera y queso parmesano recién rallado y espolvoreado en la lasaña. Luego gratínala al horno hasta que quede ligeramente dorada y el queso fundido.

Pasta con sofrito

El ingrediente
Entendemos como sofrito una base de verduras picadas y cocinadas a fuego lento hasta que adquieren el punto de cocción deseado, para emplear posteriormente en la elaboración de salsas o bien para aplicar directamente como base de infinidad de preparaciones. Un sofrito puede contener solo cebollas, ajos y puerros o bien combinar estos tipos de *alliums* con pimientos, zanahorias, etc. En muchas ocasiones ligamos las verduras con una salsa añadida que por lo general, y tratándose de platos de pasta, suele ser de tomate frito, pero también se puede ligar con un caldo de ternera, ave o verduras.

La técnica
A la hora de elaborar nuestro sofrito es importante que la verdura o verduras empleadas estén finamente picadas o, al menos, cortadas a un tamaño regular para que no se doren unas y queden crudas otras. No todas las verduras tienen el mismo tiempo de cocción; si empleamos puerro, por ejemplo, deberemos dejar que el resto de las verduras estén ya tiernas antes de incorporarlo, ya que este tiene un textura muy fina y se cocina con rapidez. En el caso de utilizar tomate fresco o elementos ricos en agua (como el calabacín), esperaremos a que las verduras "secas" se doren antes de agregarlos, pues el agua desprendida por el tomate cortaría de algún modo la cocción del resto de verduras.

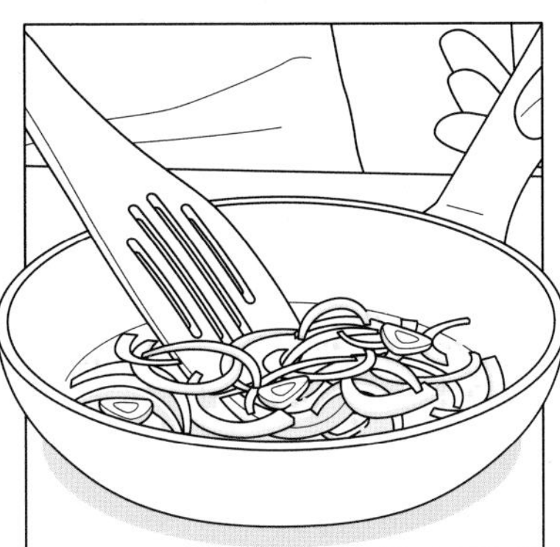

Plato a plato

Nivel **1** ***Rigatoni* gratinados al horno con bechamel.** Empieza con un básico de pasta con sofrito y el toque cremoso de la bechamel. Puedes elegir las verduras a tu gusto.

Nivel **2** **Canelones de tomate, cigala y olivas griegas.** Sorprende a tus comensales con unos canelones con sorpresa. La pasta *won-ton* los hace muy ligeros.

Nivel **3** **Nidos de espaguetis con vieiras al horno.** Para el tercer nivel prueba a acompañar la pasta con vieiras, cuya textura combina a la perfección con los espaguetis.

Nivel 1 *Rigatoni* gratinados al horno con bechamel

- 400 g de *rigatoni*
- 1 cebolla
- 1 puerro
- 2 dientes de ajo
- 75 g de mantequilla
- 125 g de harina
- 400 ml de leche
- Queso rallado
- Aceite de oliva
- Sal y pimienta

20 min
20 min
2 €/persona
Esta receta no está indicada para personas con intolerancia a la lactosa.

- Cuece la pasta siguiendo las indicaciones del fabricante hasta que esté *al dente*. Por lo general, tratándose de pasta seca, el tiempo de cocción será de aproximadamente 16 minutos. Una vez cocida, enfría la pasta bajo el chorro de agua fría. Resérvala.
- Sofríe la cebolla, el puerro y el ajo en un cazo o una sartén con un chorrito de aceite de oliva a fuego lento, hasta que la verdura se ablande. Añade entonces los *rigatoni* y mezcla bien. Salpimienta y dispón la pasta en una bandeja de horno.
- Para hacer la bechamel derrite la mantequilla en un cazo a fuego lento, añade la harina y mezcla bien. Vierte entonces la leche poco a poco, integrándola a la harina con la ayuda de unas varillas de cocina, sin dejar de remover y a fuego muy lento, hasta obtener una salsa lisa y homogénea, sin grumos. Deja cocer 3-4 minutos y salpimienta.
- Vierte la bechamel sobre los *rigatoni* y espolvorea queso rallado por encima. Gratina al horno a 180 °C, durante 8-10 minutos.

Trucos

No cabe decir que puedes emplear la pasta corta que desees. Aquí hemos calculado 100 g de pasta por persona para obtener un primer plato copioso; en el caso de agregar otros ingredientes a la receta, como carne picada, pollo o marisco, deberás reducir la cantidad de pasta utilizada y cocer 75 g por persona.

Finalmente, no olvides que la salsa bechamel puede resultar algo pesada si no se elabora correctamente.

Nivel **2** Canelones de tomate, cigalas y olivas griegas

- 8-12 láminas de pasta *won-ton*
- 8-12 cigalas
- 4 tomates rojos de rama
- 1 cebolleta tierna
- 2 dientes de ajo
- 2 cucharadas de miel
- 150 g de olivas griegas de Kalamata
- 100 g de tirabeques
- 1 manojo de cebollino
- Aceite de oliva
- Sal y pimienta

20 min
10 min
6 €/persona
Sin contraindicaciones.

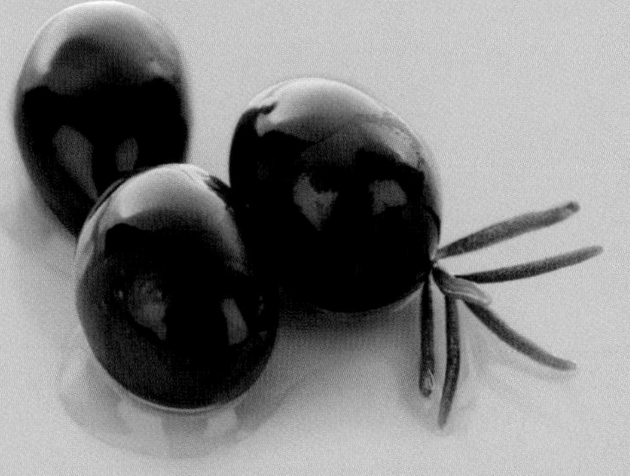

- Cuece las hojas de pasta *won-ton* en un cazo con agua hirviendo y sal durante 2-3 minutos. Pasado este tiempo saca las hojas del agua caliente y enfríalas en un recipiente con abundante agua y hielo.
- Lamina los dientes de ajo y corta en juliana la cebolleta y los tirabeques. Sofríelo todo en una sartén o un cazo, con un chorrito de aceite de oliva, a fuego lento. Una vez la verdura se ablande, añade las cigalas peladas y retira de inmediato del fuego, dejando que estas se cocinen muy brevemente. Reserva.
- Pela los tomates, elimina las semillas, córtalos en gajos o estrújalos y reserva.
- Prepara una olivada con la mitad de las olivas deshuesadas y trituradas y la miel hasta obtener una crema o puré. Reserva.
- Estira las hojas de pasta *won-ton* sobre una mesa de trabajo y dispón en un extremo una cigala con una cucharadita de la verdura salteada, un par de pétalos de tomate y un par de olivas deshuesadas. Cierra la pasta formando un canelón y calienta al horno durante 3-4 minutos.
- Una vez los canelones estén calientes sírvelos con una cucharada de olivada y cebollino picado. Salpimienta con moderación, ya que las olivas al horno ofrecen un punto salado a nuestra preparación.

Trucos

Pon una fina capa de agua en la bandeja de horno para calentar los canelones sin que estos se peguen a la bandeja. Si los dejas más tiempo en el horno, la pasta se gratinará y quedará ligeramente crujiente.

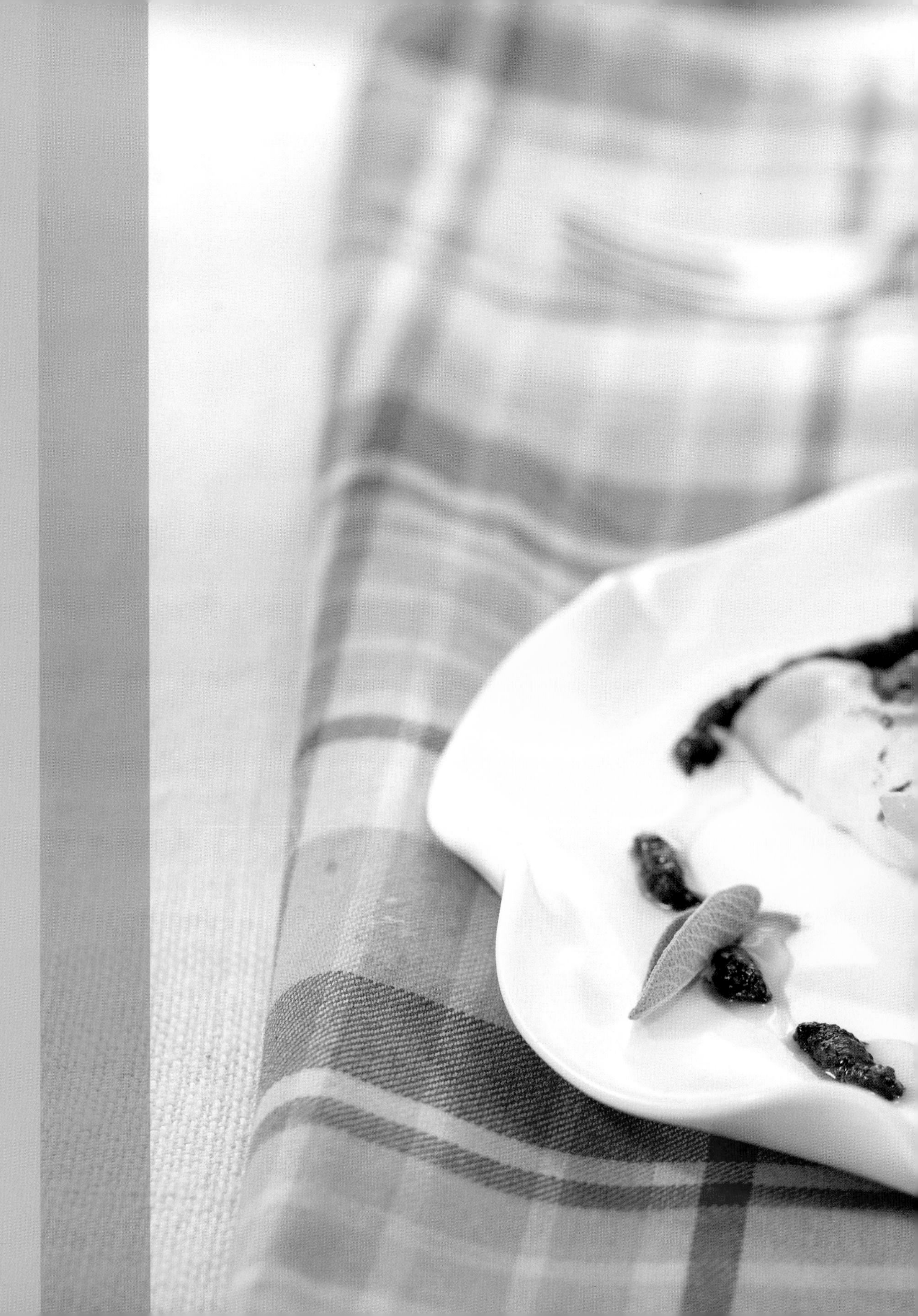

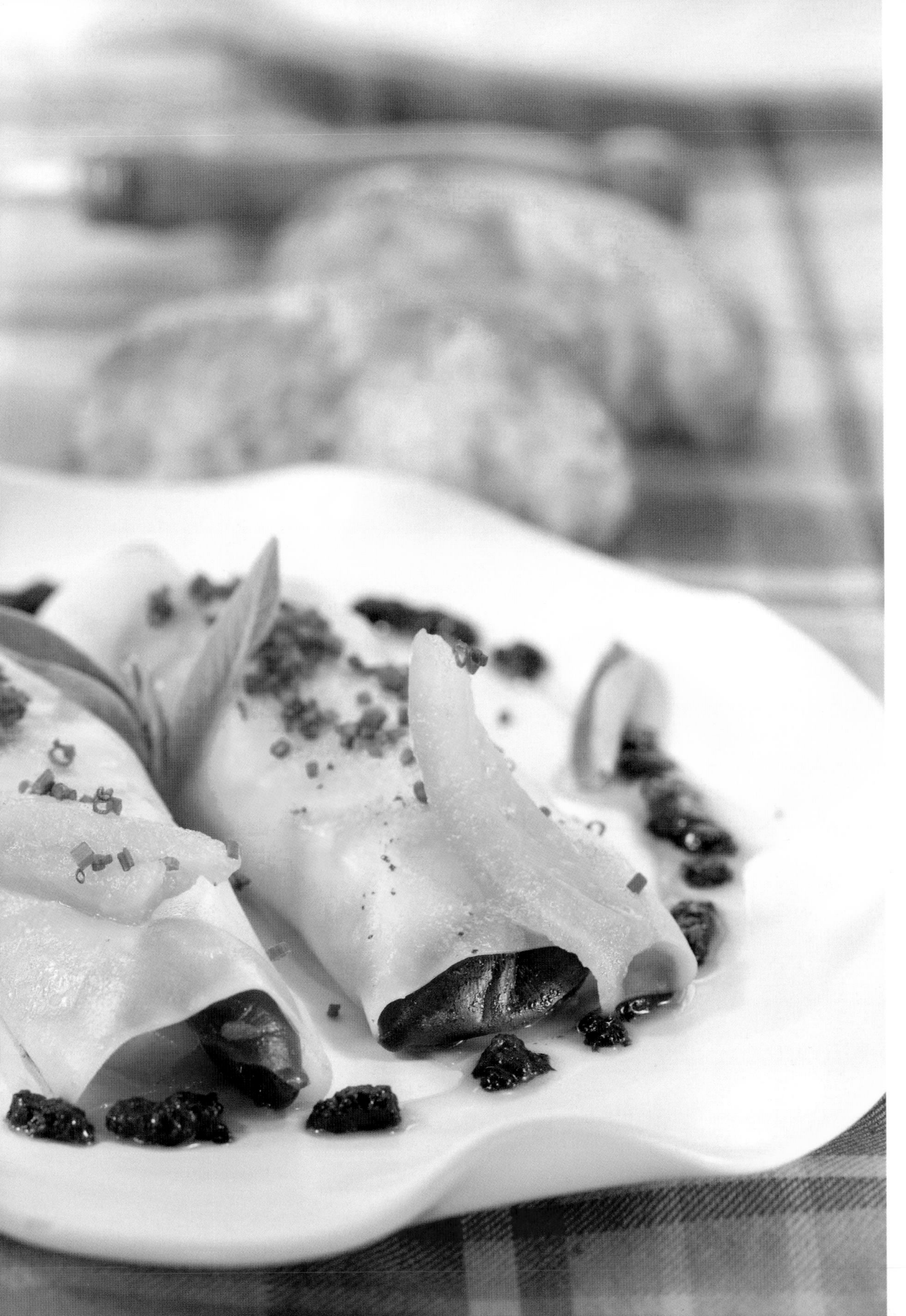

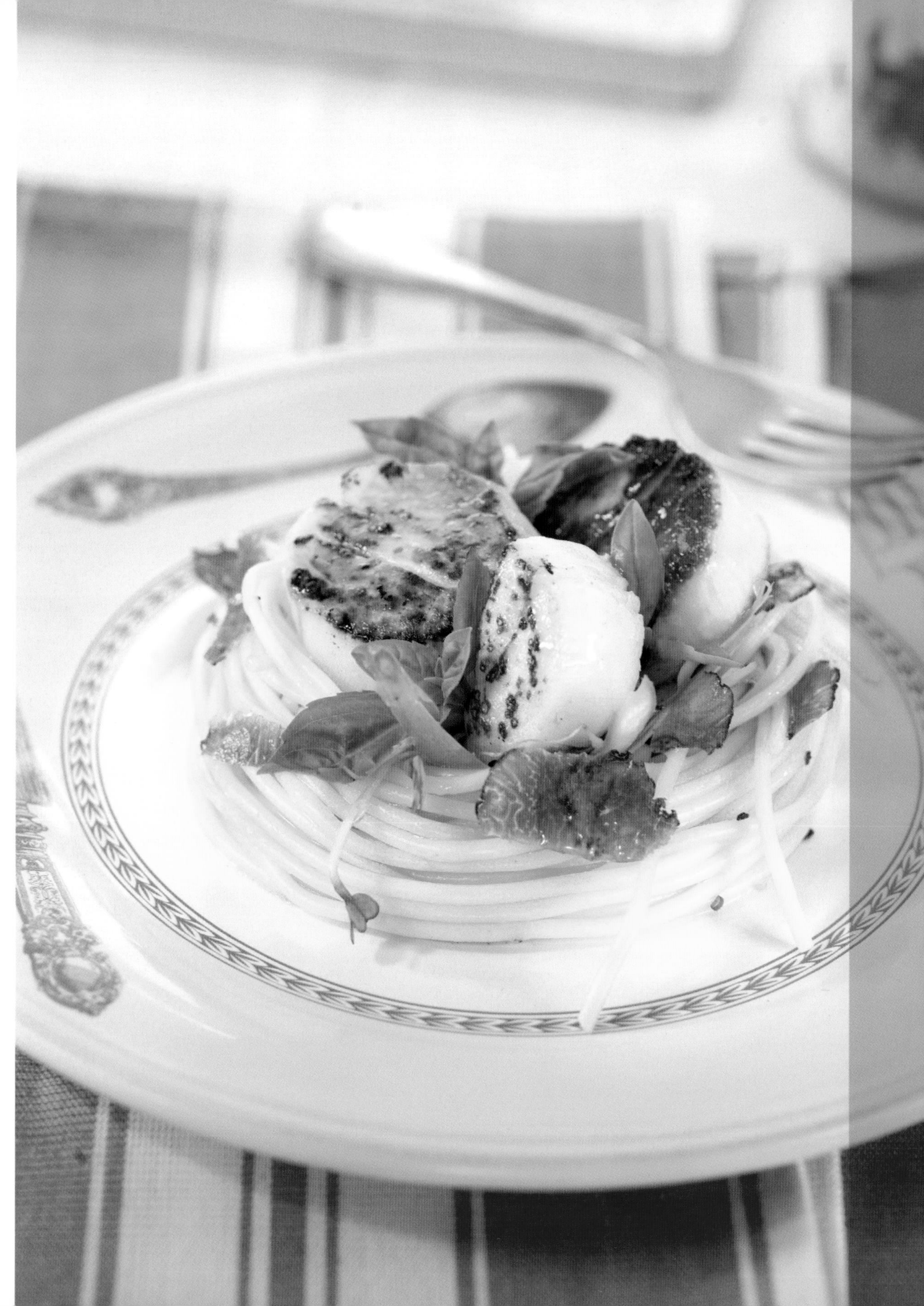

Nivel **3**

Nidos de espaguetis con vieiras al horno

- 12 vieiras limpias
- 300 g de pasta fresca de tipo espagueti
- 2 yemas de huevo
- 2 cebollas tiernas
- 2 manojos de espárragos trigueros
- 1 trufa de temporada (10 g)
- Aceite de oliva
- Sal y pimienta

15 min
20 min
6 €/persona
Sin contraindicaciones.

■ Cuece la pasta siguiendo las indicaciones del fabricante hasta que esté *al dente*. Una vez cocida la pasta, enfríala bajo el chorro de agua fría. Resérvala.

■ Sofríe la cebolla cortada en juliana en una sartén o en un cazo con un chorrito de aceite a fuego lento. Una vez se ablande, añade los espárragos cortados en cuartos y saltea. Reserva.

■ Con la ayuda de un molde metálico de cocina forma nidos con los espaguetis. Píntalos con la yema de huevo batida, dispón en su interior el salteado de cebolla y espárragos y salpimienta. Hornea a 180 °C durante 8-10 minutos, hasta que la pasta esté bien caliente.

■ Sácala del horno, retira el molde metálico y sírvela acompañada de las vieiras, que freirás en una sartén con una pizca de sal y un chorrito de aceite de oliva. Ralla la trufa en el instante de servir y agrega si lo deseas un chorrito de aceite de oliva.

Trucos

Puedes enriquecer aún más esta preparación añadiendo al sofrito unas cigalas, gambas, mejillones, navajas, etc. También bañando la pasta con una bechamel muy ligera.

Arr

oces

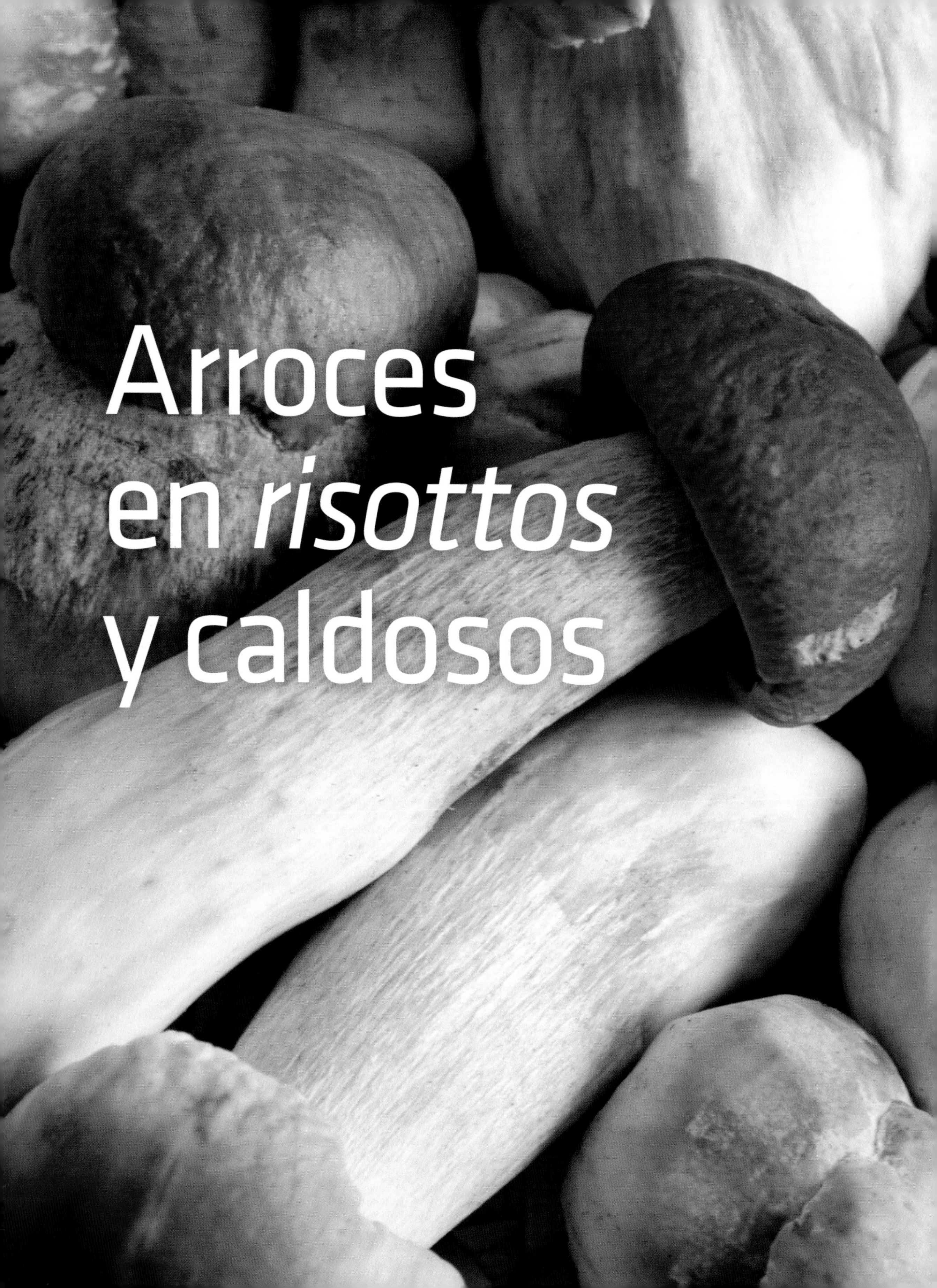

Arroces en *risottos* y caldosos

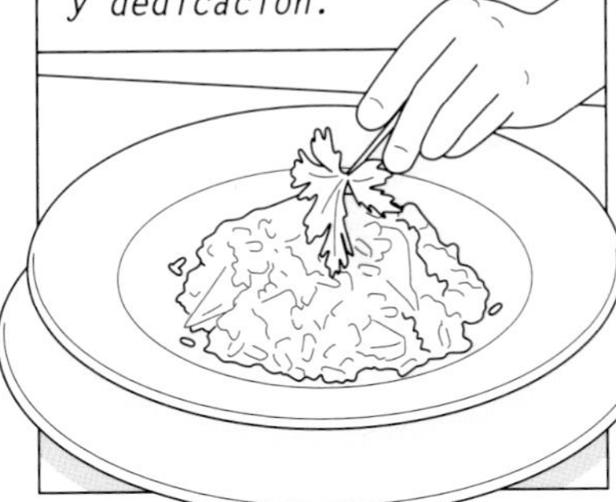
Para preparar risottos no hace falta ser un chef ni una mamma italiana, solo hace falta cariño y dedicación.

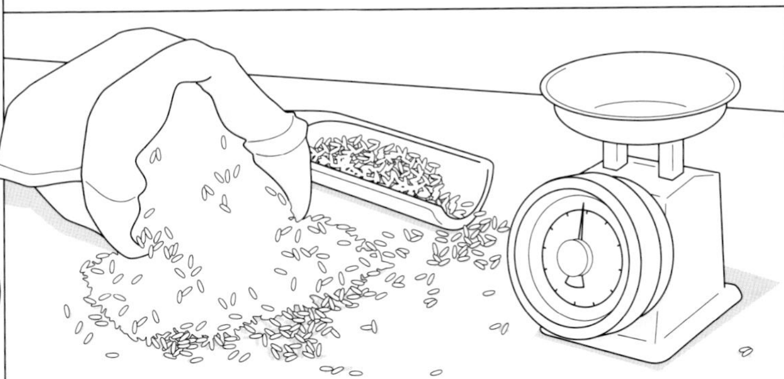
Se suele utilizar arroz de grano corto, que tiene un alto contenido en almidón.

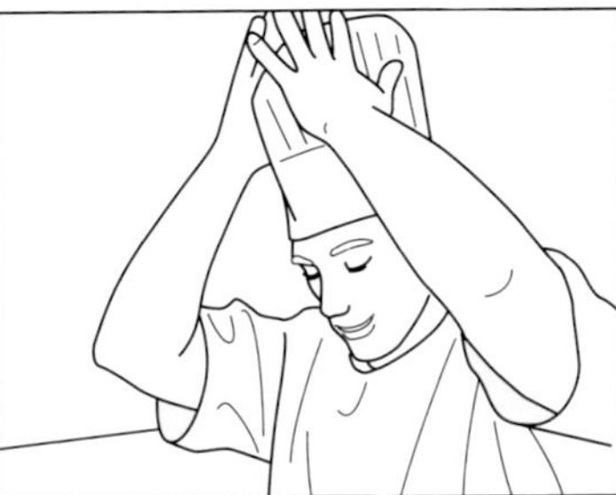
Es este almidón bien trabajado el que da la melosidad característica al risotto.
¡Manos a la obra!

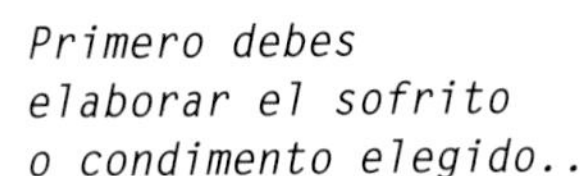
Primero debes elaborar el sofrito o condimento elegido...

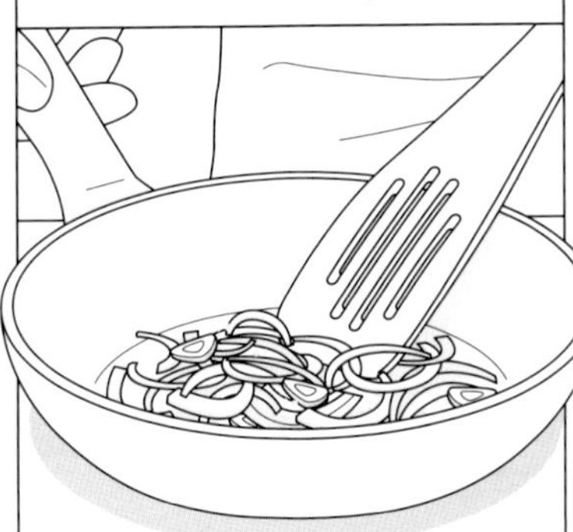

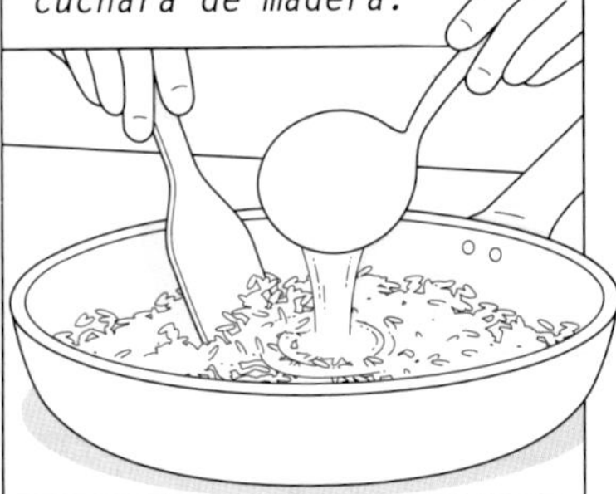
Después, agregar el arroz e ir "regándolo" poco a poco con caldo, mientras lo remueves con una cuchara de madera.

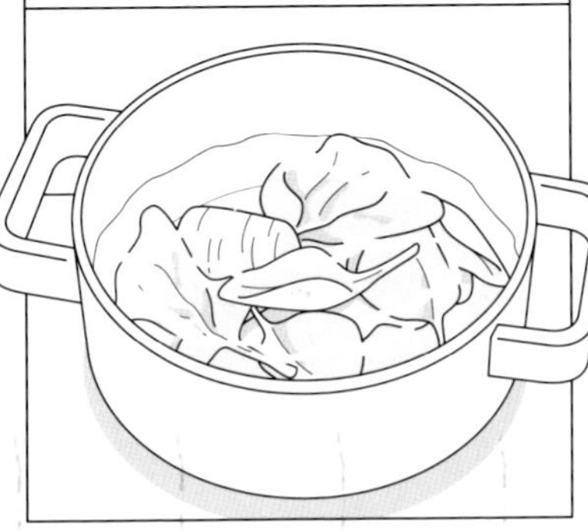
Por supuesto que también te voy a enseñar a hacer caldo para arroces...

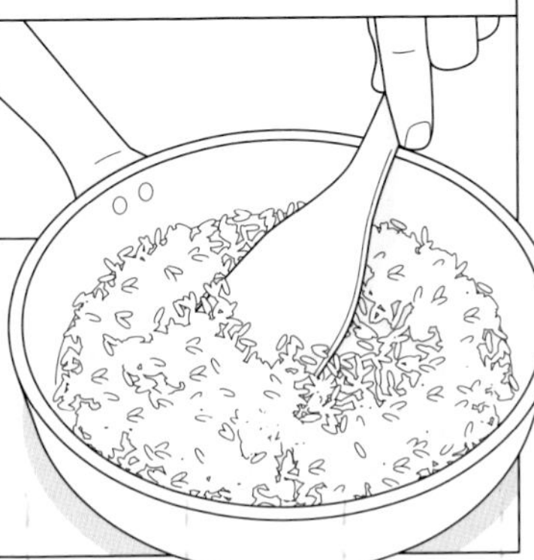
Debes ir moviendo el arroz para que libere el almidón.

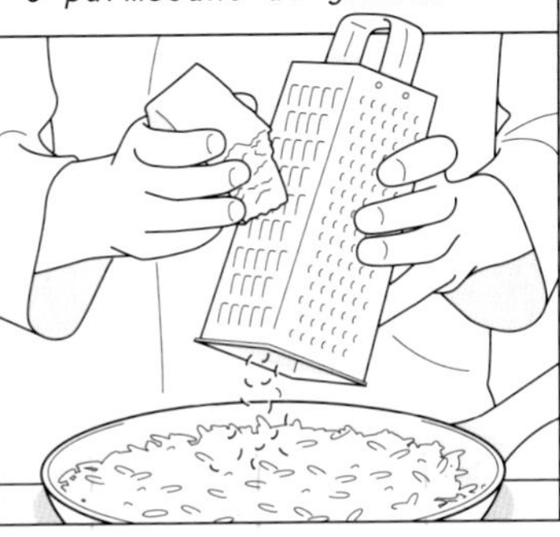
Cuando el arroz esté cocido, solo tienes que agregar crema de leche, mantequilla o parmesano al gusto.

Risottos

El ingrediente

Cuando vayamos a adquirir arroz para *risotto* y solicitemos información o consejo, muy probablemente nos dirijan hacia las variedades de arroz italiano, de tipo Vialone, Carnaroli, Arborio, etc. Se trata sin duda de una sugerencia acertada, pero no por eso debemos descuidar los excelentes arroces nacionales de grano corto, por ejemplo el de tipo bomba como el del Delta del Ebro, que resulta excepcional para la elaboración de arroces melosos y *risottos*.

La técnica

El *risotto* debe "trabajarse" durante todo el proceso de cocción. Con esta afirmación nos referimos a que es aconsejable remover cuidadosa y constantemente el arroz durante el proceso de cocción, si es con una cuchara de madera, mejor. El movimiento que conferimos al guiso provoca que el arroz desprenda almidón, espesando así nuestro caldo y resultando un arroz con textura cremosa sin la necesidad de agregar mantequillas, cremas o quesos para ligar el arroz.

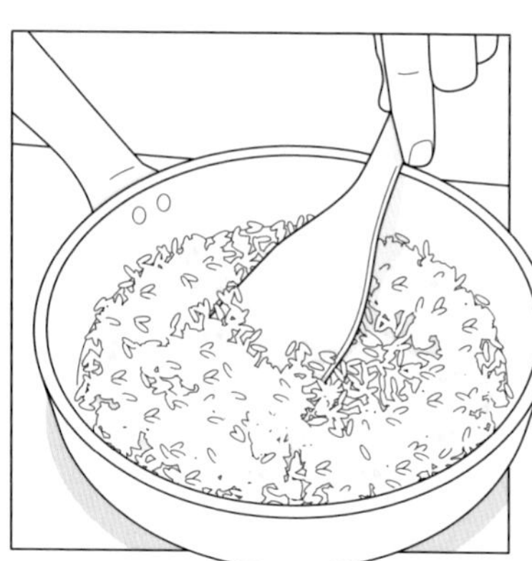

Plato a plato

Nivel **1** ***Risotto* a la milanesa.** Estrénate en el mundo del *risotto* con una receta básica, en la que el arroz se cuece en caldo y se le da un toque cremoso con mantequilla y parmesano.

Nivel **2** ***Risotto* de *ceps* y aceite de trufa.** Da un paso más aromatizando el arroz con los aristócratas de la familia de las setas. Obtendrás un arroz meloso y con sabor otoñal.

Nivel **3** ***Risotto* al azafrán del Líbano servido dentro de una camisa de gambas.** Atrévete a coronar tu *risotto* con un envoltorio de gambas en *carpaccio*. Obtendrás una combinación de sabores y texturas que no te dejará indiferente.

Nivel **1** *Risotto* a la milanesa

- 300 g de arroz bomba
- 50 g de queso parmesano
- 1 nuez de mantequilla (75g)
- 1 l de caldo de verduras o pollo
- Una pizca de azafrán (2 g)
- Sal y pimienta

10 min
20 min
3 €/persona
Esta receta no está indicada para personas con intolerancia a la lactosa.

- En un cazo o una sartén a fuego medio rehoga los granos de arroz y el azafrán con la mitad de la mantequilla. Deja que el arroz se sofría durante 4-5 minutos.
- Transcurrido este tiempo cubre con el caldo bien caliente y deja que se consuma absorbido por el arroz. Vuelve a cubrir el arroz con caldo y así sucesivamente, hasta cocer el arroz por completo (aproximadamente 16 minutos). No podemos parar de remover el arroz durante todo el proceso de cocción.
- Por último, deja que el caldo se evapore por completo y agrega el resto de la mantequilla y el parmesano, mezcla bien y déjalo reposar un par de minutos. Corrige el punto de sal y sirve.

Trucos

Es conveniente calentar ligeramente el azafrán antes de proceder a su utilización, pues de esta manera obtendremos un sabor intenso y todas las propiedades de tan deliciosa especia. Puedes hacerlo en el sofrito previo o bien en un platito al horno.

Nivel **2** # *Risotto* de *ceps* y aceite de trufa

- 200 g de arroz bomba
- 600 g de *ceps* (*Boletus edulis*)
- 1 trufa fresca de temporada (10 g)
- 6 cebollas tiernas
- 1 manojo de cebollino
- 50 ml de nata líquida
- Aceite aromatizado de *ceps*
- Aceite de oliva
- Sal y pimienta

30 min
20 min
6 €/persona
Esta receta no está indicada para personas con intolerancia a la lactosa.

- Prepara un caldo de *ceps*. Para ello, dora en un cazo 3 cebollas cortadas en juliana con un buen chorro de aceite de oliva. Cuando la cebolla esté dorada, añade 300 g de *ceps* troceados y deja que se doren igualmente. Una vez dorados, llena el cazo con agua (1,5 l) y deja que las setas infusionen durante unos 20-25 minutos a fuego lento. Salpimienta, cuela el caldo y reserva.
- En una sartén sofríe a fuego lento las cebollas restantes picadas muy finas. Cuando empiecen a dorarse añade el resto de las setas y deja que se doren, añade el arroz y sofríe durante un par de minutos.
- Transcurrido este tiempo, añade el caldo de *ceps* poco a poco, sin dejar de remover y en pequeñas cantidades, dejando que el arroz absorba el caldo antes de agregar más. Deja que el arroz se cueza durante unos 16-18 minutos.
- Transcurrido este tiempo deja que el arroz se seque y añade la nata líquida. Cuece durante 2-3 minutos, añade el cebollino picado y deja reposar.
- Corrige el punto de sal y sirve el arroz. En el momento de servir ralla trufa fresca encima y rodea el plato con un chorrito de aceite de *ceps*.

Trucos

Puedes preparar este *risotto* fuera de temporada empleando setas deshidratadas. Ten en cuenta que antes de usarlas deberás hidratarlas en agua caliente o caldo durante un par de horas. Conserva esta agua de remojo para elaborar el caldo de *ceps*.

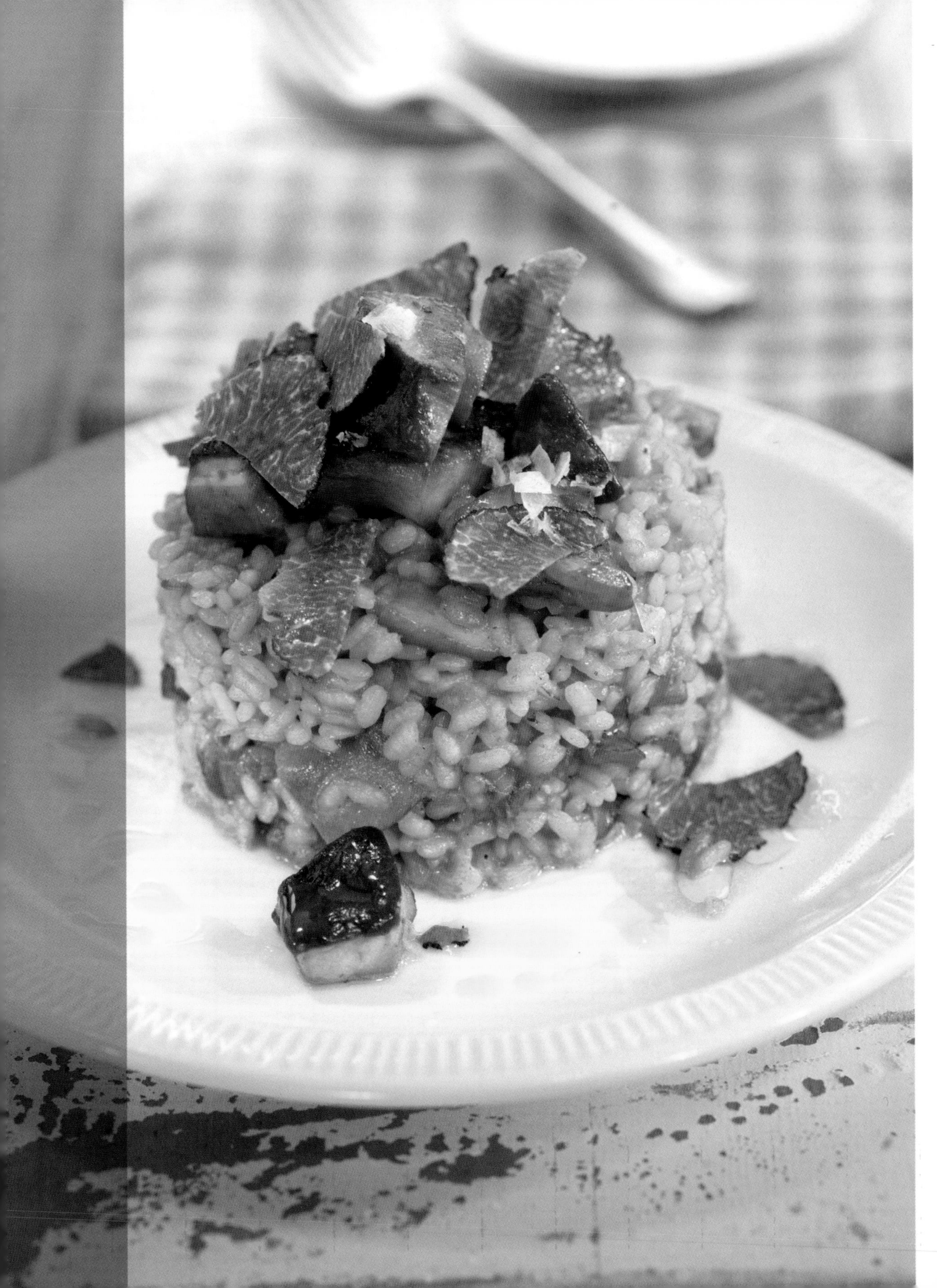

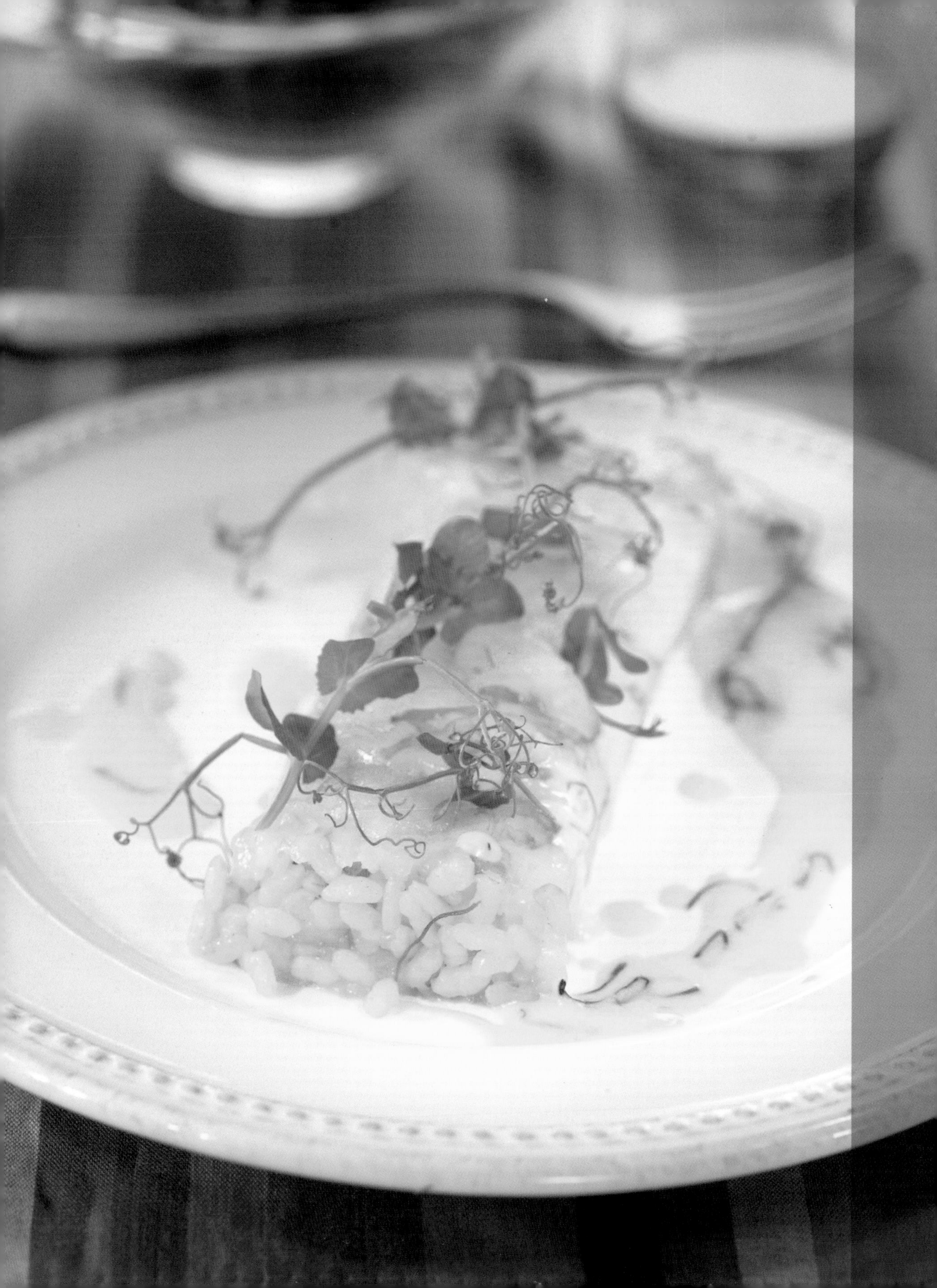

Nivel **3** *Risotto* al azafrán del Líbano servido dentro de una camisa de gambas

- 200 g de arroz bomba
- 24 gambas rojas
- 2 g de azafrán del Líbano
- 600 ml de caldo de ave
- Mantequilla
- 1 manojo de cebollino
- Aceite de oliva
- Sal fina y en escamas y pimienta
- Germinados

30 min
20 min
6 €/persona
Esta receta no está indicada para personas alérgicas al marisco.

■ Limpia las gambas y disponlas sobre un papel antiadherente, puede ser papel de horno o papel film; con la ayuda de un pincel de cocina unta ligeramente la hoja con aceite de oliva y dispón las gambas sobre esta formando un cuadrado, abiertas en medias lunas. Pliega la hoja hasta cubrir las gambas y aplástala con la ayuda de un rodillo de cocina u otro instrumento de superficie plana. Deberás obtener un *carpaccio* de gamba muy fino. Congélalo.

■ Sofríe el arroz junto al azafrán en una sartén con un chorrito de aceite de oliva. Rehoga durante un par de minutos y vierte el caldo caliente poco a poco, sin dejar de remover y esperando que el arroz absorba el caldo antes de seguir agregando más. Realiza esta operación durante 14-16 minutos, hasta que el arroz esté bien cocido. Deja por último que el arroz se seque bien.

■ Una vez seco el arroz, agrega una nuez de mantequilla y un buen puñado de cebollino picado muy fino, salpimienta y deja reposar un par de minutos.

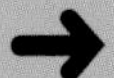

Nivel 3 *Risotto* al azafrán del Líbano servido dentro de una camisa de gambas

➜ ■ Mientras tanto, saca el *carpaccio* de gambas del congelador.
■ Sirve el arroz en un plato alargado, formando algo similar a un canelón o una forma cilíndrica. Dispón el *carpaccio* sobre el arroz y moldéalo ayudándote de una espátula. Agrega una pizca de sal en escamas y un chorrito de aceite de oliva antes de servir. Puedes acompañarlo también con un puñado de germinados.

Trucos

☛ Si te resulta más fácil, dispón el *carpaccio* de gambas sobre una mesa de trabajo, sirve el arroz sobre él y con la ayuda de una espátula cierra el *carpaccio* hasta encerrar el arroz en él.

☛ También puedes acompañar con una crema de azafrán. Para prepararla, derrite en un cazo a fuego lento una nuez de mantequilla con una pizca de azafrán, deja que se cueza un minuto y agrega la nata. Déjalo cocer hasta que espese ligeramente y salpimienta.

Arroces caldosos

El ingrediente

El caldo es, junto con el sofrito o los ingredientes integrados en nuestra preparación, el responsable del sabor final de nuestro arroz, por ello debes cuidar esta preparación con mimo y esmero. Puedes elaborar caldos de carne, pescado, verduras, setas o aves, pero todos ellos deben potenciar el sabor de nuestro arroz, por lo que deben ser elaborados con productos nobles, ya sean huesos, carcasas o verduras tiernas. No debes emplear la verdura atrasada o las carnes, ya sean de ternera, pollo o pescado al límite de su caducidad, ya que otorgarías un sabor ácido o amargo al caldo que luego se verá reflejado en el resultado final del arroz.

La técnica

Elabora un sofrito de verduras que potencie el sabor de nuestro caldo. Además, como hemos dicho anteriormente, para preparar los caldos se precisan carcasas de ave, espinas de pescado o huesos de vaca. Conviene asar al horno hasta dorar estos elementos para extraer un intenso aroma de ellos. En el caso del pescado, es suficiente cocerlos en agua con las verduras apropiadas.

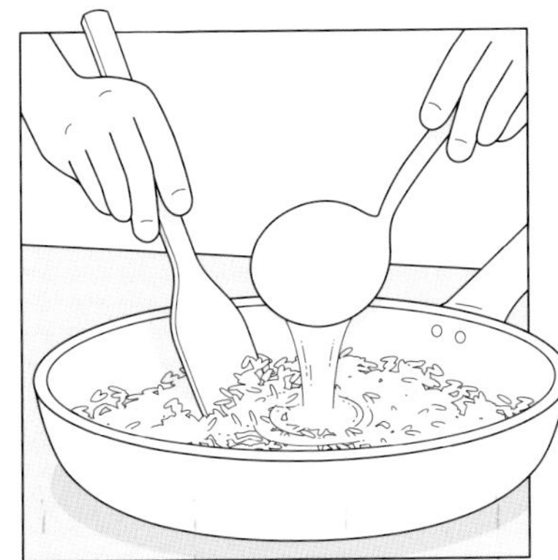

Plato a plato

Nivel **1** **Arroz caldoso con guisantes y alcachofas.** Un arroz con todo el verde de la huerta. Con él descubrirás que el arroz caldoso es tan fácil que te preguntarás por qué no lo has hecho antes.

Nivel **2** **Arroz caldoso con ñoras y espinacas.** Una versión un poco más original con el toque único del bacalao, que en esta ocasión se acompaña del aroma de la ñora, con la que casa a la perfección.

Nivel **3** **Arroz caldoso con bogavante.** Atrévete con un plato con mucha tradición en la cocina de pescadores. El selecto bogavante es una pieza clave con todas las garantías de éxito.

Nivel 1 Arroz caldoso con guisantes y alcachofas

- 300 g de arroz bomba
- 300 g de guisantes frescos
- 6 alcachofas
- 1 cebolla
- 1 puerro
- 1 zanahoria
- 2 dientes de ajo
- 2 tomates de rama
- Aceite de oliva
- Sal y pimienta

10 min (+ 2 h caldo)
20 min
2 €/persona
Sin contraindicaciones.

- En una olla o una cazuela reparte la cebolla, el puerro, la zanahoria, los dientes de ajo y los tomates troceados. Cúbrelo con 3 litros de agua mineral, agrega un chorrito de aceite de oliva y deja cocer, primero a fuego vivo hasta que arranque a hervir, y luego a fuego lento durante un par de horas, hasta que el caldo reduzca a dos tercios del volumen inicial. Cuela el caldo, salpimienta y consérvalo caliente.
- Limpia y corta las alcachofas a cuartos o a sextos, dependiendo del tamaño. Sofríelas en una cazuela, a ser posible de barro, a fuego lento y con un chorrito de aceite de oliva. Una vez empiecen a dorarse, agrega los guisantes y el arroz y sofríe todo junto durante un par de minutos.
- Vierte 1 litro de caldo caliente sobre el arroz y deja que arranque a hervir, en ese momento baja el fuego y deja que el arroz se cueza durante 15-16 minutos a fuego lento.
- Transcurrido este tiempo comprueba la cocción del grano y agrega un cucharón de caldo si fuera necesario. Salpimienta y sirve al instante.

Trucos

Puedes elaborar el caldo en la olla a presión: en apenas 25 minutos lo tendrás listo para su empleo. También puedes trocear las verduras y agregarlas al arroz.

Nivel **2** Arroz caldoso con ñoras y espinacas

- 300 g de arroz bomba
- 100 g de espinacas frescas
- 2 lomos de bacalao
- 1 espina de bacalao
- 1 cebolla
- 1 puerro
- 1 pizca de azafrán (1 g)
- 2 dientes de ajo
- 2 tomates de rama
- 8 ñoras
- Aceite de oliva
- Sal y pimienta

20 min (+ 2 h caldo)

20 min

4 €/persona

Sin contraindicaciones.

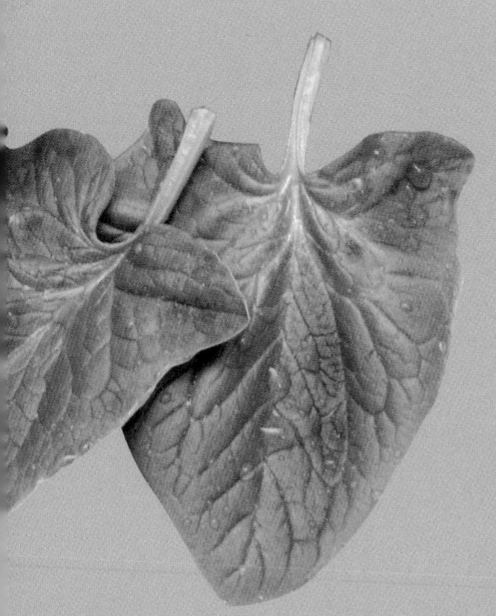

■ Hidrata las ñoras sumergiéndolas en un recipiente con agua caliente. Mientras tanto, sofríe la cebolla y el puerro cortados en trozos regulares en una olla o una cazuela con un chorrito de aceite de oliva. Una vez estén blancos, añade la carne de las ñoras, el azafrán y el tomate troceado, mezcla bien, incorpora la espina de bacalao y cúbrelo con 2 litros de agua. Déjalo cocer a fuego medio durante una hora.

■ Rehoga los dientes de ajo laminados en una sartén o una cazuela con un chorrito de aceite de oliva. Cuando se ablanden añade los lomos de bacalao y el arroz, mezcla bien y báñalo con 1 litro de caldo de ñoras. Deja que arranque a hervir y cuece a fuego lento durante aproximadamente 16 minutos. El resultado deberá ser un arroz muy caldoso; si se ha secado agrega más caldo.

■ Dos minutos antes de retirar del fuego añade las espinacas, mezcla bien y deja que se cuezan. Salpimienta.

Trucos

Comprueba la cocción del arroz partiendo un grano por la mitad, si aún le falta cocción, su núcleo se presentará con un punto blanco en el centro, que será crocante al paladar. El arroz estará tierno cuando este punto haya desaparecido.

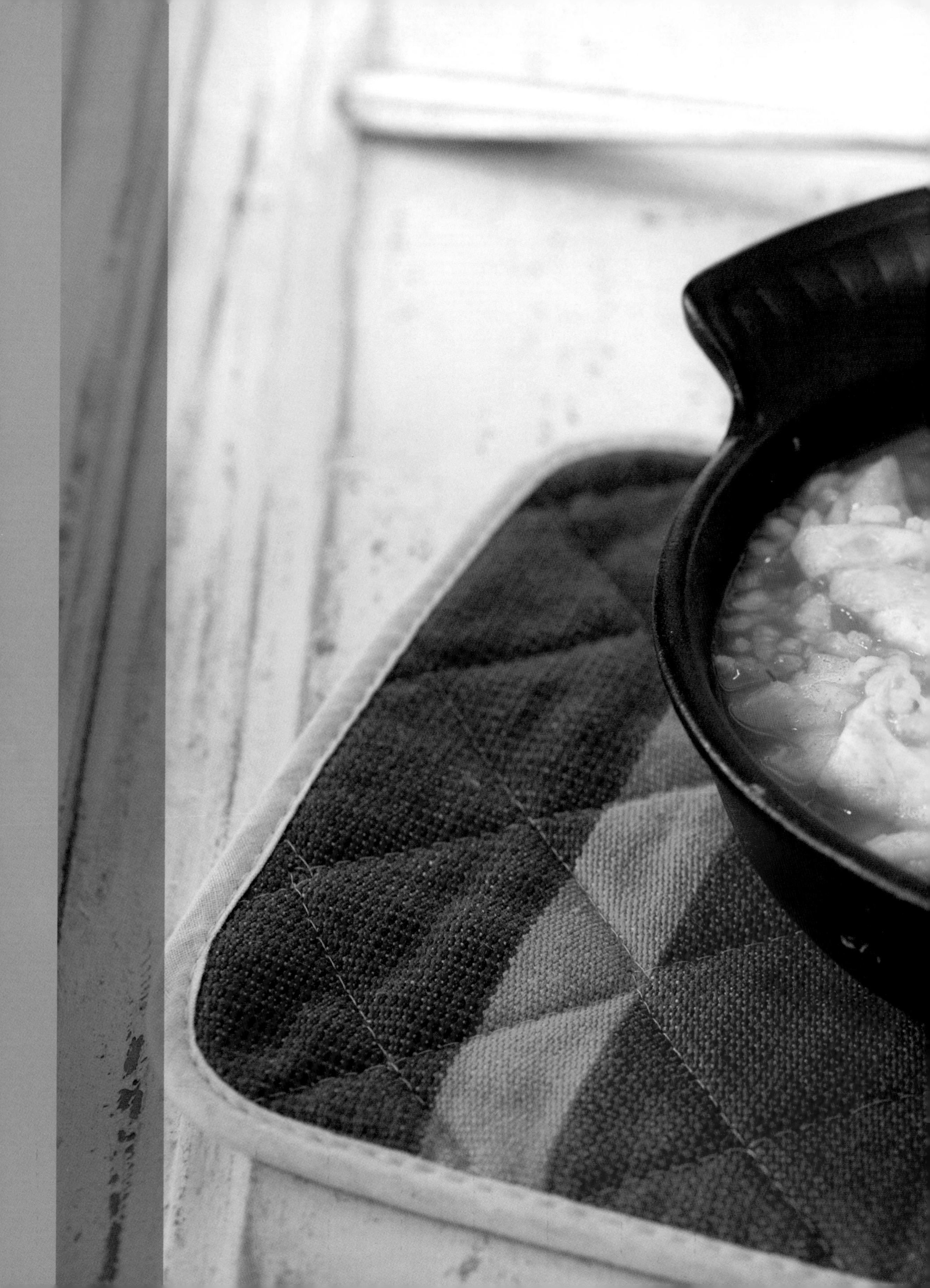

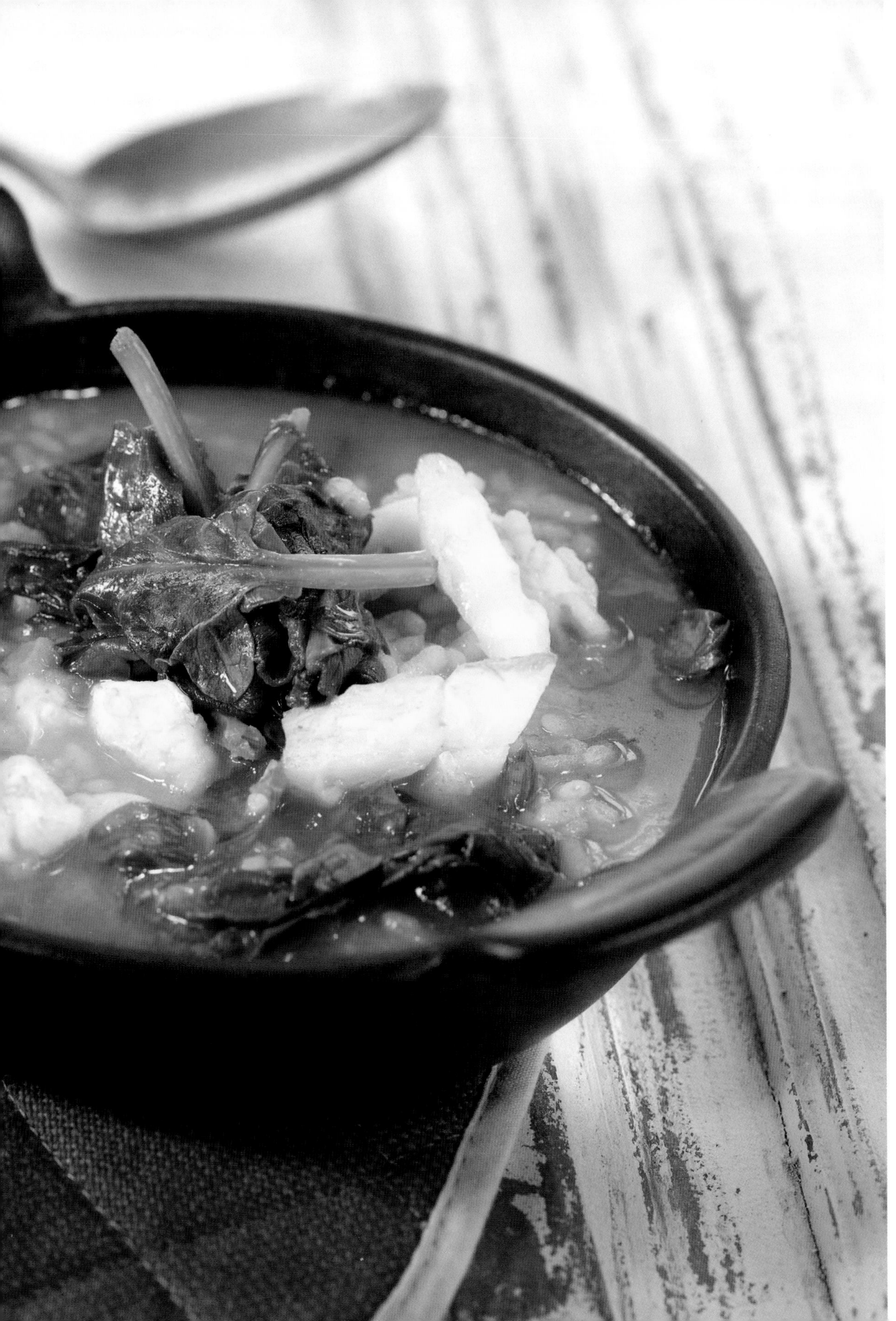

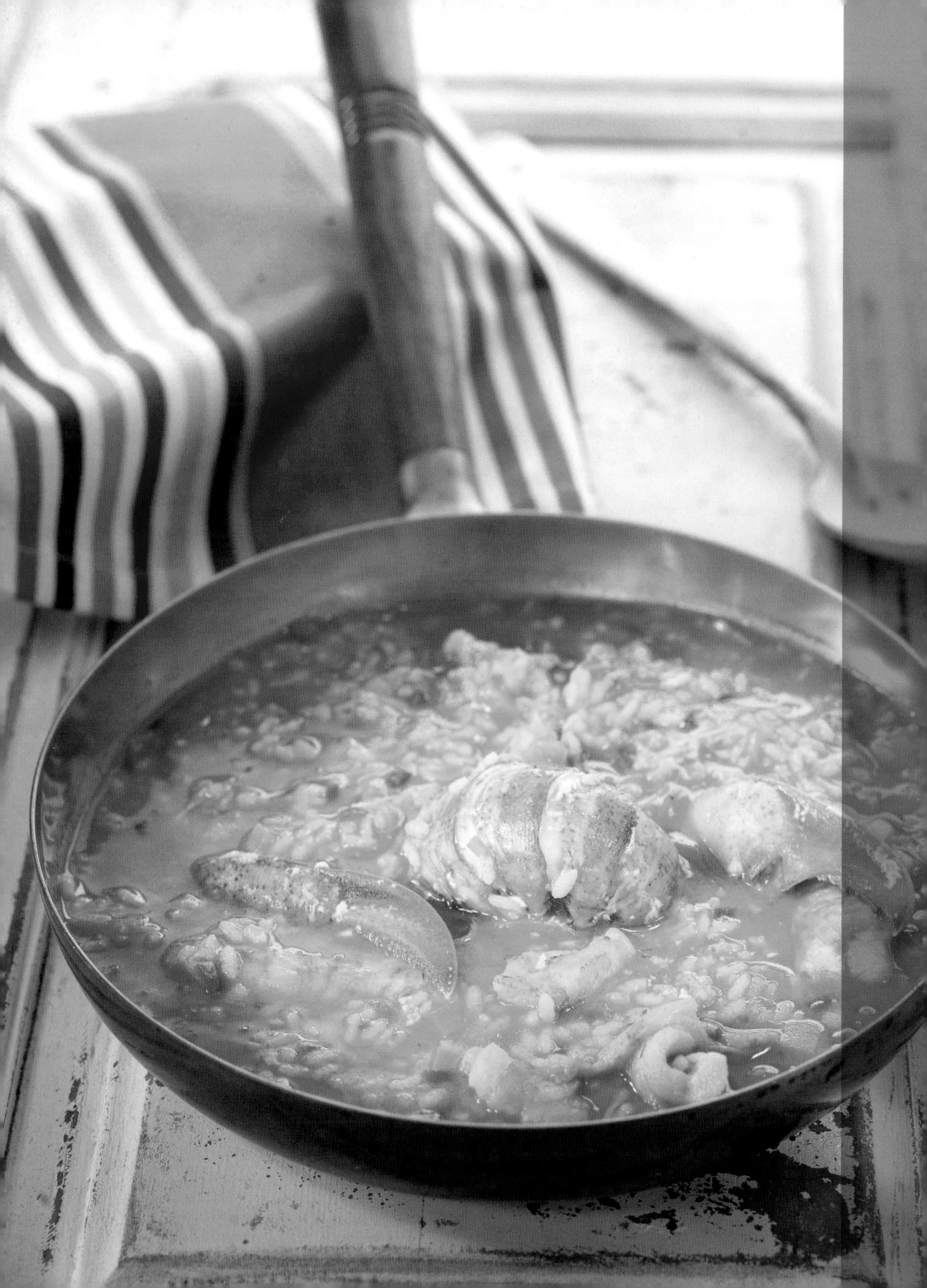

Nivel 3 Arroz caldoso con bogavante

- 400 g de arroz
- 2 bogavantes
- Gambas (opcional)
- 1 sepia
- 1 espina de rape, rodaballo o merluza
- 2 cebollas
- 2 zanahorias
- 2 dientes de ajo
- 2 pimientos verdes italianos
- 1 puerro
- 1 pimiento rojo
- 2 cucharadas de tomate frito (100 ml)
- 2 g de azafrán
- Aceite de oliva
- Sal

20 min (+ 20 min caldo)
20 min
8 €/persona
Sin contraindicaciones.

- Sofríe la cebolla junto al puerro, la zanahoria, los pimientos y el ajo picados muy finos en un cazo con un buen chorro de aceite de oliva. Tienes que dejarlo a fuego lento durante 20 minutos, hasta que la verdura empiece a caramelizar.
- Añade entonces la sepia y cuece durante 15 minutos más, luego agrega el tomate frito y cuece otros 5 minutos.
- Fríe los bogavantes abiertos por la mitad en una cazuela con un chorrito de aceite de oliva y una pizca de sal. Una vez empiecen a dorarse y se forme una costra, retíralos de la cazuela y resérvalos. Añade entonces el sofrito de verdura a la cazuela, y luego el arroz y el azafrán. Rehógalo todo durante un par de minutos.
- Pon en una olla con 3 litros de agua una cebolla y un puerro troceados con un manojo de perejil y la espina de pescado. Cuece durante 20 minutos y reserva.
- Cubre el arroz con 1 litro de caldo de pescado e introdúcelo al horno a 200 °C. Deja cocer durante 15 minutos, añade los bogavantes y deja cocer 5 minutos más (si quieres también puedes añadir unas gambas). Corrige el punto de sal y sirve al instante.

Trucos

Para obtener un caldo de pescado limpio deberás "espumar" el caldo durante la cocción; ello supone retirar la espuma que aparece en la parte superior del caldo mientras hieve.

Arroces en ensalada y aromatizados

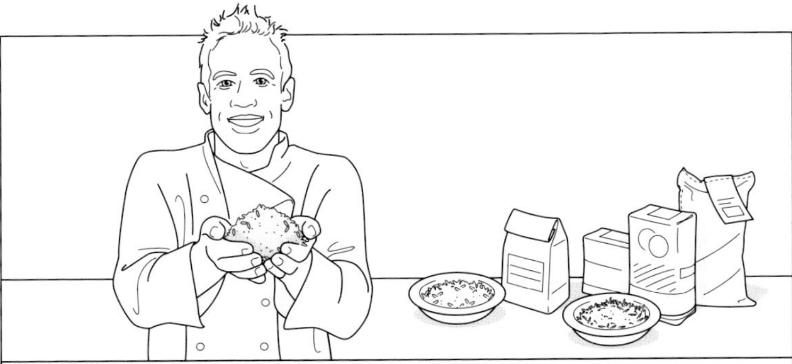

El arroz es un alimento fundamental para una dieta equilibrada: aporta energía, es beneficioso para la digestión, y bajo en colesterol. Un alimento básico para gran parte de la humanidad.

Para las ensaladas de arroz utilizaremos arroz de grano largo, que además no se pasa.

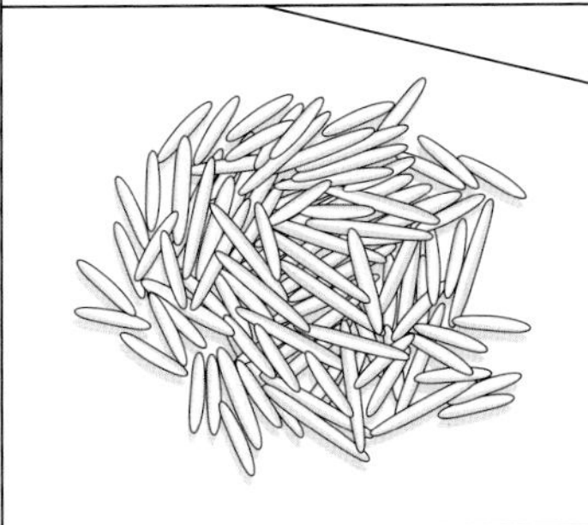

Después de cocerlo podemos enfriarlo bajo el grifo y así quitar los restos de almidón y dejarlo más suelto.

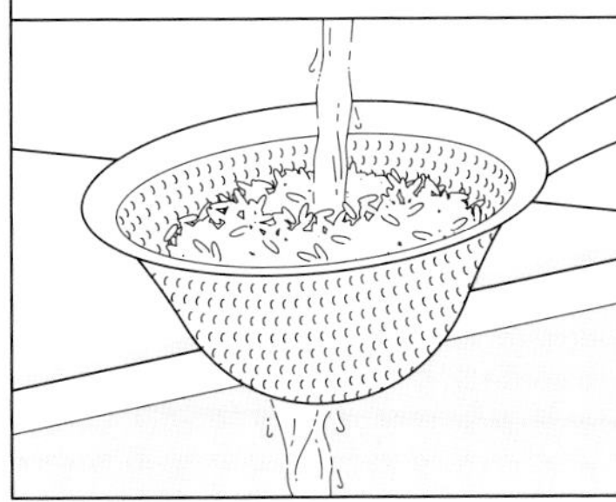

Puedes acompañarlo de frutas o verduras...

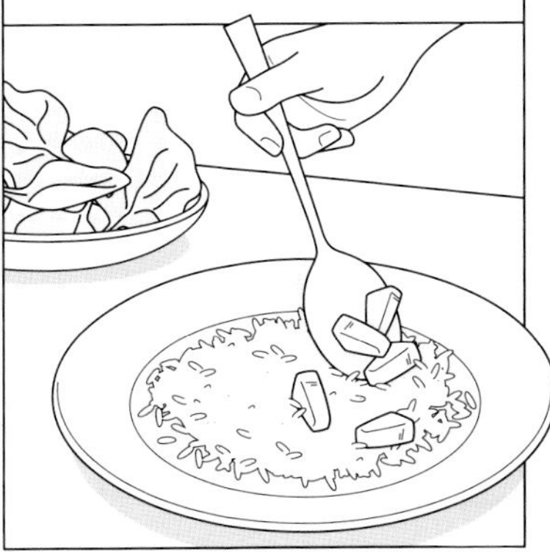

... o bien de carnes, pescados o mariscos.

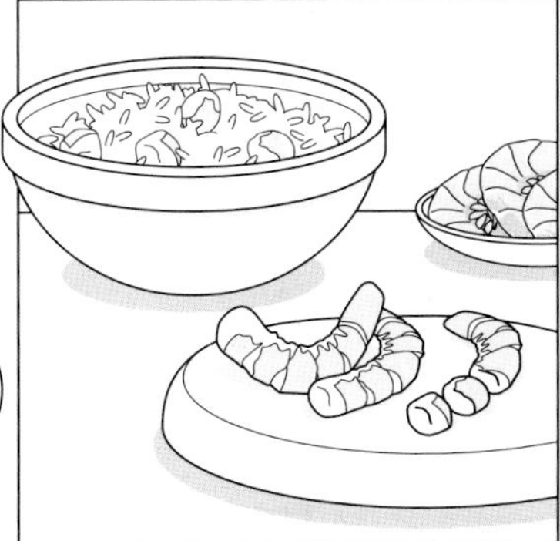

Emplearás arroces aromatizados...

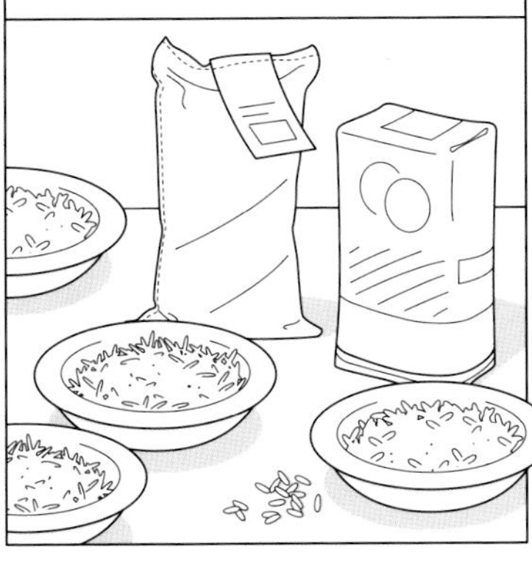

... con tofu para los vegetarianos...

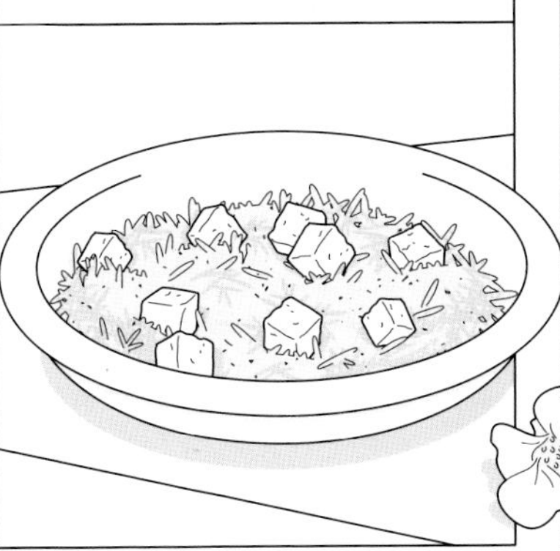

... y diferentes aderezos y acompañamientos, ¡incluso flores!

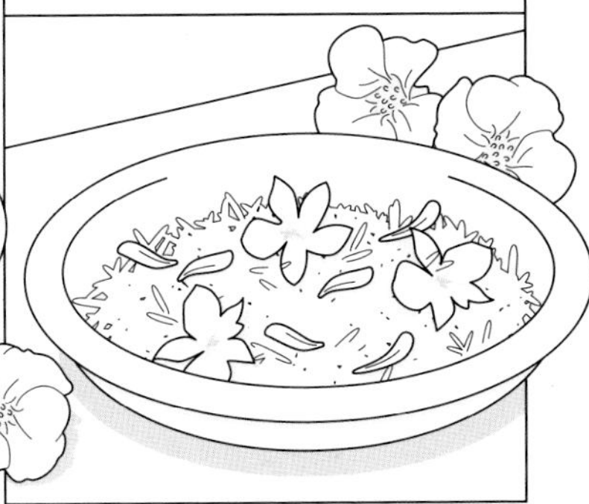

Arroces en ensalada

El ingrediente

Existen arroces o, mejor dicho, granos de arroz, que se adaptan a cada necesidad, ya sean más o menos glutinosos, de grano más o menos largo o incluso de un color u otro. Para elaborar ensaladas podemos emplear varios tipos de granos, pero el más recomendado es, sin duda, el arroz *basmati*, de grano largo, muy fino y con muy poca presencia de almidón, por lo que obtendremos con facilidad un arroz suelto y muy tierno. También podemos emplear otras variedades de arroz de grano alargado, como los arroces vaporizados, que, como están precocidos se preparan en un tiempo récord, y cómo no, el arroz salvaje, aunque este, así reconocido, no sea propiamente un grano de arroz sino una semilla de una graminácea, es decir, un cereal.

La técnica

Si queremos obtener arroces sueltos para la composición de ensaladas, es recomendable acudir a las variedades citadas anteriormente: *basmati*, vaporizado, salvaje, etc., pero también debemos adoptar la precaución de lavar el grano de arroz bajo el chorro de agua fría para eliminar así parte del almidón que pudiera contener y obtener un grano más suelto si cabe.

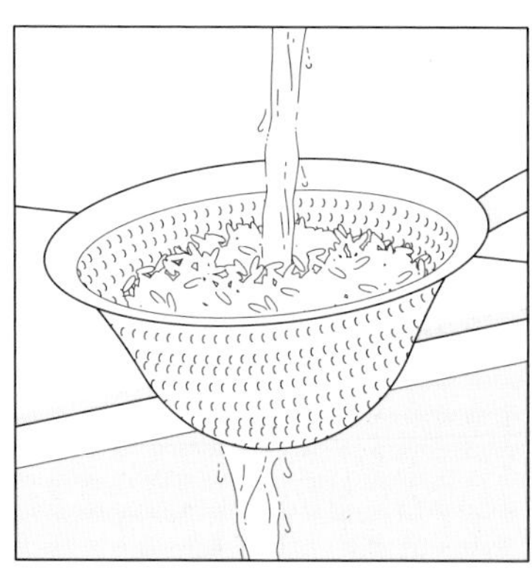

Plato a plato

Nivel **1** **Ensalada de arroz 5 delicias.** Un arroz enriquecido con lo mejor de las verduras y el bonito amarillo de la tortilla. Fácil, rápida y deliciosa.

Nivel **2** ***Taboulé* de arroz, sémola y verduritas tiernas.** Aproxímate a los sabores de Oriente con un arroz frío repleto de color y sabor. Una receta muy saludable, a medio camino entre lo básico y lo sofisticado.

Nivel **3** **Ensalada de arroz en concha de vieiras con marisco y vinagreta de ajo tierno.** Sorprende a tus comensales con un arroz con todo el sabor del mar y una presentación muy original.

Nivel 1 Ensalada de arroz 5 delicias

- 200 g de arroz vaporizado
- 100 g de jamón cocido
- 100 g de maíz cocido
- 100 g de guisantes frescos
- 100 g de *mezclum*
- 100 g de brotes de soja
- 1 cebolleta
- 1 zanahoria
- 1 lechuga
- 2 huevos
- 2 rodajas de piña fresca
- Aceite de oliva
- Vinagre de Jerez
- Sal y pimienta

10 min
15 min
2 €/persona
Sin contraindicaciones.

- Cuece el arroz siguiendo las instrucciones del fabricante (puede recomendarte que cuezas el arroz al vapor, al horno o ¡incluso al microondas!). Una vez cocido, enfríalo bien y reserva.
- Cuece también los guisantes en agua hirviendo durante 15-16 minutos, hasta que queden tiernos, y enfríalos en agua con hielo.
- Bate los huevos y prepara una tortilla en una sartén a fuego medio con un chorrito de aceite de oliva. Una vez esté bien cuajada, retírala del fuego y reserva. Deja enfriar.
- Pica finamente la cebolleta, la zanahoria, el jamón cocido, la tortilla, la piña, los brotes de soja y la lechuga y mézclalo todo en un recipiente con el arroz, los guisantes y el maíz. Adereza con un buen chorro de aceite de oliva, un chorrito de vinagre de Jerez y una pizca de sal y pimienta.

Trucos

Si lo prefieres puedes prescindir de la propuesta de ensalada y saltear esta misma preparación para degustarla como un entrante caliente. Puedes añadir también otros ingredientes de tu agrado.

Nivel **2** *Taboulé* de arroz, sémola y verduritas tiernas

- 200 g de arroz vaporizado
- 100 g de guisantes
- 50 g de tirabeques
- 50 g de bayas de Goji
- 50 g de uvas pasas
- 50 g de pipas de calabaza
- 100 g de germinados de rábano
- 1 zanahoria
- 1 cebolleta tierna
- Aceite de oliva
- Vinagre de Jerez
- Sal y pimienta

10 min
15 min
2 €/persona
Sin contraindicaciones.

■ Cuece el arroz siguiendo las instrucciones del fabricante (al vapor, al horno o al microondas). Una vez cocido, enfríalo bien y reserva.
■ Cuece también los guisantes en agua hirviendo durante 15-16 minutos, hasta que queden tiernos, y enfríalos en agua con hielo.
■ Pica la cebolleta, la zanahoria y los tirabeques tan finos como te sea posible y mézclalos en un recipiente con el arroz cocido, los germinados, las bayas, las uvas y las pipas.
■ Adereza la ensalada con un chorrito de aceite de oliva, otro chorrito de vinagre y una pizca de sal y de pimienta. Ya lo puedes servir.

Trucos

Para preparar el *taboulé* puedes combinar granos de arroz con sémola de trigo. También puedes añadir una cucharadita de azúcar glas y canela en polvo a la presentación para darle un toque más exótico.

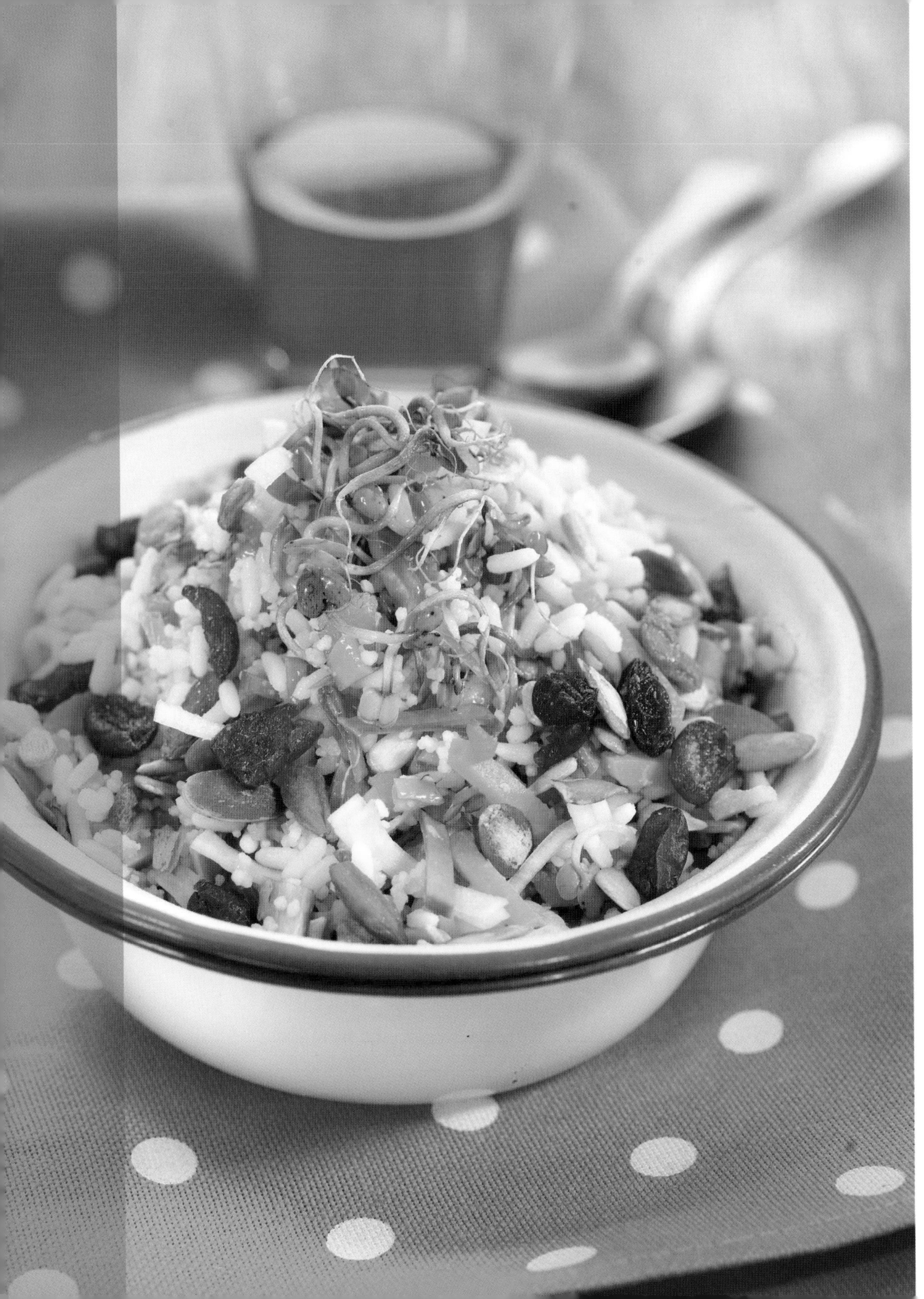

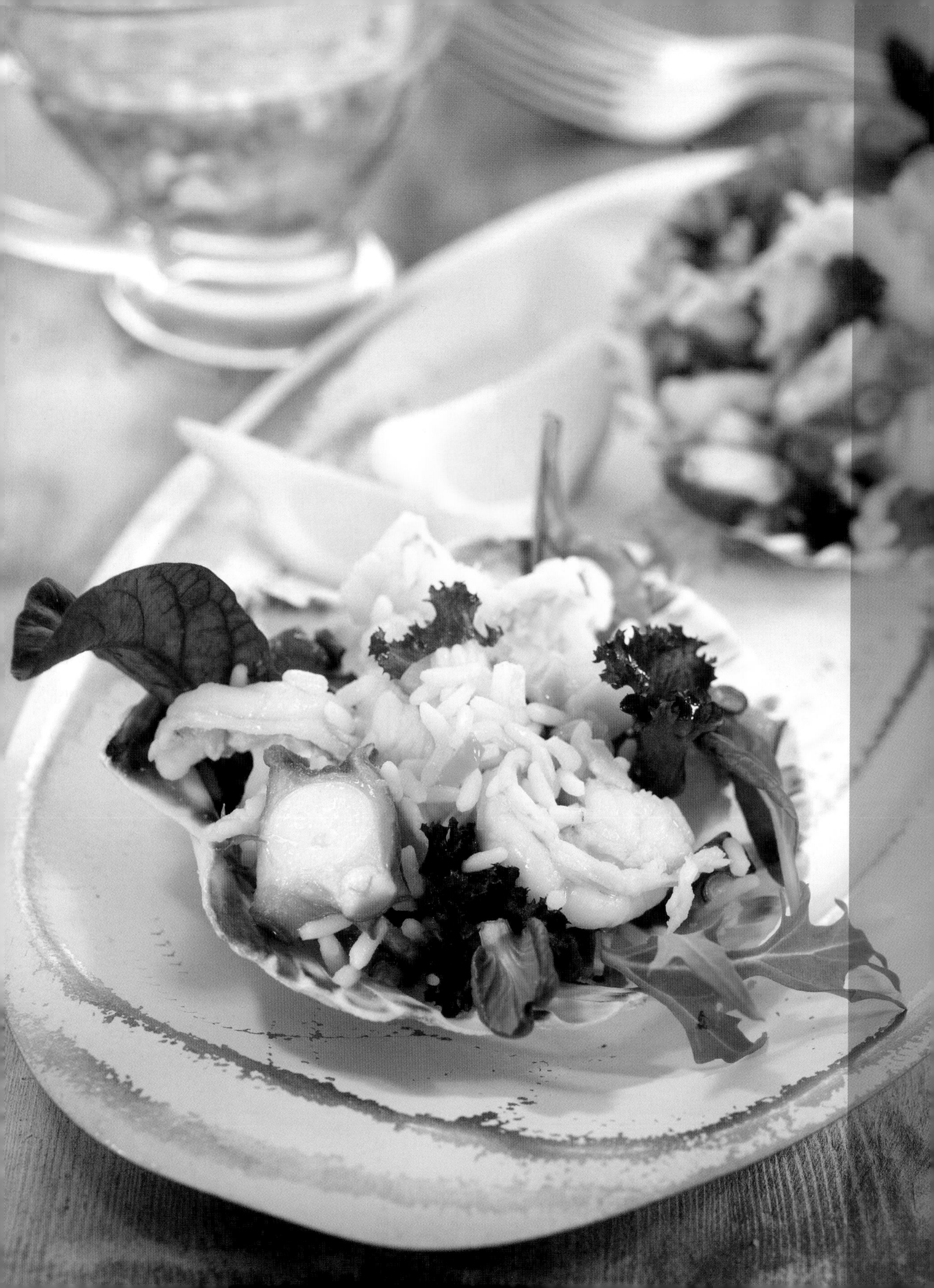

Nivel **3**
Ensalada de arroz en concha de vieiras con marisco y vinagreta de ajo tierno

- **200 g de arroz vaporizado**
- **12 langostinos**
- **4 vieiras**
- **1/2 limón**
- **1 pata de pulpo cocida**
- **1 medallón de rape**
- **2-3 ajos tiernos**
- **100 g de *mezclum***
- **Aceite de oliva**
- **Vinagre de Jerez**
- **Sal y pimienta**

10 min

10 min

8 €/persona

Esta receta no está indicada para personas alérgicas al marisco.

■ Cuece el arroz siguiendo las instrucciones del fabricante (al vapor, al horno o al microondas). Una vez cocido, enfríalo bien y reserva.

■ Limpia bien las vieiras hasta tener la carne limpia. Lava también con un cepillo sus conchas, pues nos servirán para presentar la ensalada.

■ En una olla al vapor o en un cazo con medio vaso de agua y el zumo de medio limón, cuece los langostinos pelados y abiertos por la mitad, las vieiras y el rape cortado en trocitos. Retira del fuego y deja enfriar.

■ Prepara un aceite de ajos tiernos. Para ello calienta a fuego lento el aceite, agrega el ajo tierno cortado en medallones y deja que enfríe. Añade un chorrito de vinagre cuando esté bien frío.

■ Mezcla las lechugas troceadas con el pulpo cortado en finos medallones, el rape, los langostinos, la carne de vieira troceada y el arroz hervido. Sirve sobre las conchas, salpimienta y adereza con aceite de ajos tiernos.

Trucos

Puedes acompañarlo también con una mayonesa de ajos tiernos o con una salsa rosa, y añadir mejillones, almejas, un bogavante troceado o el marisco que quieras.

Arroces aromatizados

El ingrediente

El arroz aromatizado por excelencia es el llamado "jazmín", que posee un fresco aroma floral y que resulta delicioso tanto en ensaladas como en salteados. Se trata de un arroz de grano largo, de cocción breve, muy similar al *basmati*. Pero el arroz aromatizado no está disponible solo en las tiendas, podemos aromatizarlo nosotros mismos cociendo el arroz al vapor. Para conferirle el aroma deseado, enriqueceremos la base de agua de nuestra olla a vapor con hierbas aromáticas, flores, verduras o raíces. Así, podemos añadir al agua una raíz de jengibre, una ramita de citronela, hojas de lima, laurel, romero o el ingrediente de nuestro agrado.

La técnica

Por lo general se trata de arroces cocidos al vapor que, como ya hemos indicado, aromatizamos enriqueciendo el agua de cocción. Una vez cocidos, podemos saltearlos con los ingredientes que deseemos o presentarlos en ensalada. Otra forma de aromatizar el arroz es saltearlo con las hierbas o especias deseadas, también con aceites aromatizados, con frutos secos, hierbas, setas, etc.

Plato a plato

Nivel **1** **Ensalada de arroz con fruta y verduritas de temporada.** El punto de partida es un básico de las ensaladas de arroz aromatizadas, donde las frutas y verduras que tu imaginación y preferencias elijan aportan un toque único y colorista.

Nivel **2** **Ensalada de arroz silvestre con tofu.** Prueba a cocinar dos arroces y mézclalos con albahaca, una hierba aromática de sabor suave, y unos daditos de tofu pasado por la sartén.

Nivel **3** **Ensalada de arroz jazmín con flores y otros acompañamientos.** En el tercer nivel atrévete a preparar un sorprendente plato de arroz aromático con flores comestibles que dejará al comensal atónito.

Nivel 1 Ensalada de arroz con frutas y verduritas de temporada

- 200 g de arroz jazmín
- 100 g de maíz cocido
- 1 zanahoria
- 1 pepino
- 1 escarola
- 1 cebolleta
- 1 aguacate
- 1 mango
- 1 granada
- 1 manzana
- 2 rodajas de piña fresca
- Aceite de oliva
- Vinagre de Jerez
- Sal y pimienta

10 min
15 min
2 €/persona
Sin contraindicaciones.

- Cuece el arroz siguiendo las instrucciones del fabricante (al vapor, al horno o al microondas). Una vez cocido, enfríalo bien y reserva.
- Pica todas las frutas y verduras tan finamente como te sea posible (lo ideal sería en dados pequeños), y mézclalas en un recipiente con el arroz, la escarola y un buen chorro de aceite de oliva y otro de vinagre de Jerez. Salpimienta y sirve.

Trucos

Si no tienes alguna fruta o verdura no te preocupes, adapta la ensalada a las que dispongas: peras, fresas, calabacín, brotes de soja, naranja, etc.

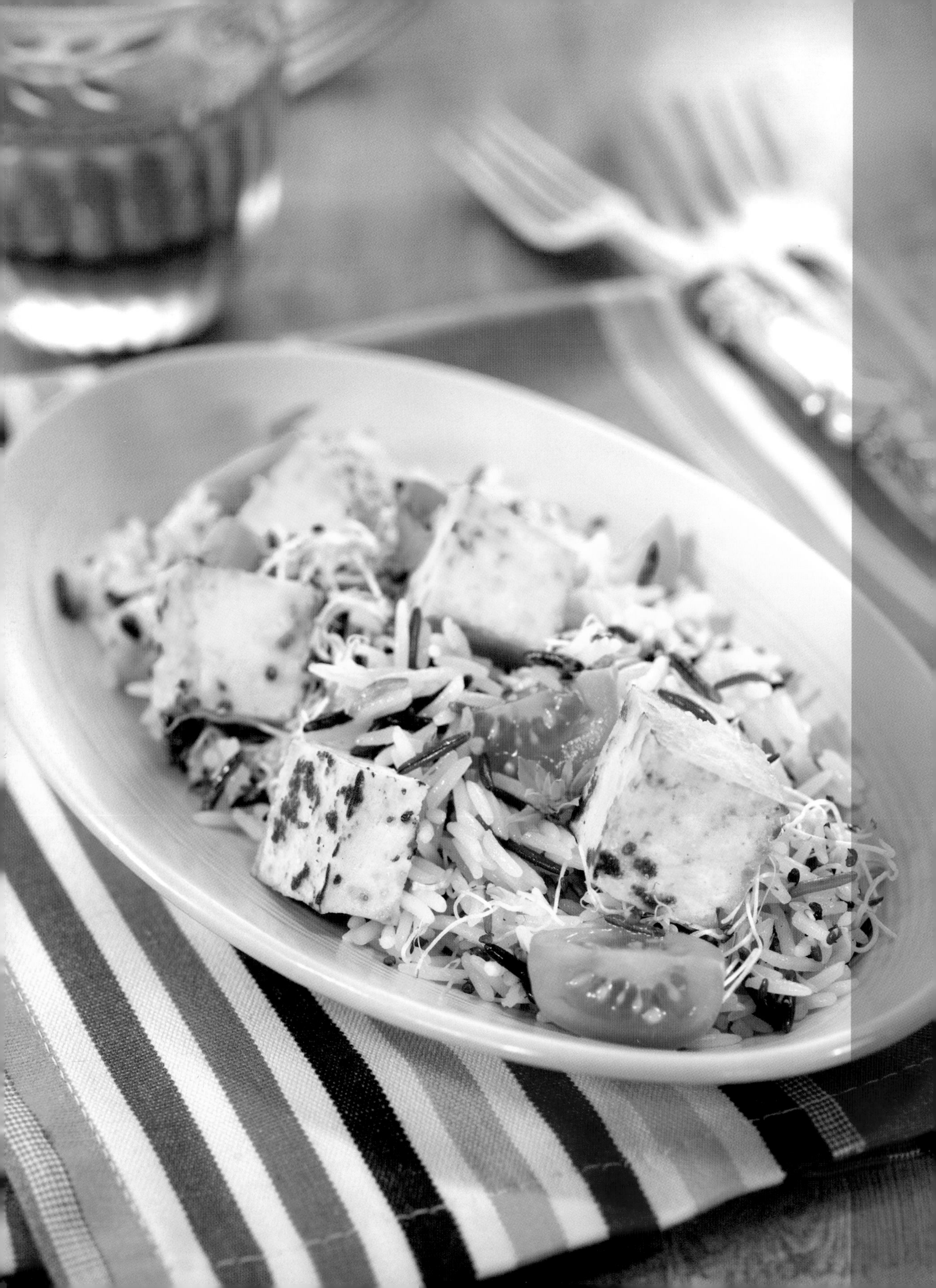

Nivel **2**

Ensalada de arroz silvestre con tofu

- 100 g de arroz *basmati*
- 100 g de arroz salvaje
- 200 g de tofu
- 50 g de germinados de alfalfa
- 1 bandeja de tomates cherry
- Albahaca
- Aceite de oliva
- Sal y pimienta

10 min
15 min
2 €/persona
Sin contraindicaciones.

■ Cuece los arroces siguiendo las instrucciones del fabricante (al vapor, al horno o al microondas). Una vez cocidos, enfríalos bien y reserva.

■ En un recipiente mezcla los arroces con los brotes de alfalfa, los tomates cherry y unas hojitas de albahaca. Remueve bien y aderézalo con un chorrito de aceite de oliva y otro de vinagre de Jerez. Salpimienta y repártelo en platos individuales.

■ En el momento de servir, corta el tofu en dados y fríelos en una sartén con un chorrito de aceite de oliva y una pizca de sal. Cuando empiece a dorarse disponlo sobre la ensalada.

Trucos

Existen bolsitas de cocción al vapor que contienen la mezcla de estos arroces, *basmati* y salvaje; puedes utilizarlas para preparar esta ensalada.

Nivel **3** Ensalada de arroz jazmín con flores y otros acompañamientos

- 200 g de arroz jazmín
- 2 rosas comestibles
- 1 manojo de puntas de espárragos trigueros
- 1 bandeja de frambuesas
- 30 g de pistachos verdes pelados
- Vinagre de frambuesa
- Sal en escamas
- Aceite de oliva
- Sal y pimienta

10 min
15 min
2 €/persona
Sin contraindicaciones.

- Cuece el arroz siguiendo las instrucciones del fabricante (al vapor, al horno o al microondas). Una vez cocido, enfríalo bien y reserva.
- Con la ayuda de un pelador, extrae finas láminas de espárrago triguero y déjalas reposar durante media hora en abundante agua con hielo. Reserva.
- Tritura en un mortero una pizca de sal en escamas con la mitad de las frambuesas, unos pétalos de rosa, los pistachos y un chorrito de aceite que deberás verter de forma paulatina, como si fueses a preparar un alioli. Una vez la vinagreta presente una textura de crema ligera, añade un chorrito de vinagre de frambuesa y una pizca de pimienta.
- Mezcla el arroz con las láminas de espárrago, las rosas cortadas en juliana y las frambuesas restantes. Sírvelo en platos individuales y adereza con la vinagreta.

Trucos

Puedes utilizar otras flores de temporada como violetas, flores de azahar, hibisco, jazmín, etc. Y si no encuentras vinagre de frambuesa puedes utilizar vinagre de Jerez o bien rociar la ensalada con un chorrito de reducción de vinagre balsámico.

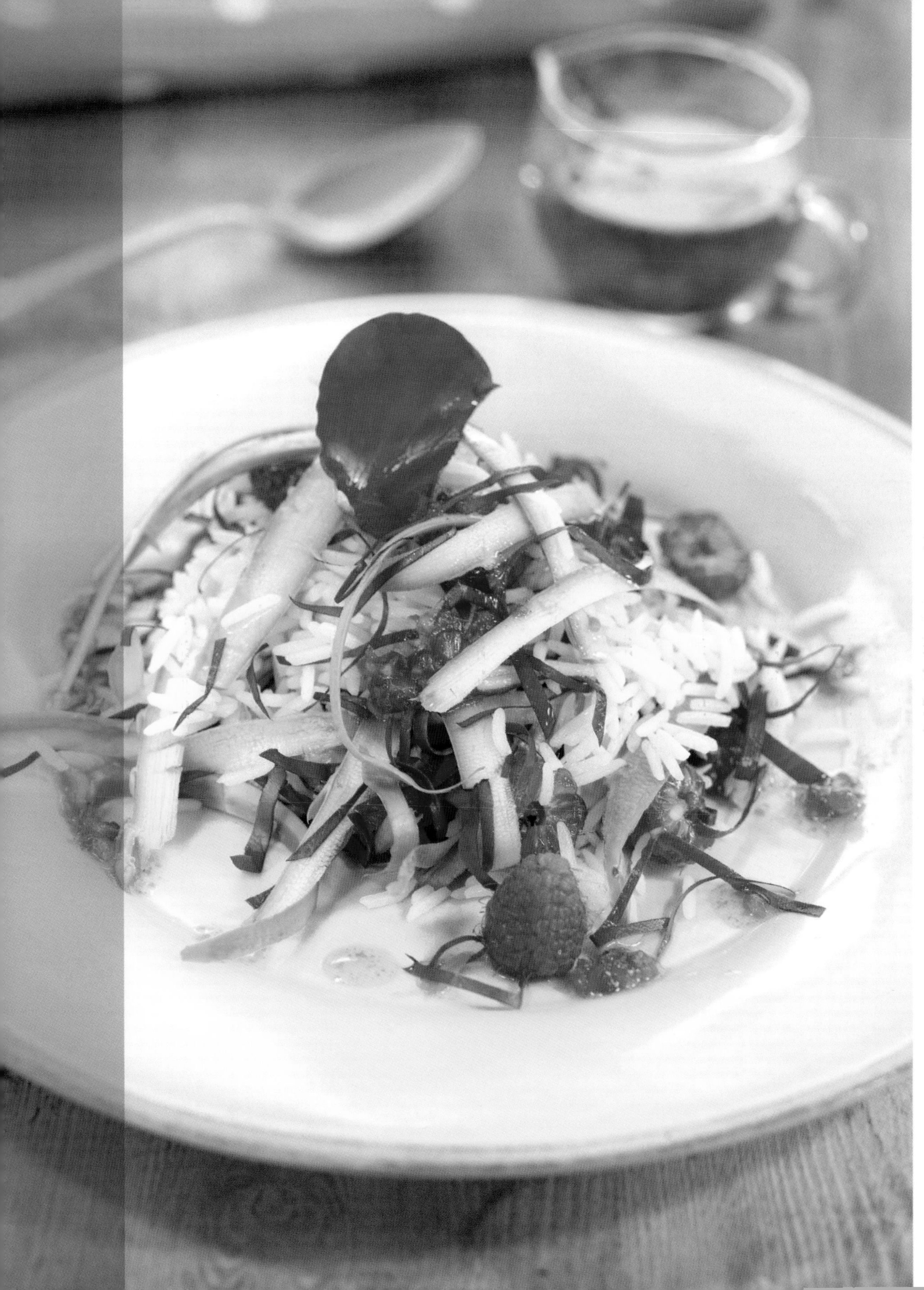

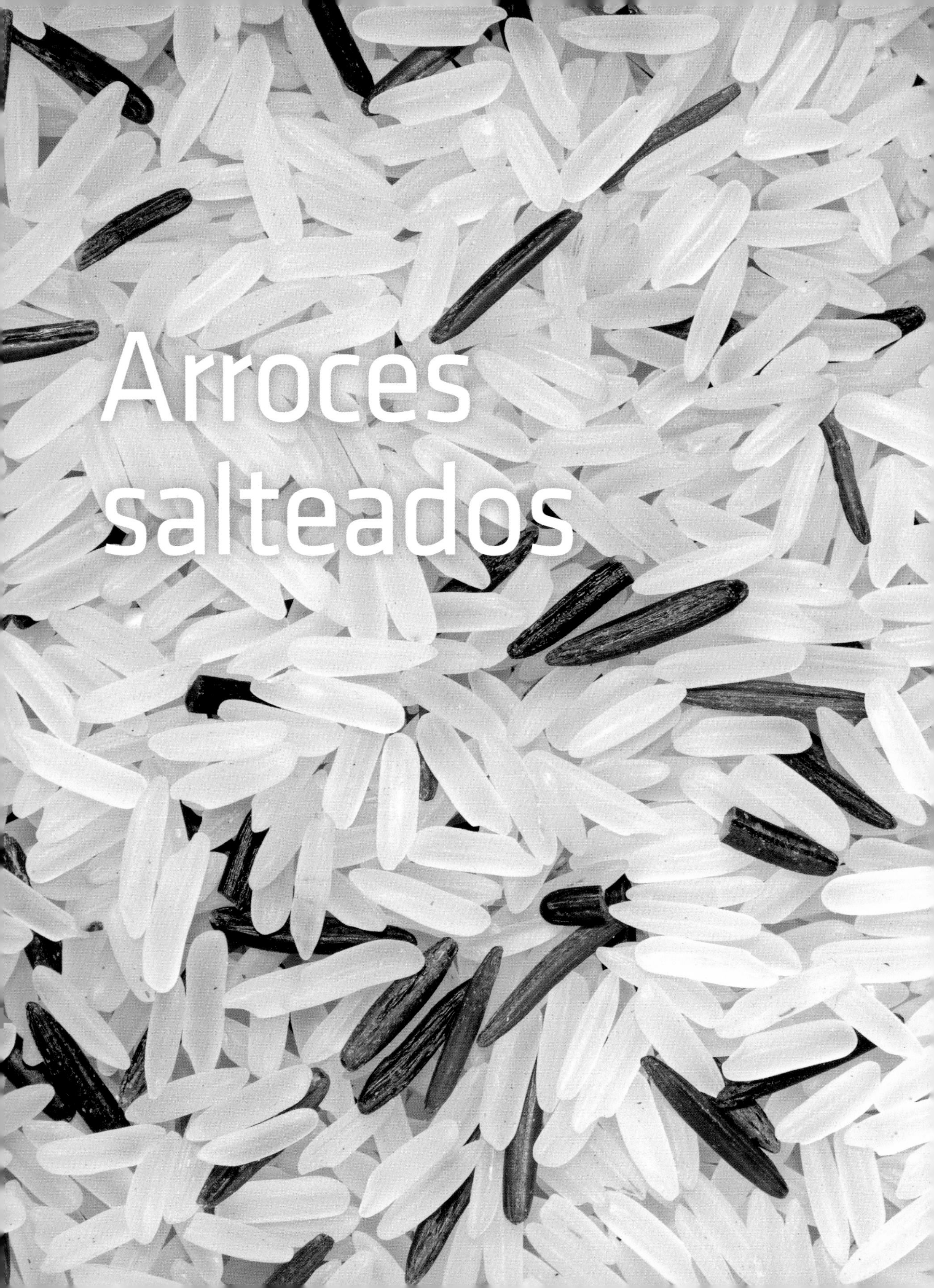

Arroces salteados

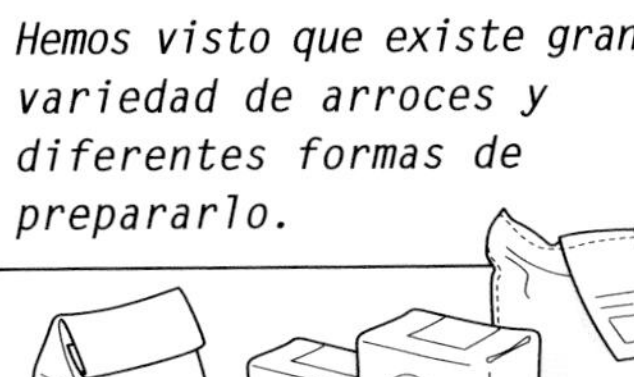
Hemos visto que existe gran variedad de arroces y diferentes formas de prepararlo.

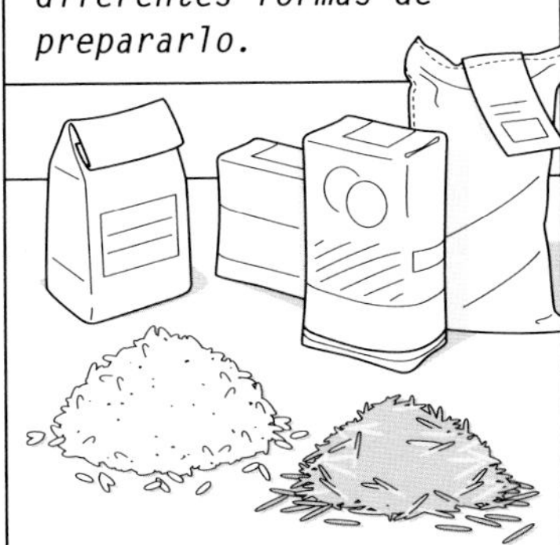

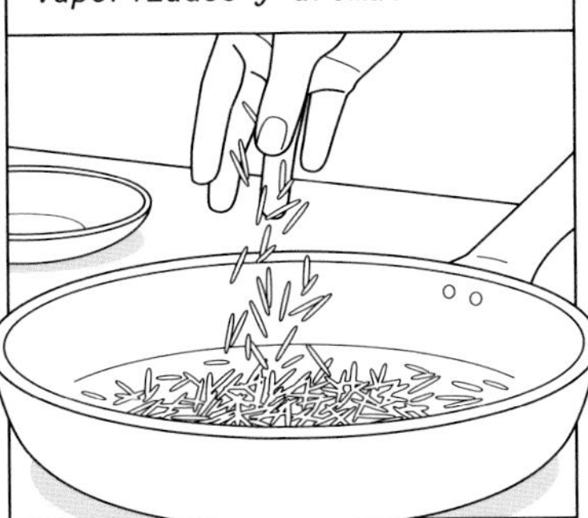
Para los salteados se emplean arroces de grano largo, salvajes, vaporizados y aromatizados.

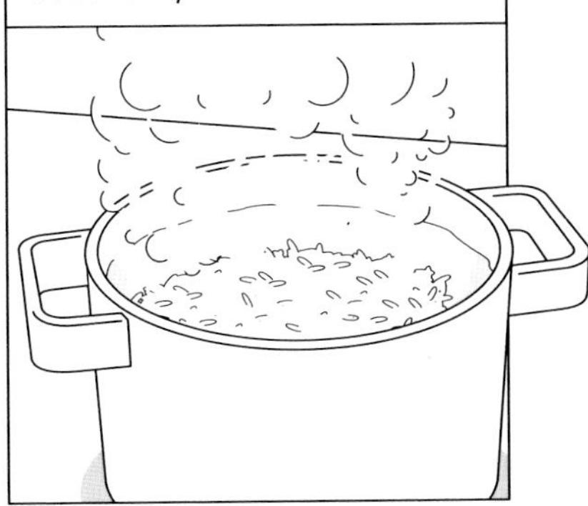
Todos los arroces que se saltean deben cocerse previamente.

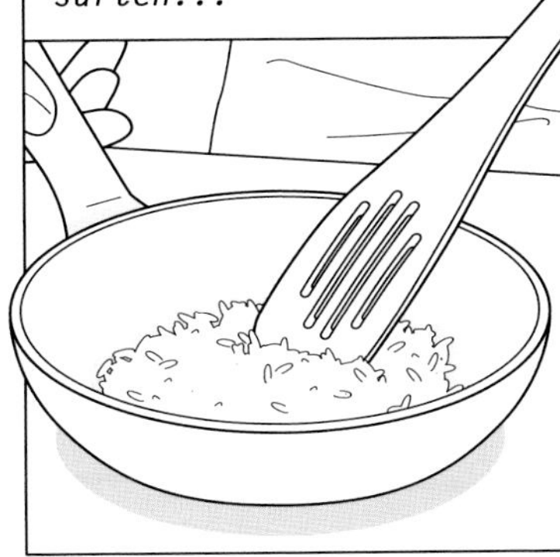
Podemos saltear el arroz por sí solo en un wok o sartén...

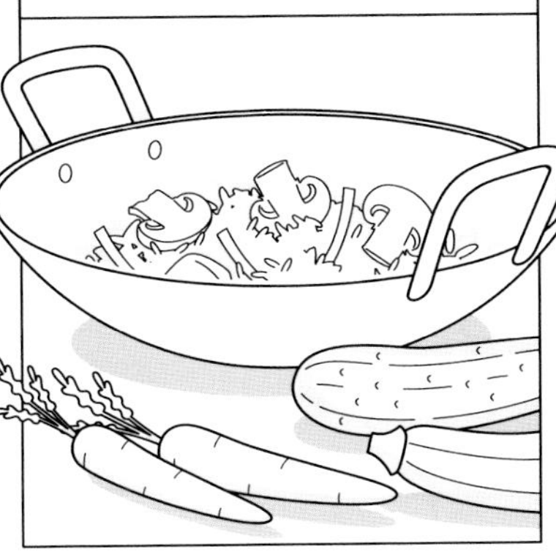
... o saltearlo con verduras...

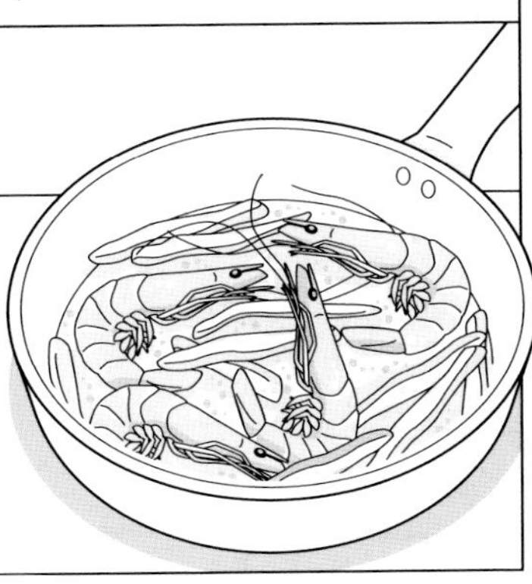
... carnes, pescados o mariscos...

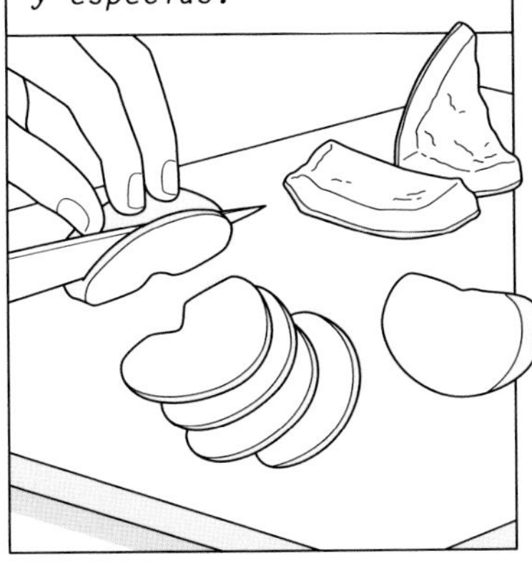
... e incluso frutas y especias.

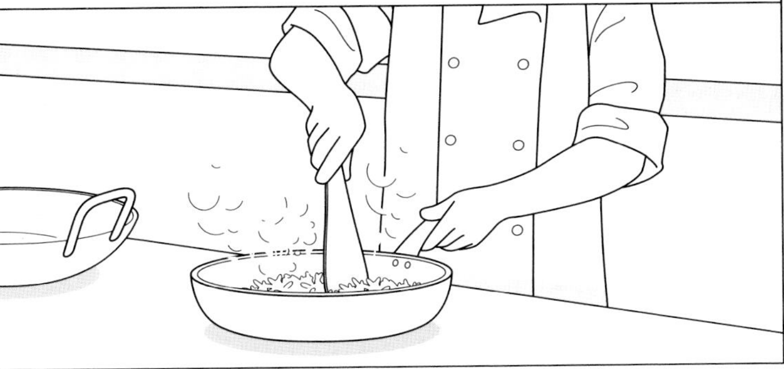
Como el arroz ya está cocido, saltearemos brevemente y a alta temperatura, para que no absorba aceite en exceso y se mantenga ligero.

Arroces vaporizados

El ingrediente

Por lo general los arroces vaporizados se presentan en bolsitas de cocción. Este tipo de arroces resultan muy prácticos, ya que no suelen precisar de cantidades exactas de agua y no se pasan. Se trata de arroces que ya han sido cocidos al vapor y que "regeneramos" ofreciéndoles una segunda cocción, por lo general muy breve. Estamos ante arroces que se cuecen en un tiempo récord, por lo que resultan extremadamente prácticos.

La técnica

Sumerge las bolsitas de cocción en abundante agua hirviendo, siguiendo las recomendaciones y consejos del fabricante hasta obtener un arroz tierno y listo para degustar.

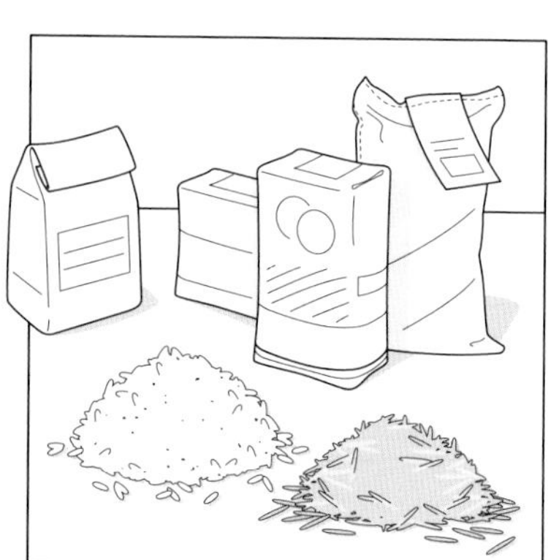

En el caso de presentarse en terrinas, caliéntalas al microondas o bien al baño María durante el tiempo que indique el fabricante.

Plato a plato

Nivel **1** **Arroz salteado con setas de temporada.** Una receta ideal para guisar las setas de una forma distinta, acompañándolas de un delicioso arroz aromatizado con trufa.

Nivel **2** **Salteado de arroz con gambas, coco, lima y brotes de soja.** Dale un toque novedoso al clásico salteado con el inconfundible sabor y textura del coco.

Nivel **3** **Arroz al *wok* con pato caramelizado y otros acompañamientos.** Atrévete a acompañar el arroz de un peso pesado de las aves de corral. Con el caramelizado que le aplicarás, el plato final tendrá un sabor único.

Nivel 1 Arroz salteado con setas de temporada

- 200 g de arroz vaporizado
- 500 g de setas de temporada
- 3-4 ajos tiernos
- 1 trufa o aceite de trufa (opcional)
- 1 manojo de perejil
- Aceite de oliva
- Sal y pimienta

15 min
15 min
4 €/persona
Sin contraindicaciones.

■ Cuece el arroz siguiendo las instrucciones del fabricante (al vapor, al horno o al microondas). Una vez cocido, enfríalo bien y reserva.
■ Lava bien las setas eliminando la tierra o las hojas que pudieran contener. Para esta receta puedes utilizar níscalos, carreretas, *ceps*, colmenillas o tu seta preferida.
■ Sofríe un minuto los ajos tiernos limpios y cortados en rodajas en una sartén muy caliente con un chorrito de aceite de oliva. Agrega las setas troceadas y saltea hasta que empiecen a dorarse. Luego añade el arroz cocido y mezcla bien. Saltea y sálalo, agrega una pizca de pimienta y un buen puñado de perejil recién picado.
■ Si te apetece, sirve el salteado acompañado de trufa fresca rallada o con un chorrito de aceite de trufa.

Trucos

Fuera de temporada puedes elaborar este arroz con setas de cultivo como las gírgolas o los champiñones. También con setas deshidratadas, pero recuerda que antes de cocinarlas deberás hidratarlas a tu gusto.

Nivel **2**

Salteado de arroz con gambas, coco, lima y brotes de soja

- 200 g de arroz vaporizado
- 16 gambas o langostinos
- 6-8 hojas de lima
- 1 cebolleta
- 1 bolsa de brotes de soja (200 g)
- 1/2 coco fresco
- Aceite de oliva
- Sal en escamas

15 min
15 min
4 €/persona
Sin contraindicaciones.

■ Cuece el arroz siguiendo las instrucciones del fabricante (al vapor, al horno o al microondas). Una vez cocido, enfríalo bien y reserva.

■ Ralla finamente la mitad del medio coco y reserva. Corta también las hojas de lima y el resto del coco en una juliana muy finita.

■ En una sartén o en un *wok* bien caliente, y con un chorrito de aceite de oliva, saltea la cebolleta cortada en juliana con las hojas de lima y el coco picado. Una vez la verdura empiece a ablandarse agrega las gambas peladas, los brotes de soja y el arroz y saltéalo todo bien hasta que los ingredientes se mezclen. Añade una buena pizca de sal en escamas y el coco rallado, y sirve al instante.

Trucos

Si no encuentras hojas de lima puedes saltear este arroz con ramitas de citronela o jengibre picado. También puedes "refrescar" el salteado rallando piel de lima encima antes de servirlo.

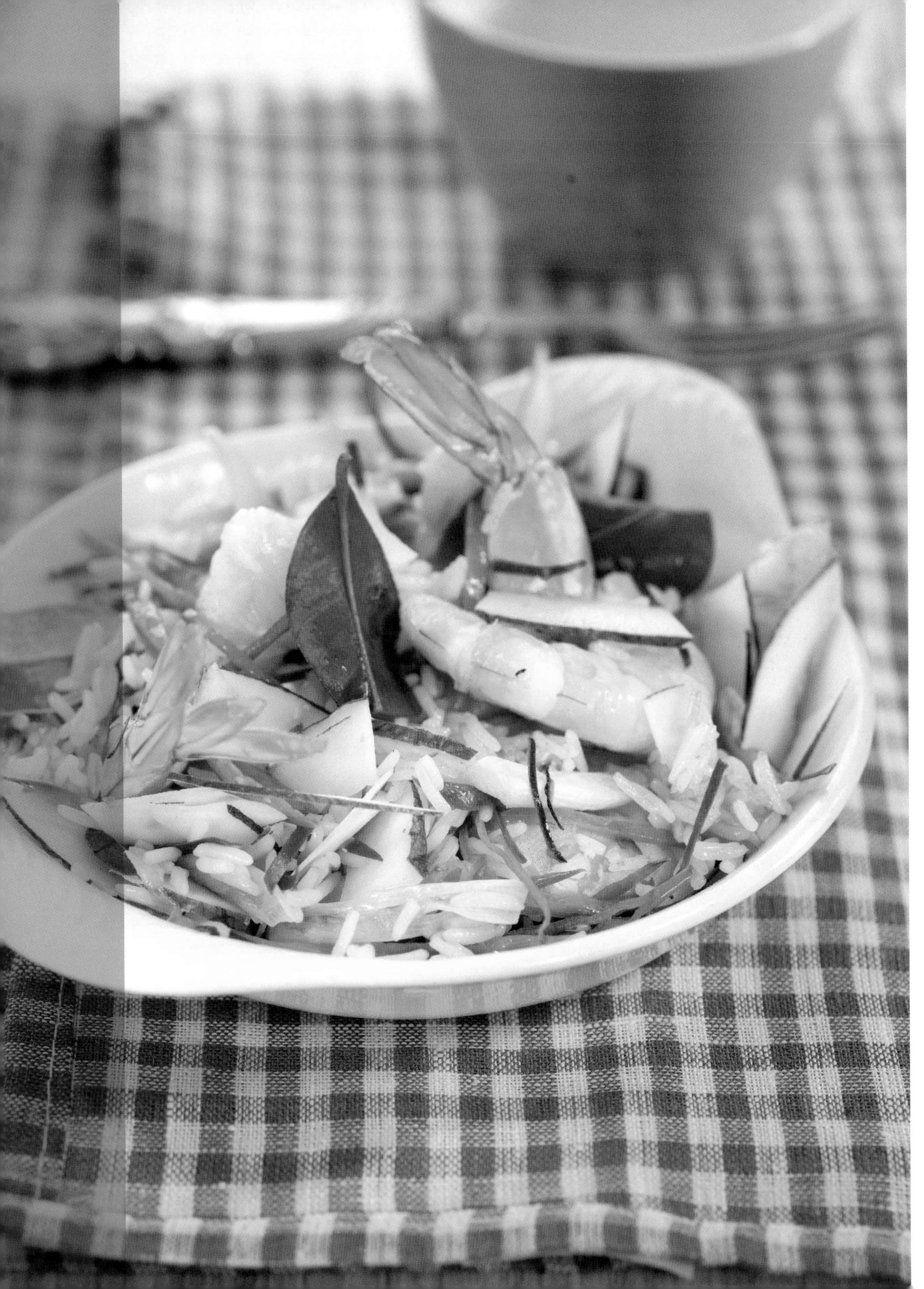

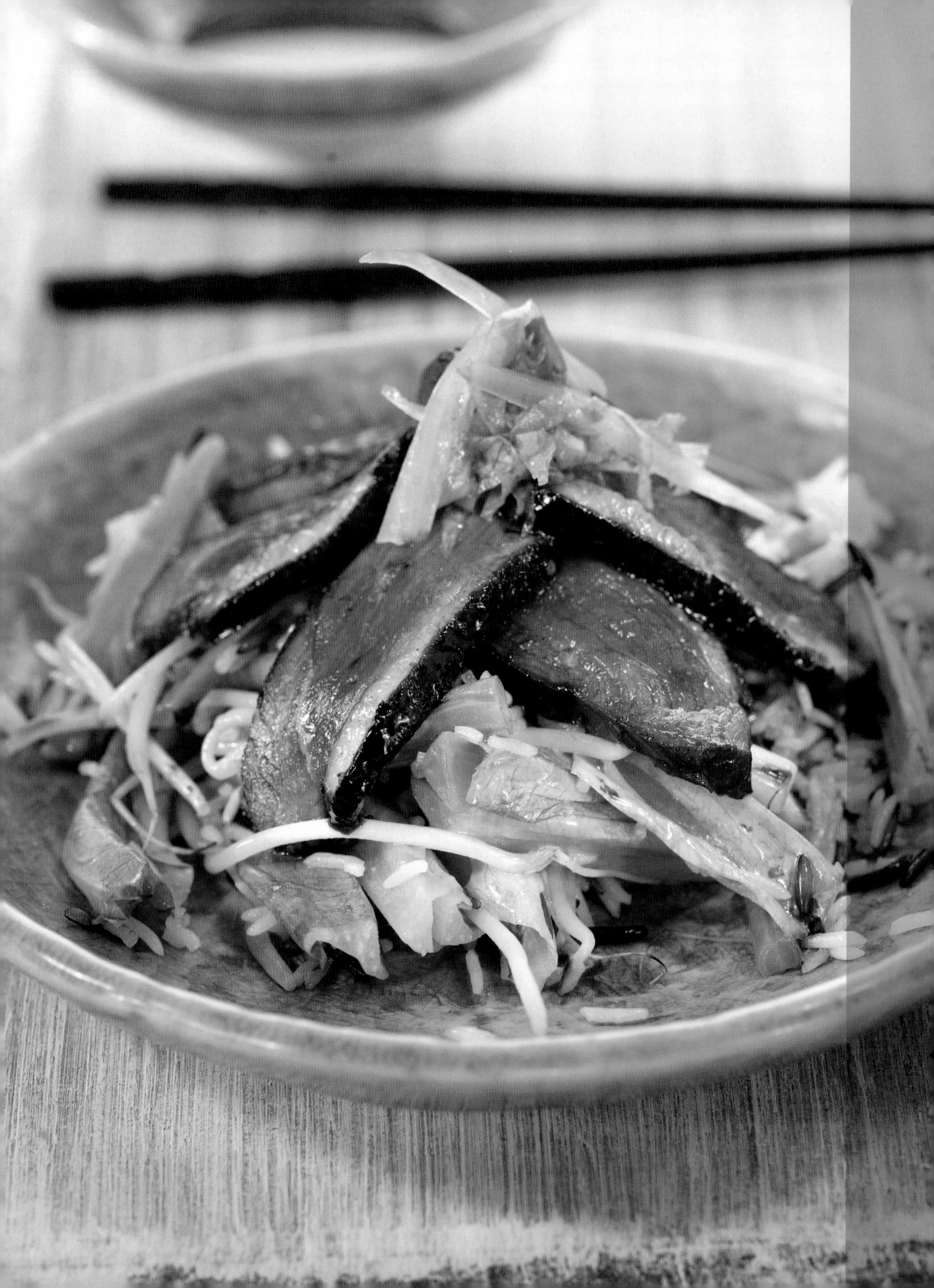

Nivel **3** Arroz al *wok* con pato caramelizado y otros acompañamientos

- 200 g de arroz vaporizado (mezcla de *basmati* y salvaje)
- 1 *magret* (pechuga) de pato
- 2 cucharadas de miel
- 2 cogollos de lechuga
- 1 cucharada de salsa de soja
- 1 bolsa de brotes de soja (200 g)
- 1 cebolleta
- 1 puerro
- Aceite de sésamo
- Sal en escamas

30 min
15 min
5 €/persona
Sin contraindicaciones.

- Cuece el arroz siguiendo las instrucciones del fabricante (al vapor, al horno o al microondas). Una vez cocido, enfríalo bien y reserva.
- Fríe el *magret* de pato entero y sin aceite en una sartén, primero por la parte de la piel, que desprenderá la suficiente grasa para cocinar la pechuga. Fríelo durante 6 minutos a fuego medio, hasta que la piel quede bien crujiente (para ello es necesario que vayas retirando el aceite desprendido por el pato). Transcurrido este tiempo da la vuelta a la pechuga y déjala cocer 3-4 minutos más.
- Una vez el pato esté cocinado, y aún en la sartén, añade la miel y la salsa de soja, deja que caramelice durante un par de minutos y retira del fuego. Deja enfriar el *magret* en el caramelo.
- Una vez frío, córtalo en finas láminas y reserva. Corta los cogollos en juliana o en cuartos.
- Corta en juliana la cebolleta y el puerro y saltéalos en una

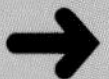

Nivel 3 Arroz al *wok* con pato caramelizado y otros acompañamientos

➔ sartén o en un *wok* con un chorrito de aceite de sésamo. Cuando se ablanden añade los cogollos y los brotes de soja, saltéalo todo bien y agrega el arroz y el pato laminado. Saltea de nuevo hasta mezclar bien todos los ingredientes, añade una pizca de sal y sirve al instante.

Trucos

☛ Para que la pechuga se impregne del caramelo, deja que se enfríe fuera del fuego. Cuanto más frío esté, más fácil será cortar el *magret* en láminas finas. Si no encuentras aceite de sésamo utiliza aceite de oliva.

Arroces en sartenes o *woks*

El utensilio

Tan importante como los ingredientes son los instrumentos que utilizaremos para cocinar nuestros platos, más aún tratándose de salteados. El *wok* tiene la peculiaridad de que ofrece una forma muy apropiada para saltear verduras, carnes, pescados, etc. Sus paredes son anchas y reparten bien el calor, lo que permite que durante el salteado, los jugos que pudieran desprender los alimentos se evaporen de forma instantánea al contacto con el calor de dichas paredes. De este modo no se forman en la base del *wok* jugos y líquidos (que, en lugar de saltear, cuecen los alimentos), con lo que éstos adquieren una textura crujiente y no acuosa. El fuego directo es también el mejor método de cocinado para este tipo de platos, ya que su llama se reparte mejor por sus paredes.

La técnica

Si queremos preparar un salteado y no tenemos *wok* podemos emplear una sartén, pero debemos procurar que sea lo más grande posible y que esté siempre bien caliente, y no saturar el calor de la sartén añadiendo demasiados ingredientes. Es preferible saltear ración a ración para evitar, como ya hemos dicho, que se acumule un exceso de líquidos en la misma y cueza los ingredientes, pues estos se ablandarían y no tendrían su característica textura crujiente.

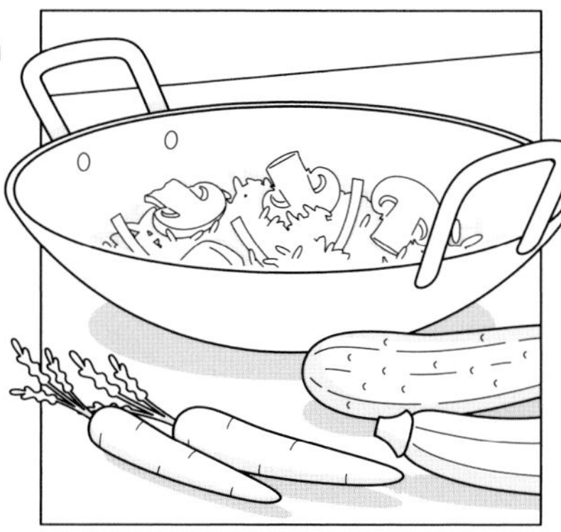

Plato a plato

Nivel **1** **Salteado de arroz con pollo y langostinos.** Si no has usado nunca un *wok*, estrénate con esta receta. Con pocos ingredientes y poco tiempo lograrás unos resultados espectaculares.

Nivel **2** **Salteado de arroz con frutas y especias.** Si sientes que ya dominas un poco el *wok* atrévete a dar sabor al arroz con un jardín de verduritas y frutas; verás como aciertas.

Nivel **3** **Salteado de arroz con cangrejo real.** Prepara en tan solo 15 minutos un arroz de cocina profesional, digno del mejor restaurante marinero.

Nivel **1** Salteado de arroz con pollo y langostinos

- 200 g de arroz jazmín o salvaje
- 16 langostinos
- 1 pechuga de pollo
- 1 cebolla tierna
- 2 dientes de ajo
- 1 cucharada de semillas de sésamo
- Aceite de oliva
- Sal y pimienta

15 min
15 min
4 €/persona
Sin contraindicaciones.

■ Cuece el arroz siguiendo las instrucciones del fabricante (al vapor, al horno o al microondas). Una vez cocido, enfríalo bien y reserva.
■ Limpia bien la pechuga de pollo y córtala en tiras. Pela los langostinos.
■ Saltea la cebolla cortada en juliana y los dientes de ajo laminados en una sartén grande o en un *wok* bien caliente con un chorrito de aceite de oliva. Cuando la verdura empiece a dorarse añade las tiras de pollo y saltea. Cuando el pollo empiece a dorarse agrega los langostinos y sigue salteando.
■ Cuando los langostinos estén cocidos, añade el arroz y una buena cucharada de semillas de sésamo. Salpimienta y sirve al instante.

Trucos

Puedes acompañar este salteado con fruta como piña, manzana, pera o naranja. Agrega también otros brotes o verduras como soja, zanahoria rallada, etc., para enriquecer la preparación.

Nivel **2** Salteado de arroz con frutas y especias

- 200 g de arroz jazmín o salvaje
- 100 g de guisantes frescos
- 50 g de coco rallado
- 1 cebolla tierna
- 1 bandeja de frambuesas
- 1 mango
- 1 rodaja de piña
- 2 dientes de ajo
- 2 hojas de lima
- 100 ml de vino blanco
- 1 cucharada de curry (no demasiado picante)
- 1 rama de romero
- 1 rama de tomillo
- Las semillas de 1 granada
- Aceite de oliva
- Sal en escamas

20 min
15 min
4 €/persona
Sin contraindicaciones.

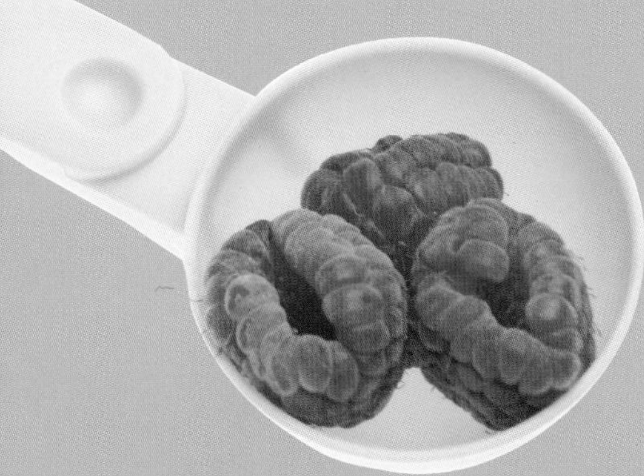

■ Cuece el arroz siguiendo las instrucciones del fabricante (al vapor, al horno o al microondas). Una vez cocido, enfríalo bien y reserva.

■ Cuece los guisantes en un cazo con agua hirviendo durante 12-14 minutos, hasta que queden bien tiernos. Reserva.

■ En un *wok* o sartén bien caliente, y con un chorrito de aceite de oliva, saltea la cebolla y el ajo cortados en daditos. Una vez la verdura empiece a dorarse agrega la piña y el mango cortado en dados, los guisantes hervidos y las hojas de lima picadas. Saltea bien y agrega el vino blanco, deja que se evapore y añade entonces los granos de granada, las hojas de tomillo y romero y el arroz. Saltéalo mientras espolvoreas una buena cucharada de curry.

■ En el último instante añade las frambuesas y el coco rallado, mezcla bien, corrige el punto de sal y sirve.

Trucos

Puedes añadir a este salteado trocitos de carne o de pescado a tu gusto: gambas, rape, pollo, pato, ternera, etc. Agrega también brotes de soja o germinados. Una cucharadita de canela en polvo le otorgará un carácter delicioso.

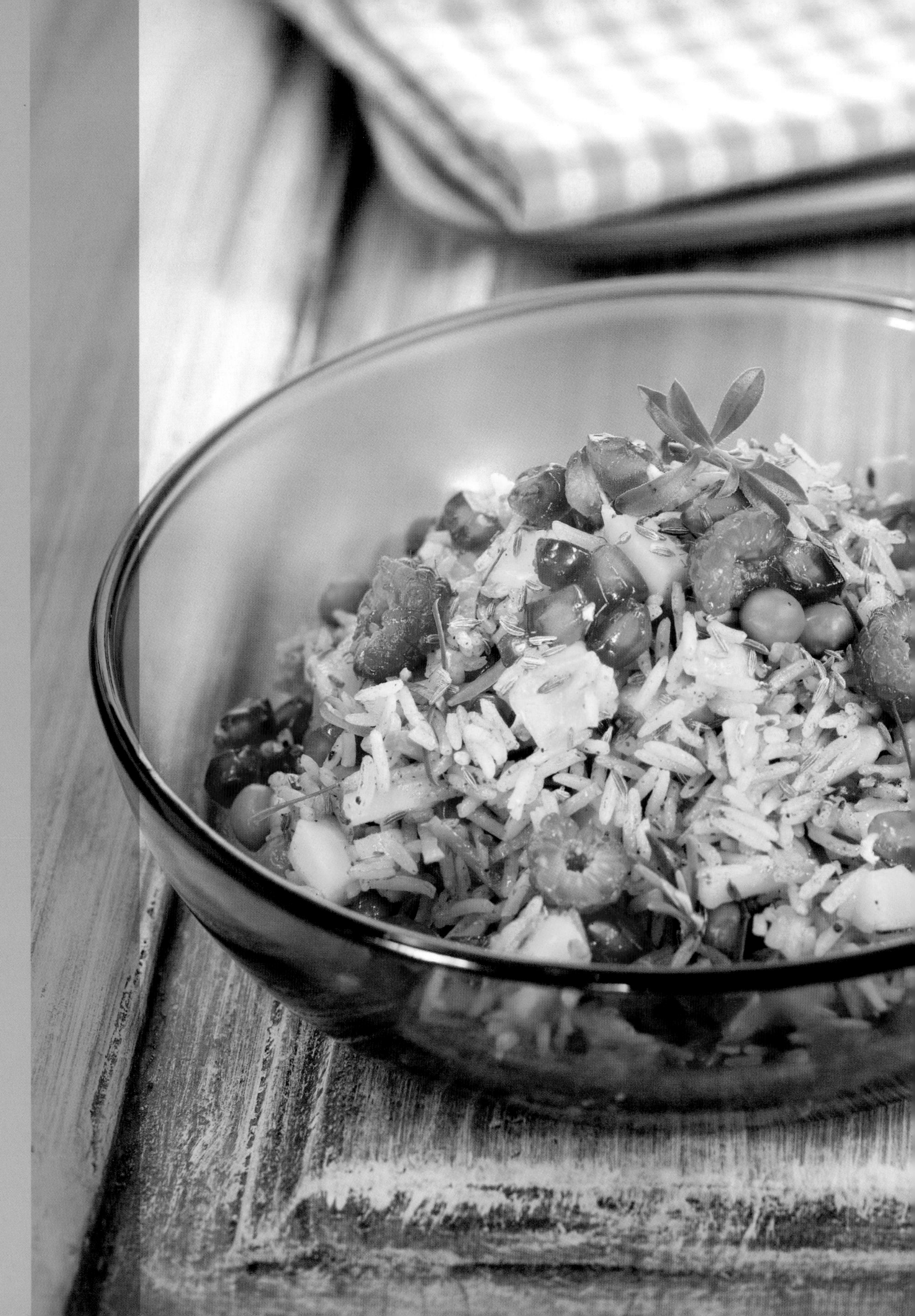

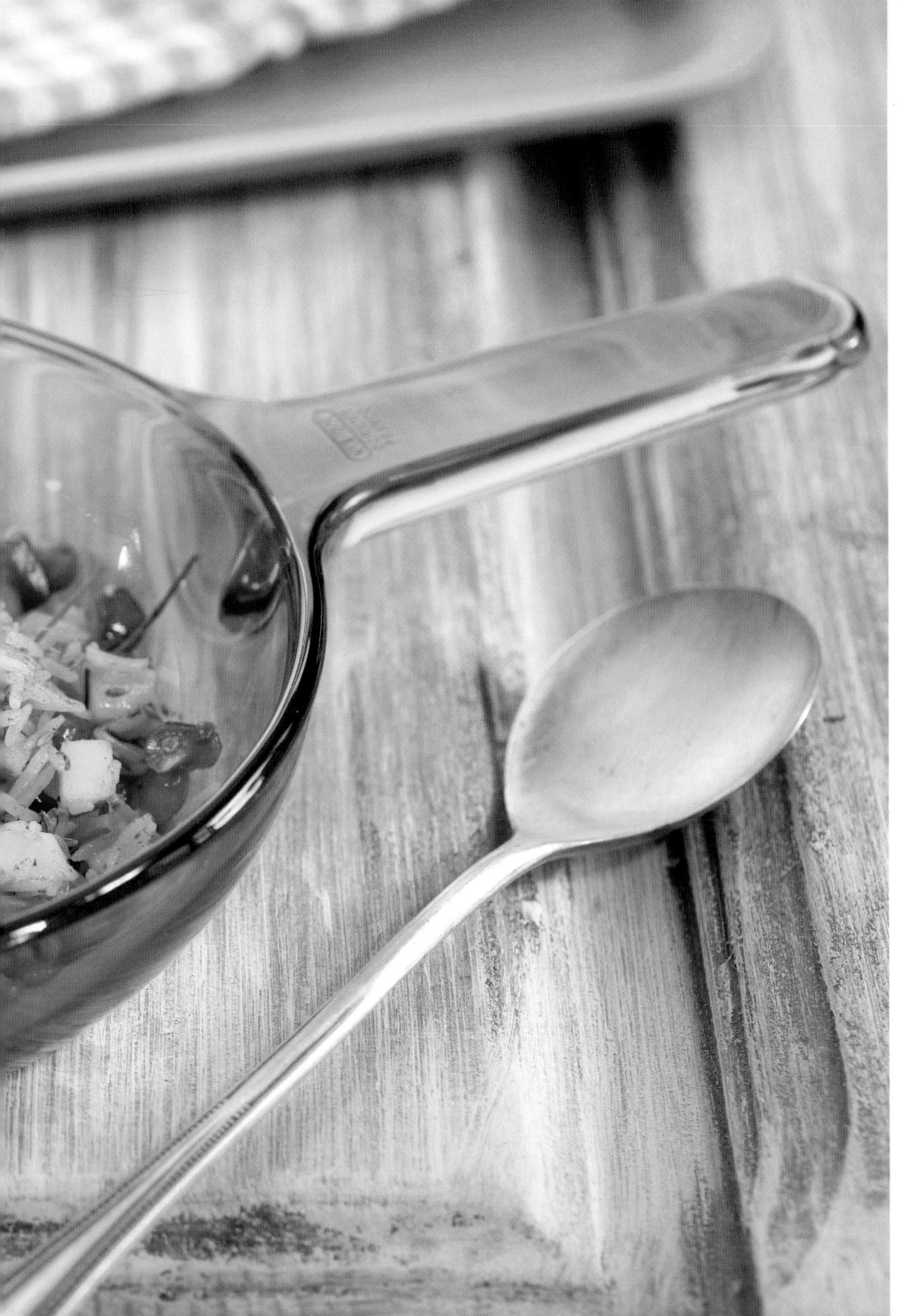

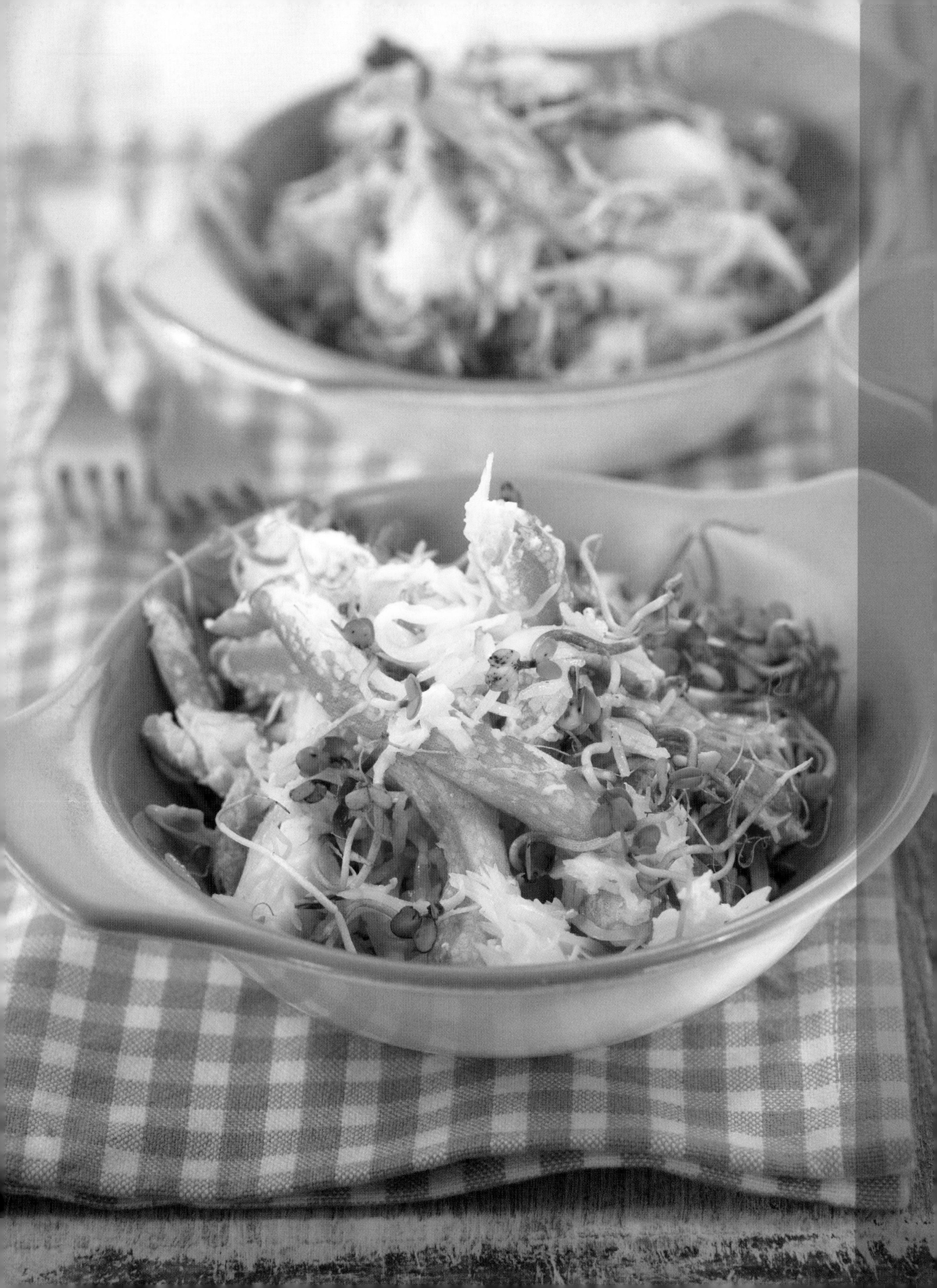

Nivel **3**

Salteado de arroz con cangrejo real

- 200 g de arroz vaporizado
- 8 patas de cangrejo real cocido
- 200 g de brotes de soja
- 100 g de germinados de rábano
- 1 cebolla tierna
- 1 puerro
- 1 raíz pequeña de jengibre
- Aceite de oliva
- Sal y pimienta blanca

15 min
15 min
8 €/persona
Esta receta no está indicada para personas alérgicas al marisco.

- Cuece el arroz siguiendo las instrucciones del fabricante (al vapor, al horno o al microondas). Una vez cocido, enfríalo bien y reserva.
- Pela las patas de cangrejo y recupera su carne. Reserva.
- Saltea la cebolla y el puerro en un *wok* o una sartén bien caliente y con un chorrito de aceite de oliva hasta que se ablanden y empiecen a dorarse. Añade entonces la carne de cangrejo, el arroz, los brotes de soja, la raíz de jengibre pelada y cortada en bastones muy finitos (como cerillas) y los germinados. Saltea durante 3-4 minutos a fuego vivo, salpimienta y sirve al instante.

Trucos

Si no encuentras cangrejo real puedes saltear langostinos, bogavante o langosta. Sustituye igualmente los germinados o brotes de rábano por alfalfa o brotes de espárrago. Si no tienes jengibre fresco puedes espolvorear jengibre en polvo al finalizar el salteado.

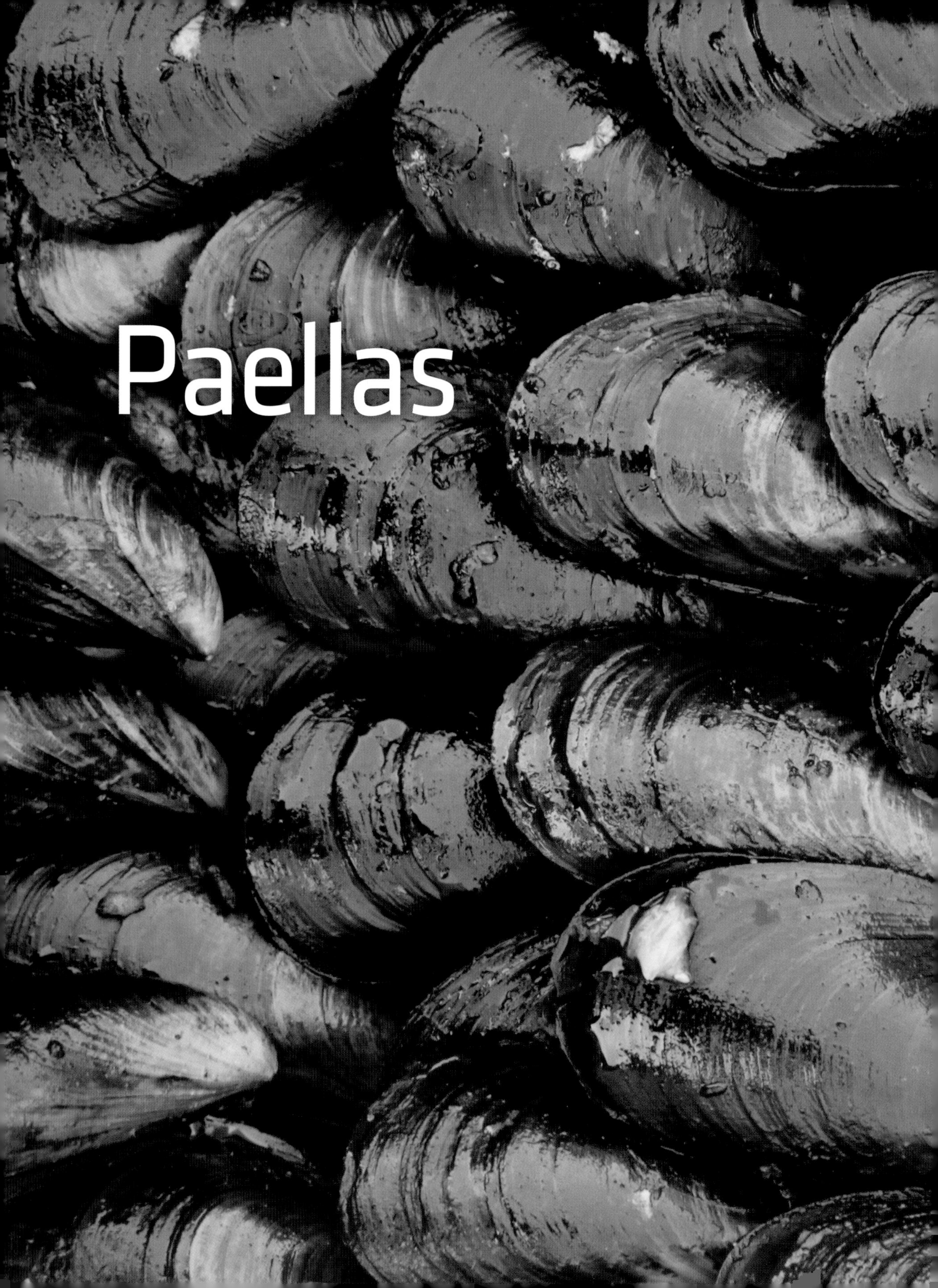

Paellas

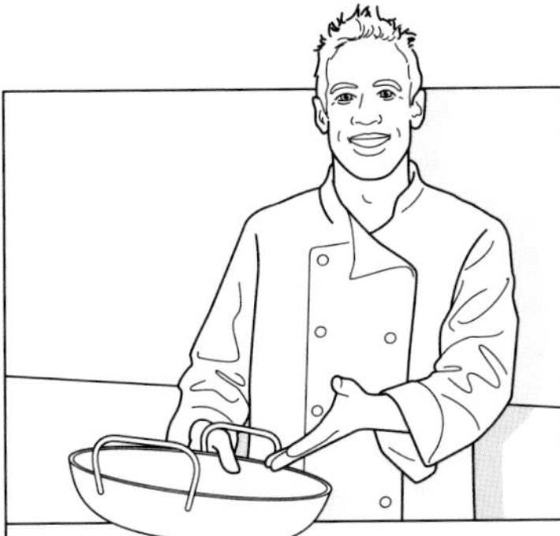
La paella es, además de una receta tradicional, el recipiente en el que se cocina nuestro plato más internacional.

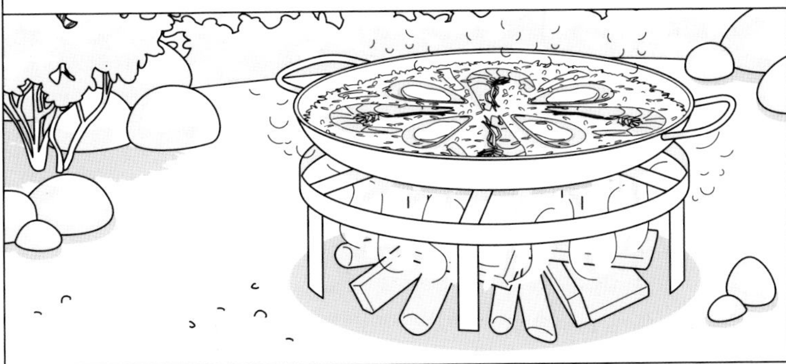
Tradicionalmente se elaboraba sobre un fuego de brasas y se empleaban productos de la huerta, el campo y la montaña.

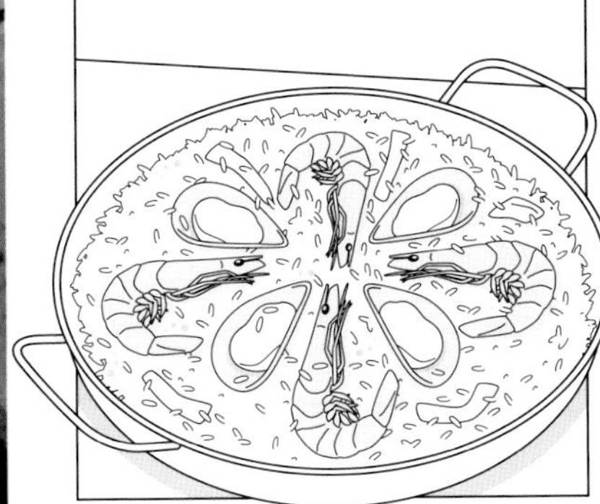
Después se incorporaron pescados y mariscos.

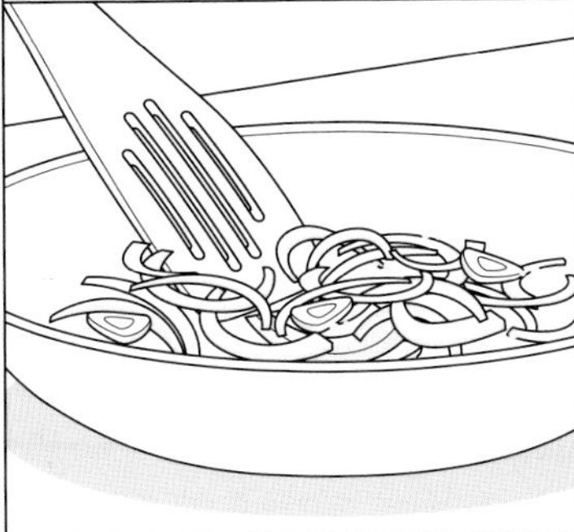
Es fundamental preparar un buen sofrito de verduras a nuestro gusto.

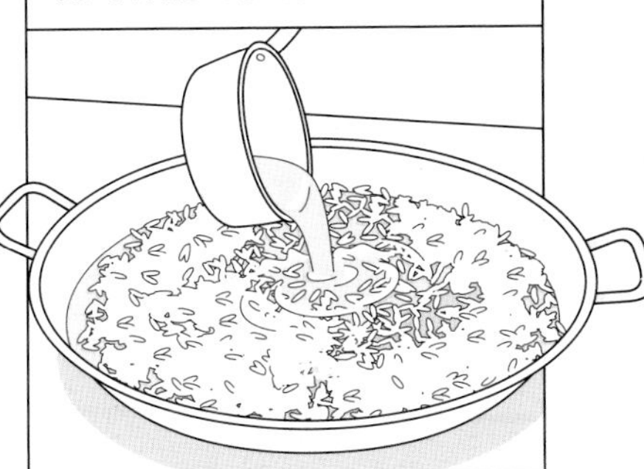
Y añadiremos el arroz y el caldo necesario, dejando cocer sin mover para que se forme la costra.

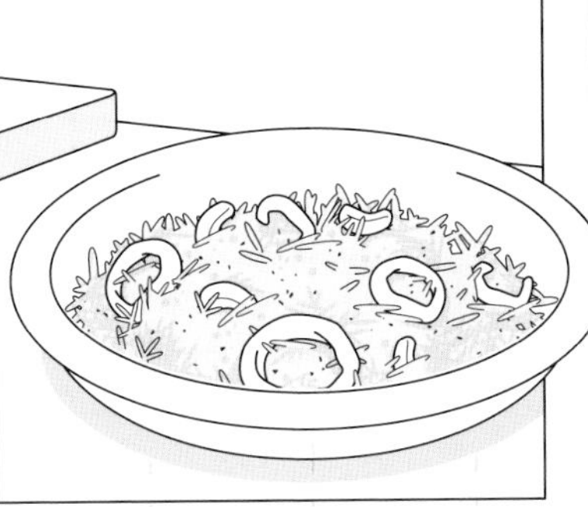
Aprenderás a preparar diversos arroces: arroz negro...

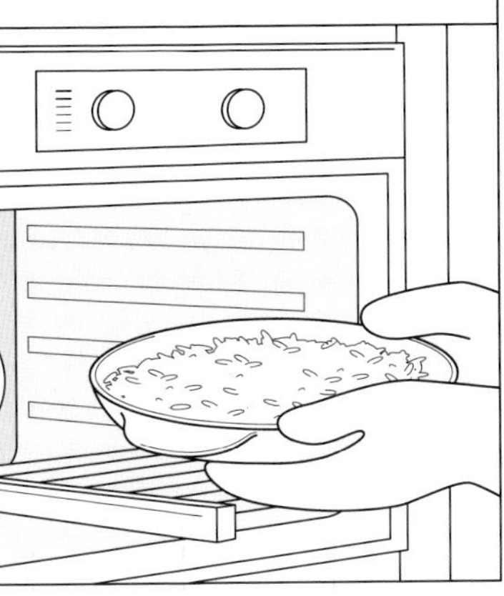
... arroz al horno...

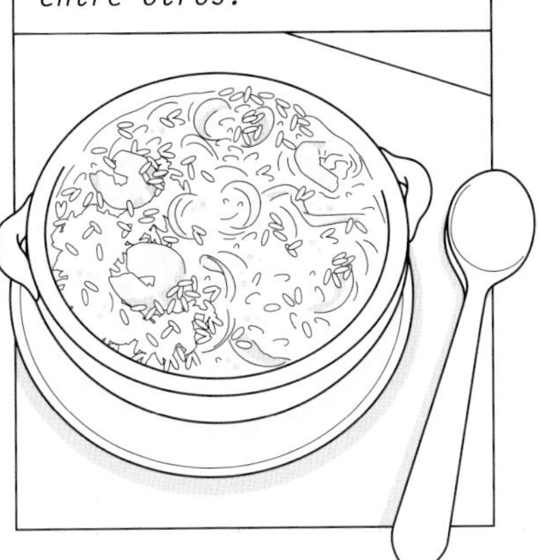
... y arroz caldoso, entre otros.

Paellas de arroz

El utensilio

La paella que relacionamos con el plato más internacional de nuestra cocina, la receta española por excelencia, debe su nombre al instrumento empleado para su elaboración: la paella o paellera. Se trata de una sartén con dos asas y paredes bajas, pero con amplio fondo o superficie de cocinado. Tradicionalmente las paellas se cocinaban sobre brasas, por lo que solo recibían calor por la parte baja del elemento. De ahí la necesidad de ofrecer una superficie amplia en la que tuvieran cabida los productos de la huerta, el arroz y el caldo. Hay regiones donde se cocina al horno, pero se sigue conservando la paella como elemento fundamental.

La técnica

Partiendo de un sofrito de verduras procede a preparar la paella, ya sea de carne, verduras o marisco, agregando los ingredientes deseados al sofrito. Tras dorar convenientemente los elementos agrega el arroz y el caldo deseado y cocina la paella, "estofando" la misma durante el tiempo adecuado. La cantidad y proporciones de agua y arroz se calculan en función de los ingredientes. No existe una regla para ello.

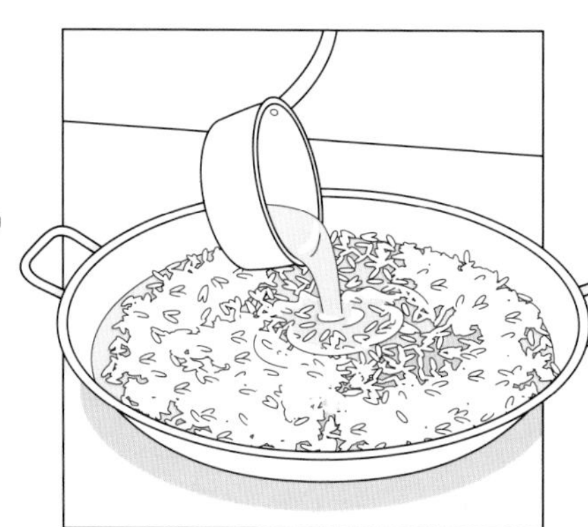

Plato a plato

Nivel **1** **Paella de verduras.** Supera el miedo a las paellas con una fórmula sencilla y muy resultona. Con la selección de ingredientes propuestos lograrás sublimar sabor y color sin esfuerzo.

Nivel **2** **Arroz negro.** En el segundo paso descubrirás que los clásicos tienen una fama merecida. Prueba a hacer este arroz y pasará a formar parte de tu recetario personal.

Nivel **3** **Paella de marisco.** Ya estás preparado para atacar la paella con mayúsculas. Prepárala con tiempo y cariño y tendrás el éxito asegurado.

Nivel 1 Paella de verduras

- 250 g de arroz bomba
- 100 g de judías verdes
- 100 g de guisantes
- 3-4 alcachofas
- 2 dientes de ajo
- 1 zanahoria
- 1 cebolla
- 1 manojo de espárragos trigueros
- 1 pizca de azafrán (2 g)
- Aceite de oliva
- Sal

PARA EL CALDO DE VERDURAS

- 2 cebollas
- 2 zanahorias
- 1 puerro
- 1/2 cabeza de ajo
- 2 tomates maduros
- 1 trozo de calabaza (unos 200 g)

20 min
20 min
2 €/persona
Sin contraindicaciones.

- Prepara un buen caldo de verduras. Para ello, trocea todos los ingredientes del caldo y déjalos cocer durante un par de horas a fuego lento. Cuela y resérvalo caliente.
- Sofríe la cebolla y el ajo picados muy finos en una paella con un chorrito de aceite de oliva. Cuando se ablanden añade las judías limpias y troceadas, la zanahoria en rodajas, los guisantes, los espárragos en bastoncitos y las alcachofas limpias y cortadas en cuartos. Sofríe todo hasta que la verdura empiece a dorarse.
- Añade entonces el arroz y el azafrán, mezcla bien e incorpora el caldo de verdura (aproximadamente 1 litro). Deja cocer sin remover durante 16-18 minutos hasta que el arroz absorba todo el caldo, deja reposar 5 minutos más, corrige el punto de sal y sirve.

Trucos

Puedes cocer esta paella a la brasa, con la cocina de que dispongas en casa o al horno.

Si no quieres asumir riesgos con la cantidad de caldo, añade la mitad e incorpora el resto comprobando el punto de cocción del arroz.

Nivel 2 Arroz negro

- 400 g de arroz bomba
- 1 kg de calamar limpio
- 100 g de tinta de calamar
- 400 g de mejillones limpios con su concha
- 4 tomates maduros
- 3 cebollas
- 2 pimientos choriceros
- 2 puerros
- 1 cabeza de ajo
- 1 manojo de perejil
- Agua mineral
- Aceite de oliva

20 min
50 min
4 €/persona
No indicado para alérgicos al marisco.

■ Para cocinar un buen arroz negro es fundamental preparar previamente un buen guiso de chipirones. Para ello, pela y corta las cebollas y los puerros en juliana y la cabeza de ajo por la mitad y lleva esta verdura a una cazuela con un buen chorro de aceite de oliva. Sofríe a fuego lento hasta que se ablande, sin llegar a dorarse. Incorpora entonces el tomate cortado en mitades, el manojo de perejil, los pimientos y los calamares. Deja cocer, estofar, a fuego lento durante una media hora aproximadamente; el calamar, al igual que la cebolla, desprenderá su agua, por lo que no le añadiremos aún líquido.

■ Transcurrida la media hora añade la tinta de calamar y 2 litros de agua mineral y deja cocer hasta que el líquido reduzca a la mitad del volumen inicial. Cuela el caldo, y reserva los chipirones, el caldo y la verdura sobrante en el colador.

■ Retira el manojo de perejil y la cabeza de ajo y pica ligeramente el resto de las verduras. En una paella sofríe un diente de ajo, añade la verdura reservada y el arroz bomba, mezcla todo e incorpora una parte de caldo de chipirones. Deja que el arroz absorba el caldo y añade más, tanto como necesites, hasta que esté al punto.

■ Dos minutos antes de retirar el arroz del fuego, agrega los mejillones, corrige el punto de sal y deja reposar 3-4 minutos antes de servir.

Trucos

En Cataluña y Valencia es costumbre acompañar el arroz negro con alioli.

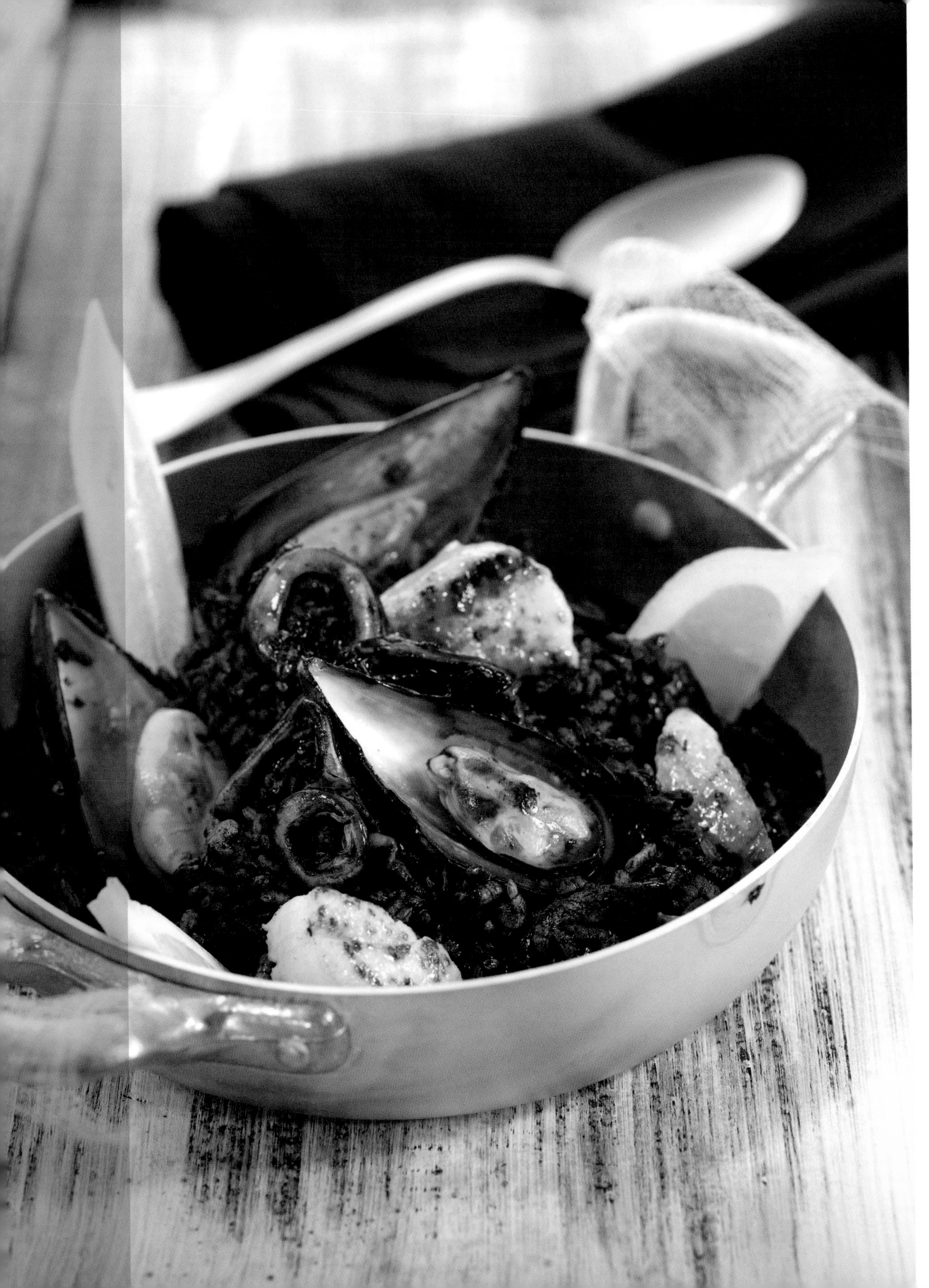

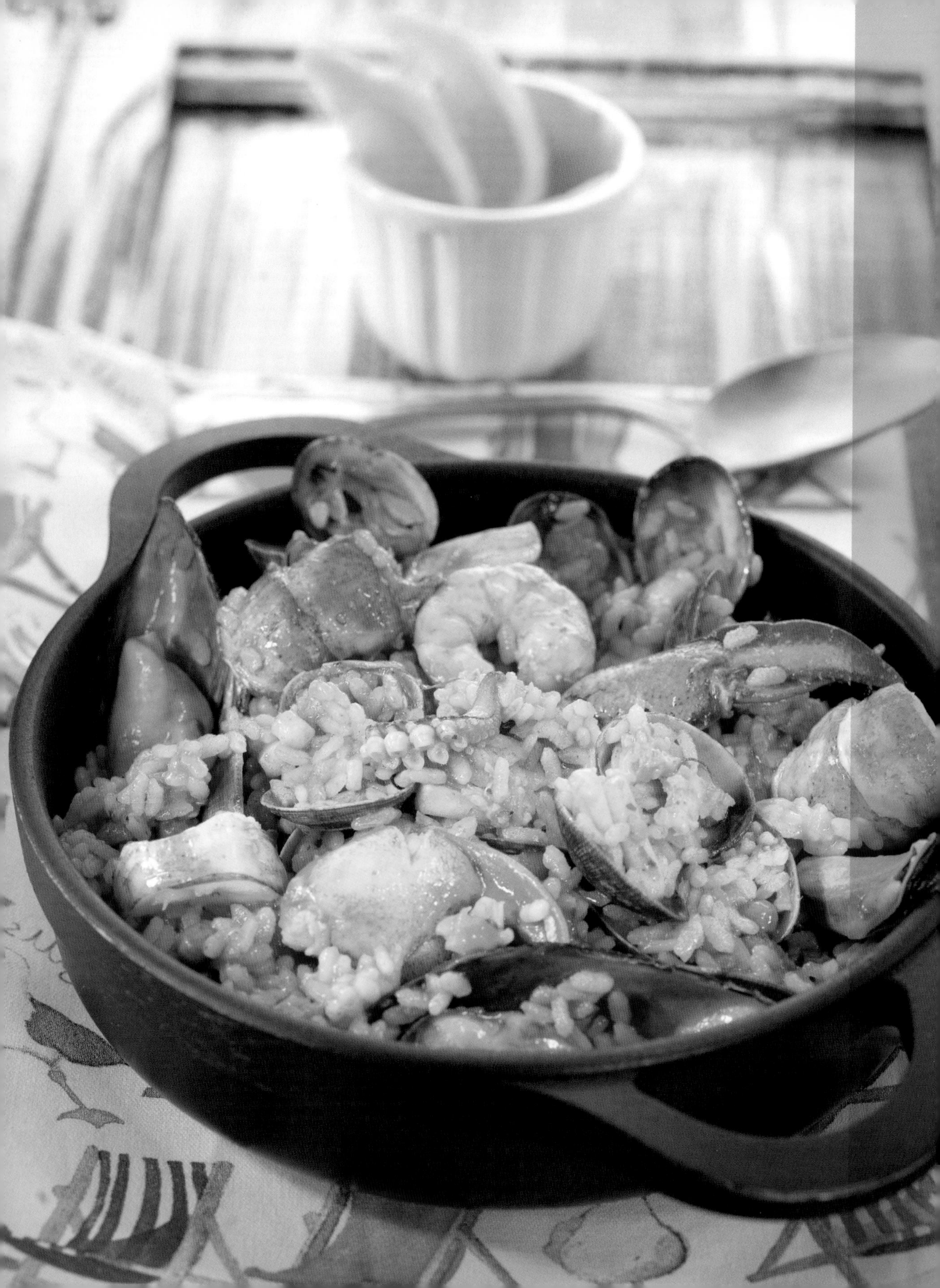

Nivel **3** # Paella de marisco

- 300 g de arroz
- 400 g de sepia
- 200 g de almejas
- 300 g de mejillones
- 16 gambas
- 8 langostinos
- 8 cigalas
- 1 cebolla
- 1 pimiento verde
- 1/2 pimiento rojo
- 2 dientes de ajo
- 2 g de azafrán
- 1 cucharada de tomate frito casero
- Aceite de oliva

PARA EL CALDO DE PESCADO

- Una espina o una cabeza de rape, rodaballo o merluza
- 1 cebolla
- 1 puerro
- 1 manojo de perejil

20 min
20 min
8 €/persona
No indicada para alérgicos al marisco.

■ Prepara el caldo de pescado cociendo una espina o cabeza de rape, rodaballo o merluza, con una cebolla, un puerro y un manojo de perejil. Deja cocer durante 20 minutos retirando la espuma que aparecerá en la superficie del caldo. Una vez cocido cuela y reserva caliente.

■ Rehoga la cebolla, el ajo, los pimientos y la sepia cortados muy finos en una paella con un buen chorro de aceite de oliva. Deja que la verdura se dore caramelizándose ligeramente a fuego muy lento.

■ Agrega entonces una buena cucharada de tomate frito, el azafrán y el arroz, mezcla bien y añade 1 litro de caldo de pescado. Deja cocer a fuego vivo hasta que la paella empiece a hervir.

■ Integra entonces las almejas y los mejillones y cuece a fuego lento durante 10 minutos. Transcurrido este tiempo incorpora las gambas, las cigalas y los langostinos. Deja cocer 5 minutos más. Retira del fuego y deja que la paella repose 3-4 minutos antes de servir. La paella debe quedar seca, el arroz debe absorber por completo el caldo de cocción.

Trucos

Es importante sofreír las verduras a fuego lento para que caramelicen. Cuanto más tiempo podamos dedicar a este paso mejor resultado obtendremos.

Arroces con sofrito

El ingrediente
El sofrito para nuestros arroces puede estar compuesto por las verduras que deseemos, aun así hay algunas de las que debemos prescindir por su intenso sabor o bien por no ser del todo óptimas para este tipo de preparaciones. Un sofrito no es otra cosa que un conjunto de verduras picadas finamente y rehogadas con aceite de oliva hasta obtener algo similar a una pasta o puré de verduras en el cual estas han perdido el agua que contienen. Cuídate de adaptar la verdura del sofrito a los ingredientes del arroz al que vayan a ser destinadas. Es importante cocinar los sofritos a fuego lento, ya que un fuego intenso puede "quemar" nuestras verduras y resultar en un sabor amargo no demasiado agradable.

La técnica
Corta las verduras tan finas como te sea posible; es importante que todas presenten un tamaño similar para que se cocinen por igual y no te encuentres unas verduras cocidas, otras quemadas y otras aún crudas. Rehógalas con abundante aceite de oliva para que no se peguen al cazo y siempre a fuego lento. Una vez el sofrito adquiera la tonalidad y textura deseadas podrás retirar con una cuchara el exceso de aceite.

Plato a plato

Nivel **1** **Arroz al horno con verduras.** Si tienes una cazuela de barro aprovéchala para esta receta, pues es un añadido a la suma de factores para triunfar.

Nivel **2** **Arroz caldoso al horno con setas.** Combina dos clásicos de la cocina del arroz: la cocción al horno y la textura caldosa. Dos ases que nunca fallan.

Nivel **3** **Cazuela de arroz al horno con costra crujiente.** El tercer paso te lleva hasta una receta original, donde el toque final es una fina capa de huevo que se cuece al final.

Nivel 1 Arroz al horno con verduras

- 300 g de arroz
- 200 g de habas o guisantes
- 1 cebolla
- 1 pimiento rojo
- 1 pimiento verde
- 1 alcachofa
- 1 zanahoria
- 3 dientes de ajo
- 2 cucharadas de tomate frito
- 2 g de azafrán
- Aceite de oliva

PARA EL CALDO DE VERDURAS

- 2 cebollas
- 2 zanahorias
- 1 puerro
- 1/2 cabeza de ajo
- 2 tomates maduros
- 1 trozo de calabaza (unos 200 g)

20 min
20 min
2 €/persona
Sin contraindicaciones.

- Prepara un buen caldo de verduras. Para ello trocea todos los ingredientes del caldo y déjalos cocer durante un par de horas a fuego lento. Cuela y resérvalo caliente.
- En una cazuela, preferiblemente de barro, rehoga la cebolla, el ajo, la zanahoria, las alcachofas limpias y cortadas en cuartos y los pimientos picados muy finos con un chorrito de aceite de oliva. Deja que la verdura se dore a fuego lento y añade entonces las habas y el azafrán, mezcla bien e incorpora el tomate frito y el arroz.
- Mezcla bien todos los ingredientes y cubre con 1 litro de caldo de verduras. Una vez el caldo arranque a hervir, introduce la cazuela en el horno precalentado a 190 °C. Deja cocer durante 20 minutos, hasta que el arroz esté en su punto. Corrige el punto de sal, deja reposar 3-4 minutos y sirve.

Trucos

Puedes añadir espárragos trigueros, también judías, trozos de calabaza o la verdura de tu agrado. También se puede combinar este arroz con legumbres cocidas para obtener un resultado más copioso y contundente.

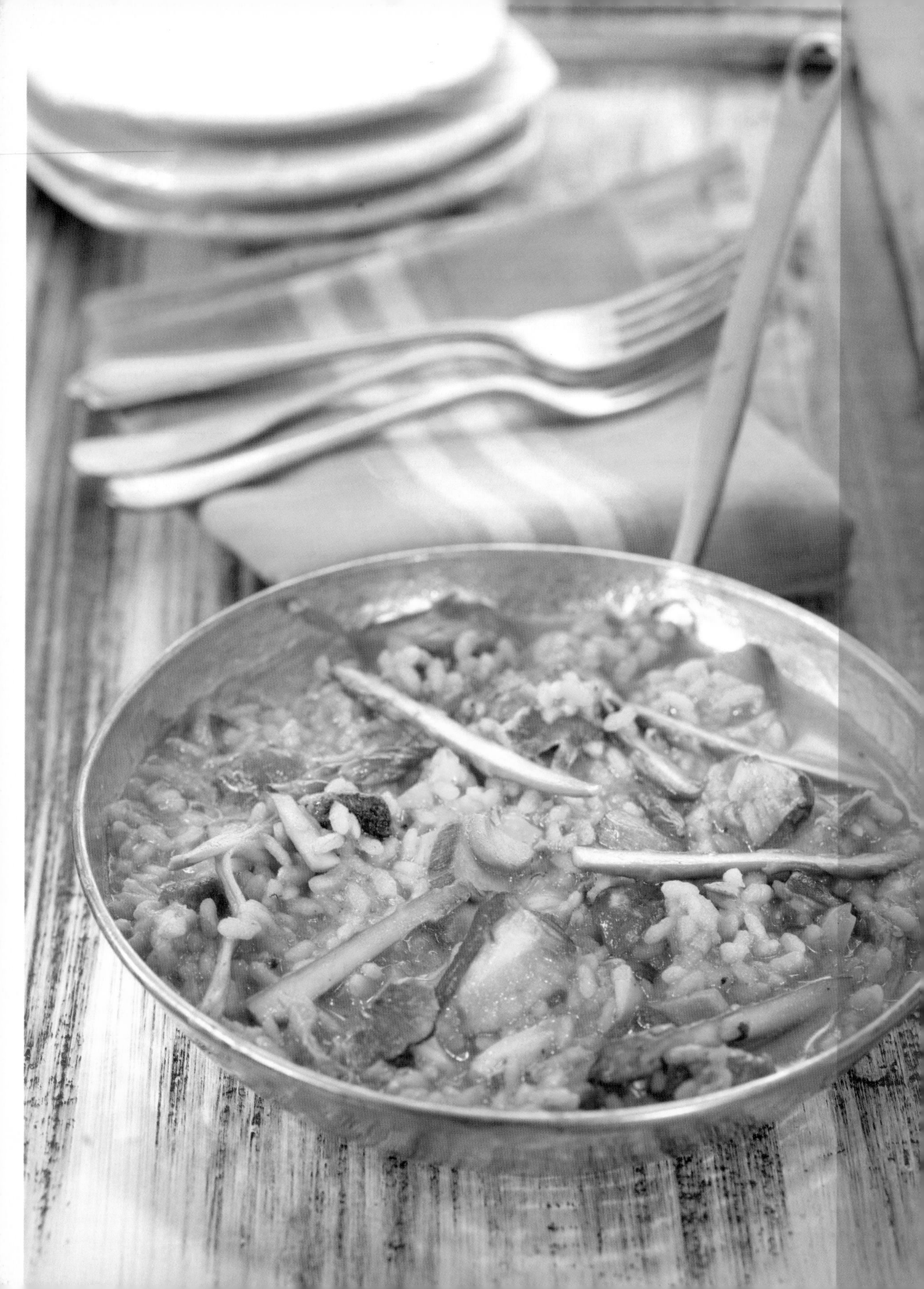

Nivel **2** Arroz caldoso al horno con setas

- 300 g de arroz bomba
- 300 g de *ceps* (*Boletus edulis*)
- 300 g de setas de temporada
- 6 cebollas tiernas
- 1 manojo de puntas de espárrago triguero
- Aceite de oliva
- Sal y pimienta

20 min
20 min
2 €/persona
Sin contraindicaciones.

- Prepara un caldo de *ceps*. Para ello, dora en un cazo 3 cebollas cortadas en juliana con un buen chorro de aceite de oliva. Cuando la cebolla esté dorada, añade los *ceps* troceados y deja que se doren igualmente. Entonces cubre el cazo con agua (2 litros) y deja que las setas se infusionen durante unos 20-25 minutos a fuego lento. Salpimienta, cuela el caldo y reserva.
- En una sartén o cazuela sofríe a fuego lento las cebollas restantes picadas muy finas. Cuando empiecen a dorarse añade las setas de temporada bien limpias y deja que se doren, añade el arroz y sofríe durante un par de minutos.
- Transcurrido este tiempo, añade 1 litro de caldo de *ceps* y deja que arranque a hervir. Introduce en ese momento en el horno y deja cocer durante 16-18 minutos, hasta que el arroz esté al punto. Añade entonces los espárragos troceados, corrige el punto de sal y pimienta, deja reposar 3-4 minutos y sirve.

Trucos

Puedes preparar este arroz con champiñones y setas de tipo gírgola, que son de cultivo y no tienen temporada, por lo que podrás disfrutar de este arroz todo el año. Espolvorea también un buen puñado de perejil picado antes de servir el arroz.

Nivel **3** Cazuela de arroz al horno con costra crujiente

- 300 g de arroz
- 1 cebolla
- 1 pimiento rojo
- 1 pimiento verde
- 3 dientes de ajo
- 2 cucharadas de tomate frito
- 2 huevos
- Aceite de oliva
- 2 g de azafrán

PARA EL CALDO

- 2 carcasas de pollo
- 1 cebolla
- 1 puerro
- 2 dientes de ajo
- 1 tomate en rama

20 min
20 min
2 €/persona
Sin contraindicaciones.

- Prepara el caldo de ave: asa en el horno a 190 °C las dos carcasas de pollo hasta que queden bien doradas (aproximadamente 45 minutos). Luego introdúcelas en una olla con 3,5 litros de agua junto al resto de ingredientes del caldo. Deja cocer durante una hora, corrige el punto de sal, cuela y reserva el caldo caliente.
- Rehoga la cebolla, el ajo y los pimientos picados muy finitos en una cazuela o una sartén con un buen chorro de aceite de oliva hasta que la verdura caramelice.
- Añade entonces las hebras de azafrán, el arroz y el tomate frito, mezcla todo bien y cubre con 1/2 litro de caldo de pollo. Espera a que el caldo arranque a hervir e introduce la cazuela en el horno precalentado a 190 °C.
- Deja cocer durante 15 minutos. Transcurrido este tiempo, el arroz estará al punto y seco y el caldo se habrá evaporado. Bate los huevos y agrégalos a la cazuela. Deja que se forme una costra al horno durante 3-4 minutos más.
- Saca del horno, deja reposar un par de minutos y sirve.

Trucos

Puedes añadir pequeños trocitos de pollo, jamón, verduras o pescado para enriquecer el sabor.

Conviene no excederse con el caldo, en este caso para que también se forme una costra o *socarrat* en la base de la cazuela.

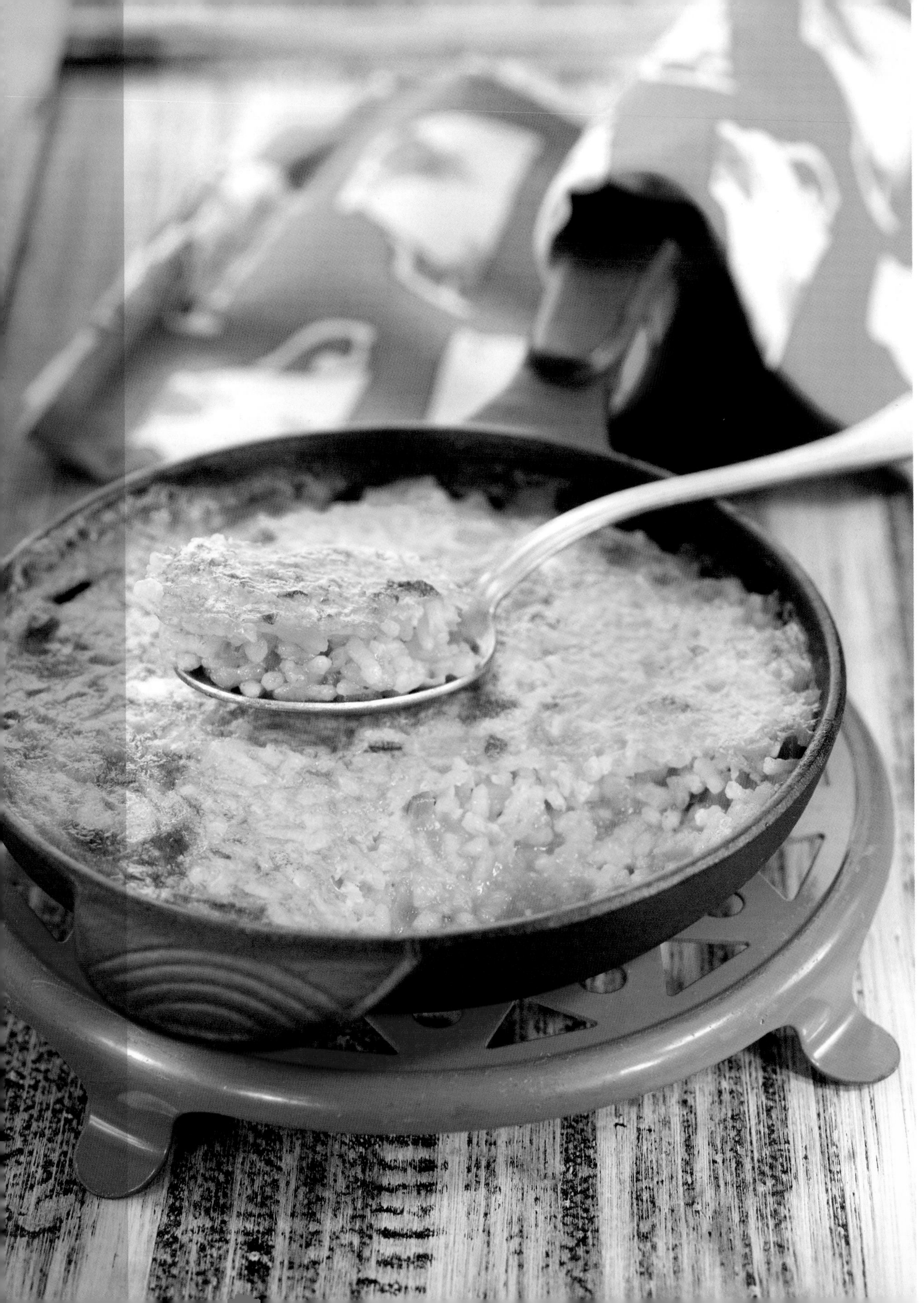

Índices de recetas

ÍNDICE POR ORDEN DE APARICIÓN

ÍNDICE POR NIVEL DE DIFICULTAD

Nivel 3

ÍNDICE POR TIPO DE PLATO

Al horno

Caldosos

Canelones y lasañas

Con salsa

En paella

Ensaladas

Risottos

Salteados